IAPSM's Textbook of
Comprehensive Research Methodology

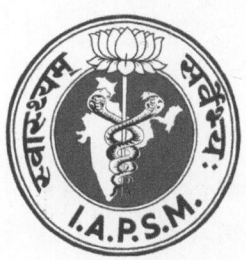

IAPSM's Textbook of Comprehensive Research Methodology

Chief Editor
Sanjay Zodpey
MBBS MD PhD DSc (Honoris Causa) Doctor of Medicine (Honoris Causa)
President
Public Health Foundation of India
New Delhi, India

Editors

Rashmi Kundapur MBBS MD
Additional Professor
Department of Community and
Family Medicine
All India Institute of Medical Sciences
Bibinagar, Hyderabad, Telangana, India

Deepthi R MBBS MD DNB
Associate Professor
Department of Community Medicine
ESIC Medical College and PGIMSR
Bengaluru, Karnataka, India

Associate Editors

Anusha Rashmi MBBS MD
Associate Professor
Department of Community Medicine
KS Hegde Medical Academy
Mangaluru, Karnataka, India

Suthanthira Kannan MBBS MD
Assistant Professor
ESIC Medical College and Hospital
Chennai, Tamil Nadu, India

Foreword
AM Kadri

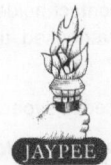

JAYPEE BROTHERS MEDICAL PUBLISHERS
The Health Sciences Publisher
New Delhi | London

Jaypee Brothers Medical Publishers (P) Ltd

Headquarters

Jaypee Brothers Medical Publishers (P) Ltd
EMCA House, 23/23-B
Ansari Road, Daryaganj
New Delhi 110 002, India
Landline: +91-11-23272143, +91-11-23272703
+91-11-23282021, +91-11-23245672
Email: jaypee@jaypeebrothers.com

Corporate Office

Jaypee Brothers Medical Publishers (P) Ltd
4838/24, Ansari Road, Daryaganj
New Delhi 110 002, India
Phone: +91-11-43574357
Fax: +91-11-43574314
Email: jaypee@jaypeebrothers.com

Overseas Office

J.P. Medical Ltd
83 Victoria Street, London
SW1H 0HW (UK)
Phone: +44 20 3170 8910
Fax: +44 (0)20 3008 6180
Email: info@jpmedpub.com

Website: www.jaypeebrothers.com
Website: www.jaypeedigital.com

© 2024, Jaypee Brothers Medical Publishers

The views and opinions expressed in this book are solely those of the original contributor(s)/author(s) and do not necessarily represent those of editor(s) and publisher of the book.

All rights reserved. No part of this publication may be reproduced, stored or transmitted in any form or by any means, electronic, mechanical, photocopying, recording or otherwise, without the prior permission in writing of the publishers.

All brand names and product names used in this book are trade names, service marks, trademarks or registered trademarks of their respective owners. The publisher is not associated with any product or vendor mentioned in this book.

Medical knowledge and practice change constantly. This book is designed to provide accurate, authoritative information about the subject matter in question. However, readers are advised to check the most current information available on procedures included and check information from the manufacturer of each product to be administered, to verify the recommended dose, formula, method and duration of administration, adverse effects and contraindications. It is the responsibility of the practitioner to take all appropriate safety precautions. Neither the publisher nor the author(s)/editor(s) assume any liability for any injury and/or damage to persons or property arising from or related to use of material in this book.

This book is sold on the understanding that the publisher is not engaged in providing professional medical services. If such advice or services are required, the services of a competent medical professional should be sought.

Every effort has been made where necessary to contact holders of copyright to obtain permission to reproduce copyright material. If any have been inadvertently overlooked, the publisher will be pleased to make the necessary arrangements at the first opportunity.

Inquiries for bulk sales may be solicited at: jaypee@jaypeebrothers.com

IAPSM's Textbook of Comprehensive Research Methodology

First Edition: **2024, Reprint: 2025**

ISBN: 978-93-5696-947-6

Printed in India

Reviewers

AM Kadri
Executive Director
State Health System Resource Centre
Ahmedabad, Gujarat, India

Bhavesh Modi
Professor and Head
Department of Community and Family Medicine
All India Institute of Medical Sciences
Rajkot, Gujarat, India

Deepak Saxena
Director
Indian Institute of Public Health
Gandhinagar, Gujarat, India

Himanshu Neghadhi
Project Director and Additional Professor
Indian Institute of Public Health
Delhi, New Delhi, India

Lalit Sankhe
Department of Community Medicine
Grant Medical College
JJ Hospital
Mumbai, Maharashtra, India

Pradeep Deshmukh
Dean (Research), Professor
Department of Community and Family Medicine
All India Institute of Medical Sciences
Nagpur, Maharashtra, India

Pradeep Kumar
Professor
Department of Community Medicine
Dr MK Shah Medical College
Ahmedabad, Gujarat, India

Purushottam Giri
Secretary General
Indian Association of Preventive and Social Medicine India

Contributors

A Akshay Subramanian MBBS MD
Assistant Professor
AJ Institute of Medical Science
Mangaluru, Karnataka, India

AM Kadri MBBS MD
Executive Director
State Health System Resource Centre
Ahmedabad, Gujarat, India

Abhishek V Raut MBBS MD DNB
Professor
Department of Community Medicine
Mahatma Gandhi Institute of Medical Sciences
Sevagram, Wardha, Maharashtra, India

Aditi Mohta MBBS MD
Assistant Professor
Department of Community Medicine
Integral Institute of Medical Sciences and Research
Lucknow, Uttar Pradesh, India

Akhil Dhanesh Goel MBBS MD
Associate Professor
Department of Community Medicine and Family Medicine and Adjunct Faculty
School of Public Health
All India Institute of Medical Sciences
Jodhpur, Rajasthan, India

Ameenah H Siraja MBBS MD
Senior Resident
Department of Community Medicine
ESICMC and PGIMSR
Bengaluru, Karnataka, India

Amir Maroof Khan MBBS MD
Professor
Department of Community Medicine
University College of Medical Sciences
Delhi, New Delhi, India

Amit Rao MBBS MD
Assistant Professor
Department of Community Medicine
KS Hegde Medical Academy, NITTE DU
Mangaluru, Karnataka, India

Amol Dongre MBBS MD FAIMER
Additional Professor
Department of Community and Family Medicine, AIIMS
Nagpur, Maharashtra, India

Anil Jacob Purty MBBS MD
Director–Principal
Pondicherry Institute of Medical Sciences
Puducherry, India

Anusha Rashmi MBBS MD
Associate Professor
Department of Community Medicine, KS Hegde Medical Academy, NITTE DU
Mangaluru, Karnataka, India

Anwita Khaitan MBBS MD
Assistant Professor
Department of Community Medicine
North DMC Medical College and Hindu Rao Hospital
Delhi, New Delhi, India

Archisman Mohapatra MBBS MD
Executive Director
Generating Research Insights for Development Council
Noida, Uttar Pradesh, India

Arvind Kasthuri MBBS MD
Professor
Department of Community Medicine
St John's Medical College
Bengaluru, Karnataka, India

Ashwath Narayan MBBS MD
Professor
Department of Community Medicine
Kempegowda Institute of Medical Sciences
Bengaluru, Karnataka, India

Ashwini Lonimath MBBS MD
Assistant Professor
Department of Community Medicine
ESICMC and PGIMSR
Rajaji Nagar, Bengaluru, Karnataka, India

Baidurjya Mahanta MBBS MD
Senior Resident
Department of Community Medicine
Assam Medical College
Dibrugarh, Assam, India

Bhavesh Modi MBBS MD
Professor and Head
Community and Family Medicine
All India Institute of Medical Sciences
Rajkot, Gujarat, India

Bhushan Kamble MBBS MD
Assistant Professor
Department of Community Medicine
All India Institute of Medical Sciences
Hyderabad, Telangana, India

Chandana H MBBS MD
Assistant Professor
Department of Community Medicine
ESICMC and PGIMSR
Bengaluru, Karnataka, India

Chandralekha Kona MBBS MD
Senior Resident
Department of Community and Family Medicine
All India Institute of Medical Sciences
Bibinagar, Hyderabad, Telangana, India

Chandrika R Doddihal MBBS MD
Associate Professor
Department of Community Medicine
BLDE(DU) Shri BM Patil Medical College
Hospital and Research Centre
Vijayapura, Karnataka, India

Chethana K MBBS MD
Associate Professor
Department of Community Medicine
Kanachur Institute of Medical Sciences
Mangaluru, Karnataka, India

Darshan BB MBBS MD
Associate Professor
Department of Community Medicine
Kasturba Medical College
Manipal, Mangaluru, India

Deepak B Saxena MBBS MD
Director
Indian Institute of Public Health
Gandhinagar, Gujarat, India

Deepthi R MBBS MD DNB
Associate professor
Department of Community Medicine
ESICMC and PGIMSR
Bengaluru, Karnataka, India

Dewesh Kumar MBBS MD
Assistant Professor
Department of Preventive and
Social Medicine
Rajendra Institute of Medical Sciences
Ranchi, Jharkhand, India

Dhanajayan MBBS MD
Assistant Professor
Department of Community Medicine
ESICMC and PGIMSR
Chennai, Tamil Nadu, India

Divya Sharma MPH
Junior Demonstrator (Health Economics)
Department of Community Medicine and
School of Public Health
Postgraduate Institute of Medical Education and Research
Chandigarh, India

Ekta Gupta MBBS MD
Scientist E
National Institute of Cancer Prevention and Research
Indian Council of Medical Research
Noida, Uttar Pradesh, India

Farah Naaz Fathima MBBS MD
Associate Professor
Department of Community Medicine
St John's Medical College
Bengaluru, Karnataka, India

Hetal Rathod (Waghela) MBBS MD
Professor and Head
Department of Community Medicine
D Y Patil Medical College
Hospital and Research Centre
Pimpri, Pune, Maharashtra, India

Ipsa Mohapatra MBBS MD
Professor
Department of Community Medicine
Kalinga Institute of Medical Sciences
Bhubaneswar, Odisha, India

Jaykaran Charan MBBS MD
Additional Professor
Department of Pharmacology and Sub Dean (Research)
All India Institute of Medical Sciences
Jodhpur, Rajasthan, India

Jeyashree Kathiresan MBBS MD
Scientist E
Institute of Indian Council of Medical Research–National Institute of Epidemiology
Chennai, Tamil Nadu, India

Kamal Kishore PhD
Assistant Professor
Department of Biostatistics
Postgraduate Institute of Medical Education and Research
Chandigarh, India

Kedar Mehta MBBS MD
Associate Professor
Gujarat Medical Education and Research Society
Vadodara, Gujarat, India

Komal Shah PhD
Assistant Professor
Indian Institute of Public Health
Gandhinagar, Gujarat, India

Mahalaqua Nazli Khatib MBBS MD
Head
Centre for Global Evidence Synthesis Initiative
Datta
Meghe Institute of Medical Sciences
(Deemed to be University)
Wardha, Faculty in Indian Council of Medical Research Cochrane affiliate Centre
New Delhi, India

Malatesh Undi MBBS MD ACME FAIMER Fellow
Assistant Professor
Department of Community Medicine
Karwar Institute of Medical Sciences
Karwar, Karnataka, India

Manish Goel MBBS MD
Professor
Department of Community Medicine
Lady Hardinge Medical College
New Delhi, India

Manish Rana MBBS MD
Assistant Professor
Department of Community Medicine
Gujarat Medical Education and Research Society Medical College
Sola, Ahmedabad, Gujarat, India

Manjula R MBBS MD
Professor
Department of Community Medicine
S Nijalingappa Medical College
Bagalkot, Karnataka, India

Manoj Kumar Gupta MBBS MD
Additional Professor
Department of Community Medicine and Family Medicine Coordinator
School of Public Health
All India Institute of Medical Sciences
Jodhpur, Rajasthan, India

Manya Prasad MBBS MD
Assistant Professor
Department of Epidemiology and Clinical research
Institute of Liver and Biliary Sciences
New Delhi, India

Maria Nelliyanil MBBS MD
Professor
Department of Community Medicine
A J Institute of Medical Sciences and Research Center
Mangaluru, Karnataka, India

Medha Mathur MBBS MD
Associate Professor
Department of Community Medicine
Geetanjali Medical College and Hospital
Udaipur, Rajasthan, India

Meely Panda MBBS MD
Assistant Professor
Department of Community Medicine
All India Institute of Medical Sciences
Hyderabad, Telangana, India

Mitasha Singh MBBS MD
Assistant Professor
Department of Community Medicine
Dr Baba Saheb Ambedkar Medical College and Hospital
Rohini, New Delhi, India

Contributors

Mohammad Waseem Faraz Ansari MBBS MD
Associate Professor
Department of Community Medicine
ESIC Medical College and Hospital
KK Nagar, Chennai, India

Mridushman Saikia MBBS MD
Junior Resident
Department of Community Medicine
Assam Medical College
Dibrugarh, Assam, India

N Nakkeeran MA (Anthropology) MPhil PhD
Professor
School of Global Affairs
Dr BR Ambedkar University
Delhi, New Delhi, India

N R Ramesh Masthi MBBS MD
Professor and Head
Department of Community Medicine
Kempegowda Institute of Medical Sciences
Bengaluru, Karnataka, India

Nirmala C J MBBS MD
Associate Professor
Department of Community Medicine
BGS Global Institute of Medical Sciences
Bengaluru, Karnataka, India

Nishanth Krishna K MBBS MD
Associate Professor
Department of Community Medicine
Father Muller Medical College
Mangaluru, Karnataka, India

Padmavathi S MBBS, MD, DNB
Senior Resident
Department of Community Medicine
ESIC Medical College and PGIMSR
KK Nagar, Chennai, Tamil Nadu, India

Pankaj Bharadwaj MBBS MD
Academic Head
School of Public Health
Professor
Community and Family Medicine
All India Institute of Medical Sciences
Jodhpur, Rajasthan, India

Pentapati Siva Santosh Kumar MBBS MD
Senior Resident
Department of Community and Family Medicine
All India Institute of Medical Sciences
Mangalagiri, Andhra Pradesh, India

Pradeep Agarwal MBBS MD
Additional Professor
Department of Community Medicine
All India Institute of Medical Sciences
Rishikesh, Uttarakhand, India

Pradeep Deshmukh MBBS MD
Dean (Research), Professor
Department of Community and Family Medicine
All India Institute of Medical Sciences
Nagpur, Maharashtra, India

Pradeep Kumar MBBS MD
Professor
Department of Community Medicine
Dr MK Shah Medical College
Ahmedabad, Gujarat, India

Preety Tanwar MBBS MD
Senior Resident
Department of Community Medicine
ESICMC and PGIMSR
Bengaluru, Karnataka, India

Prem Mony MBBS MD
Professor
Department of Community Medicine
St John's Medical College
Bengaluru, Karnataka, India

Rachana A R MBBS MD ACME
Assistant Professor
Department of Community Medicine
Karwar Institute of Medical Sciences
Karwar, Karnataka, India

Raghavendra Huchchannavar MBBS MD
Assistant Professor
Department of Community Medicine
KS Hegde Medical Academy
Mangaluru, Karnataka, India

Ramesh Holla MBBS MD
Associate Professor
Department of Community Medicine
Kasturba Medical College
Manipal, Mangaluru, India

Rashmi Kundapur MBBS MD
Additional Professor
Department of Community Medicine and Family Medicine
All India Institute of Medical Sciences
Bibinagar, Hyderabad, Telangana, India

Contributors xi

Ravish H MBBS MD
Professor Department of Community Medicine
St John's Medical college
Bengaluru, Karnataka, India

Revathi TM MBBS MD
Assistant Professor
KS Hegde Medical Academy, NITTE DU
Mangaluru, Karnataka, India

Rivu Basu MBBS MD MBA FAIMER
Assistant Professor
All India Institute of Hygiene and Public Health
Kolkata, West Bengal, India

Rock D Britto MBBS MD
Associate Professor
Department of Community Medicine
Dhanalakshmi Srinivasan Medical College
Perumbalur, Tamil Nadu, India

Roopa R Mendagudali MBBS MD PhD Scholar
Associate Professor
Department of Community Medicine
MR Medical Sciences
Kalaburagi, Karnataka, India

Rubina Saha MBBS MD
Senior Resident
Department of Community Medicine
All India Institute of Medical Sciences
Hyderabad, Telangana, India

Sanjay Zodpey MBBS MD PhD DSc (Honoris Causa)
Doctor of Medicine (Honoris Causa)
President
Public Health Foundation of India
New Delhi, India

Saranya R MBBS MD
Assistant Professor
Department of Community Medicine
ESICMC and PGIMSR
Bengaluru, Karnataka, India

Sarit Kumar Rout PhD
Additional Professor
Indian Institute of Public Health
Bhubaneswar, Odisha, India

Saritha Nair MBBS MD
Scientist E
ICMR – National Institute of Medical Statistics
New Delhi, India

Sathiabalan M MBBS MD
Assistant Professor
Department of Community Medicine
ESICMC and PGIMSR
Bengaluru, Karnataka, India

Shailaja S Patil MBBS MD
Professor
Department of Community Medicine
BLDE(DU) Shri BM Patil Medical College
Hospital and Research Centre
Vijayapura, Karnataka, India

Shambhavi Ashutosh Vaidya MBBS MD
Senior Resident
Department of Community Medicine
Bangalore Medical College and Research Institute
Bengaluru, Karnataka, India

Sivaram Kiraseni MBBS MD
Senior Resident
Department of Community and Family Medicine
All India Institute of Medical Sciences
Bibinagar, Hyderabad, Telangana, India

Somen Saha PhD
Associate Professor
Indian Institute of Public Health
Gandhinagar, Gujarat, India

Sonu Goel MBBS MD
Professor
Department of Community Medicine and School of Public Health
Postgraduate Institute of Medical Education and Research
Chandigarh, India

Soumya Swaroop Sahoo MBBS MD
Assistant Professor
Department of Community and Family Medicine
All India Institute of Medical Sciences
Bathinda, Punjab, India

Sourav Basu MBBS MD
Assistant Professor
Indian Institute of Public Health–Delhi
Public Health Foundation of India
New Delhi, India

Sridevi Kulkarni MBBS MD
Senior Resident
Department of Community Medicine
Kempegowda Institute of Medical Sciences
Bengaluru, Karnataka, India

Sudha Sharma MBBS MD
Assistant professor, MLB Medical College
Jhansi, Uttar Pradesh, India

Sudhir Prabhu H MBBS MD
Professor and Head of Department
Father Muller Medical College
Mangaluru, Karnataka, India

Sudip Bhattacharya MBBS MD
Assistant Professor
Department of Community Medicine
All India Institute of Medical Sciences
Deoghar, Jharkhand, India

Suhasini R Kanyadi MBBS MD
Assistant Professor
Department of Community Medicine
University Sains Malaysia–Karnataka Lingayat Education
International Medical Programme
Belgaum, Karnataka, India

Suhitha R Das MBBS MD
Assistant Professor
Department of Community Medicine
Sri Siddhartha Institute of Medical Sciences and Research Centre
T Begur, Nelamangala Taluk, Karnataka, India

Sumit Chawla MBBS MD
Assistant Professor
Department of Community Medicine
Shri Atal Bihari Vajpayee Government Medical College and Hospital
Chhainsa, Faridabad, Haryana, India

Sumit Malhotra MBBS MD
Professor
Department of Community Medicine
All India Institute of Medical Sciences
New Delhi, India

Sunhitha Velamala MBBS MD
Senior Resident and Project Officer
Bangalore Urban Mental Health Initiative
Department of Epidemiology, Centre for Public Health
National Institute of Mental Health and Neuro Sciences (NIMHANS)
Bangalore, Karnataka, India

Sushantha Perduru MBBS MD
Assistant Professor
Department of Community Medicine, A J Institute of Medical Sciences and Research Center
Mangaluru, Karnataka, India

Suthanthira Kannan MBBS MD
Assistant Professor
Department of Community Medicine
ESIC Medical College and Hospital
KK Nagar, Chennai, Tamil Nadu, India

Sweta Balappa Athani MBBS MD
Assistant Professor
Department of Community Medicine
ESICMC and PGIMSR
Bengaluru, Karnataka, India

Swetha Rajeshwari MBBS MD
Public Health Specialist Grade III
All India Institute of Hygiene and Public Health
Kolkata, India

Tanvi Kiran PhD
Assistant Professor of Health Economics
ESICMC and PGIMSR
Chandigarh, India

Tulika Goswami MBBS MD PhD
Professor and Head
Department of Community Medicine
Assam Medical College
Assam, India

Vikas Yadav MBBS MD
Scientist E
Indian Council of Medical Research–National Institute for Research in Environmental Health
Bhopal, Madhya Pradesh, India

Foreword

The field of Research Methodology is an ever-evolving landscape, where the rigor of scientific inquiry meets the dynamic complexities of health issues. The Indian Association of Preventive and Social Medicine (IAPSM) has consistently been at the forefront of fostering a culture of evidence-based medicine and public health practices. Recognizing the need for a comprehensive resource that encompasses the multifaceted nature of research in community medicine, we are proud to present the *IAPSM's Textbook of Comprehensive Research Methodology*.

The *IAPSM's Textbook of Comprehensive Research Methodology* is organized into six comprehensive sections, each exploring essential paradigms and methods in modern research. It begins with the foundational principles of research, progresses through the statistical rigors of quantitative methods, and unpacks the depth of qualitative research. The book then provides practical strategies for operational research, tools for economic evaluation and health technology assessment, and concludes with methodologies for systematic reviews and meta-analysis.

In crafting this textbook, we have had the privilege of collaborating with over 50 stalwarts from diverse specialties and backgrounds. Their contributions reflect the depth and breadth of knowledge that the IAPSM represents. Each author brings a wealth of experience and insight, ensuring that each chapter is not only informative but also imbued with practical wisdom. It is with great pride that we offer this textbook to the community of researchers, academicians, practitioners, and students. We believe that the *IAPSM's Textbook of Comprehensive Research Methodology* will serve as a cornerstone reference, guiding current and future generations in their quest to conduct research that informs, impacts, and illuminates the path to better health outcomes.

The *IAPSM's Textbook of Comprehensive Research Methodology*, penned by multiple authors, offers a diverse and invigorating perspective that is both refreshing and exemplary. I would like to express my sincere gratitude to the Editor, Professor Sanjay Zodpey, his editorial team, and the contributors for their tireless efforts and collective wisdom have been instrumental in bringing this textbook to life. Their dedication to the advancement of research methodology is what makes this comprehensive guide not just a repository of knowledge, but a beacon for innovation and excellence in public health research. Together, let us embark on this journey of discovery, equipped with the tools and knowledge to not only ask the right questions but also to find the answers that will shape the future of public health and medicine.

AM Kadri
National President
Indian Association of Preventive and Social Medicine

Preface

In the dynamic world of medical research, methodology acts as the compass that guides scholars through the multifaceted landscape of inquiry. It is with immense pride and a sense of responsibility toward the advancement of evidence-based public health that we present the *IAPSM's Textbook of Comprehensive Research Methodology*. This resource is a testament to the collaboration of over fifty luminaries in the field, each contributing their profound expertise to forge a text that is both foundational and forward-thinking.

Chapters in the textbooks are grouped in six sections.

Section 1: Basics of Research Methodology sets the stage for this intellectual journey, presenting the elemental concepts that underpin all research endeavors.

Section 2: Quantitative Research Methodology which aims to master the precision and objectivity that quantitative research demands.

Section 3: Qualitative Research Methodology invites readers to embrace the subtleties of human experience, enriching the quantitative perspective with depth and narrative.

Section 4: Operational Research applies these methodologies to the operational aspects of health care, emphasizing the translation of research into practice.

Section 5: Economic Evaluation and Health Technology Assessment addresses the imperative of cost-efficiency and value in health technology, an increasingly crucial aspect of healthcare decision-making.

Section 6: Systematic Review and Meta-analysis culminates the text, providing a rigorous approach to aggregating and analyzing research findings, offering a comprehensive synthesis of the available evidence.

The collective wisdom encapsulated in this textbook serves not just as a guide to research methodology but as a beacon for those who seek to illuminate the complexities of public health with the light of research. It is a bridge between theory and practice, between knowledge and application, and between the present challenges and future advancements in health research.

I extend my heartfelt gratitude to the Editor, Professor Sanjay Zodpey, and his dedicated editorial team for their exceptional efforts in orchestrating this comprehensive resource. Their commitment and expertise have been the cornerstone of this publication's success.

We trust that this textbook will inspire current and future generations of researchers, providing them with the intellectual toolkit necessary to embark upon their own quests for knowledge and to contribute meaningfully to the ongoing narrative of medical science. But, there is always a scope of improvement. We are eager to receive feedback from respected teachers and researchers.

Please share your valuable feedback/suggestions to academia.iapsm@gmail.com.

Purushottam Giri
Secretary General
Indian Association of Preventive and Social Medicine

Preface

Research is an integral pillar of public health action. Evidence informed public health decision making requires robust contextual evidence that is generated through research studies. This research must be health system informed and aligned to the future needs of the health system.

Young public health professionals and public health researchers in general, particularly those who are pursuing a doctoral program or working in a research role should be equipped with strong research skills. The research skills should be nurtured during the dissertation work undertaken by the postgraduate students. They should learn the methodology and the conduction of research.

There is a great emphasis placed upon the proper planning, handling, analysis, and reporting of data for producing a high-quality dissertation work. Within the Indian setting, we have witnessed a stronger emphasis on the conduction and publication of research work in colleges and universities.

With this textbook, the IAPSM has created a wonderful resource that has been led by experienced teachers and researchers to distil their technical knowledge for the consumption of bright and eager minds. The chapters and the content are well aligned and progress naturally for a reader. This textbook is a resource for current and future cohorts of budding researchers.

I am sure that the efforts of the Association in storing the development of this textbook will strengthen research skills among the readers.

Professor Sanjay Zodpey

Acknowledgments

We, the editors of *IAPSM's Textbook of Comprehensive Research Methodology*, hereby like to thank Dr AM Kadri, President IAPSM, and Dr. Purushottam Giri, Secretary General IAPSM for their unwavering support which has paved the way for the making of this book titled *IAPSM's Textbook of Comprehensive Research Methodology* from the modules of *IAPSM's Research Methodology Workshop*. The guiding force and inspiration for us is our Chief Editor and Former President IAPSM, Dr Sanjay Zodpey, one of the well-known eminent researchers. The book covering topics from basic research to advanced research methods has been molded with expertise, skill, hard work, passion, and dedication. It is with immense pleasure we would like to thank each and every speaker, experts in their field who gave their precious time and contributions which provided invaluable insights to participants as well as the coordinating teams. All coordinators and facilitators who balanced and put in a lot of their time have not only been the backbone for the module but also the workforce behind chapters of their modules. "Teamwork makes the dreamwork" as truly said is seen vividly in the making of this book. We, on this occasion would also like to thank our Past Presidents of IAPSM, Dr Suneela Garg and Dr Harivansh Chopra who supported the workshop, from which we could bring this book into a reality. We also thank the Secretary General IAPSM, Dr Purushottam Giri for his support.

Last but not the least, we gratefully thank Shri Jitendar P Vij (Group Chairman), Mr Ankit Vij (Managing Director), Mr MS Mani (Group President), Dr Madhu Choudhary (Director-Educational Publishing), Ms Pooja Bhandari (Director-Production), Ms Sunita Katla (Executive Assistant to Group Chairman and Publishing Manager), Mr Ajay Kumar Sharma [Deputy General Manager (Books and Journals)], for their all-round support as and when needed. We also acknowledge the help of Dr Upma Tomar (Development Editor), Mr Rajesh Sharma (Production Coordinator), Ms Neha (Cover Visualizer), Mr Kulwant Singh (Typesetter), Mr Dilip Kumar Jha (Quality Analysts), Satender Singh (Graphic Designer), and wish to thank all others of M/s Jaypee Brothers Medical Publishers (P) Ltd., New Delhi, India, who worked for this project.

Dedication in its true sense can bring wonders when likeminded people come together for a cause. The effect shall only then be exponential.

Rashmi Kundapur
Deepthi R
Anusha Rashmi
Suthanthira Kannan

Contents

SECTION 1 BASICS OF RESEARCH METHODOLOGY

Chapter 1: Title and Abstract for a Research Paper — 3
Deepthi R, Suhitha R Das, Nirmala CJ

Chapter 2: Formulation of a Research Question and Hypothesis — 10
Arvind Kasthuri, Suhitha R Das, Nirmala CJ

Chapter 3: SMART Objectives — 16
Manish Rana, Nirmala CJ, Suhasini Kanyadi, Suhitha R Das

Chapter 4: Review of Literature — 22
Farah Naaz Fathima, Suhitha R Das, Suhasini Kanyadi

Chapter 5: Methodology and Quantitative Study Designs in Research — 27
Pradeep Kumar, IPSA Mohapatra, Nirmala CJ, Meely Panda, Suhitha R Das

Chapter 6: Protocol Writing — 35
Anil Purty, Raghavendra R Huchchannavar, Suhitha R Das, Sridevi Kulkarni

Chapter 7: Manuscript Writing — 41
Sanjay Zodpey, Raghavendra R Huchchannavar, Aditi Mohta, Suhitha R Das, Manjula R

Chapter 8: Research to Health Policy — 46
AM Kadri, Somen Saha, Chandana H, Sudha Sharma, Nishanth Krishna K, Sivaram Kiraseni

SECTION 2 QUANTITATIVE RESEARCH METHODOLOGY

Chapter 9: Descriptive Studies — 55
Deepthi R, Raghavendra Huchchannavar, Suhitha R Das, Manjula R

Chapter 10: Analytical Study Designs — 59
Tulika Goswami, Nirmala CJ, Sweta Balappa Athani, Baidurjya Mahanta, Mridushman Saikia, Manjula R

Chapter 11: Cross-sectional Study Design — 61
Pradeep Aggarwal, Darshan BB, Sudip Bhattacharya, Rubina Saha, Meely Panda

Chapter 12: Case-control Study Design — 65
Amir Maroof Khan, Chandralekha Kona, Aditi Mohta, Ekta Gupta, Meely Panda

Chapter 13: Cohort Study Design — 70
Prem Mony, Bhushan Kamble, Chandralekha Kona

Chapter 14: Experimental Study Designs — 77
NR Ramesh Masthi, Ashwath Narayan, Ravish H, Shivram, Ramesh Holla, Suhasini R Kanyadi, Sweta Balappa Athani

Chapter 15:	Sample Size Estimation Manjula R, Mitasha Singh, Manish Goel, Suhasini Kanyadi, Preety Tanwar, Aditi Mohta, Meely Panda	89
Chapter 16:	Sampling Methods and Errors Rivu Basu, Mitasha Singh, Raghavendra Huchchannavar, Ameenah H Siraja, Aditi Mohta, Bhushan Kamble, Manjula R	98
Chapter 17:	Basic Statistics Rashmi Kundapur, Sumit Chawla, Archisman Mohapatra, Aditi Mohta, Suhasini Kanyadi, Preety Tanwar, Manjula R, Bhushan Kamble	107
Chapter 18:	Test of Significance Malatesh Undi, Rachana AR, Raghavendra Huchchannavar, Ameenah H Siraja, Manjula R	125
Chapter 19:	Advanced Statistics Soumya Swaroop Sahoo, Kamal Kishore, Aditi Mohta, Bhushan Kamble	136
Chapter 20:	Referencing and Discussion Rock D Britto, Raghavendra Huchchannavar, Sridevi Kulkarni, Manjula R	149

SECTION 3 QUALITATIVE RESEARCH METHODOLOGY

Chapter 21:	Introduction to Qualitative Research Roopa R Mendagudali, Amit Rao, Anusha Rashmi, Chethana K	167
Chapter 22:	Types of Qualitative Research Hethal Rathod (Waghela), Abhishek V Raut, Amol Dongre, Swetha Rajeshwari, Amit Rao, Anusha Rashmi, Revathi TM	182
Chapter 23:	Sampling in Qualitative Research Saritha Nair, Maria Nelliyanil, Anusha Rashmi, Sunhitha Velamala	194
Chapter 24:	Analysis and Ethics in Qualitative Studies Abhishek V Raut, Amit Rao, Anusha Rashmi, Sushantha Perduru	203
Chapter 25:	Report Writing in Qualitative Research Pradeep Deshmukh, Maria Nelliyanil, Roopa R Mendagudali, Amit Rao	211
Chapter 26:	Educational Research Rashmi Kundapur, Sridevi Kulkarni, Roopa R Mendagudali, Shambhavi Ashutosh Vaidya	216
Chapter 27:	Practical Applications of Qualitative Research N Nakkeeran, Sridevi Kulkarni, Roopa R Mendagudali, Amit Rao	221

SECTION 4 OPERATIONAL RESEARCH

Chapter 28:	Overview of Operational Research Shailaja S Patil, Chandrika R Doddihal, Sonu Goel	227
Chapter 29:	Introduction to Health Systems Covering WHO Building Blocks Pentapati Siva Santosh kumar, Bhavesh Modi	233
Chapter 30:	Operational Research in Health Programs Sumit Malhotra, Saranya R, Bhavesh Modi	238

Contents xxiii

Chapter 31: **Role of Stakeholders and Ethical Concerns** 249
Pentapati Siva Santosh Kumar, Anwita Khaitan, Anil Jacob Purty

Chapter 32: **Qualitative Research in Operational Research** 253
Rashmi Kundapur, Suthanthira Kannan

Chapter 33: **Quasi-experimental Studies** 256
Ashwini Lonimath, Sumit Malhotra, Sonu Goel

Chapter 34: **Qualitative Analysis in Operational Research** 268
Sathiabalan M, Jeyashree Kathiresan

Chapter 35: **Writing for Media Communication** 273
Chandana H, Rashmi Kundapur, Suthanthira Kannan

Chapter 36: **Funding Opportunities in Operational Research** 277
Siva Santosh Kumar Pentapati, Aditi Mohta, Deepak B Saxena

SECTION 5 ECONOMIC EVALUATION AND HEALTH TECHNOLOGY ASSESSMENT

Chapter 37: **Economic Evaluation and its Types** 283
Farah Naaz Fathima, Rivu Basu, Sudhir Prabhu, Chandralekha Kona

Chapter 38: **Concept of Cost and Cost Analysis** 289
Somen Saha, Kedar Mehta

Chapter 39: **Micro and Macro Health Economics** 296
Sarit Kumar Rout, Sudhir Prabhu H, Chandralekha Kona

Chapter 40: **Introduction to HTA and Steps in HTA Protocol Development** 299
Suthanthira Kannan, Komal Shah, Chandrlekha Kona

Chapter 41: **Outcome Assessment in Economic Evaluation Studies** 302
Tanvi Kiran, Divya Sharma, Mohammad Waseem Faraz Ansari

Chapter 42: **Sensitivity Analysis and Modeling** 307
Komal Shah, A Akshay Subramanian, Sunhitha Velamala, Mohammad Waseem Faraz Ansari

Chapter 43: **Budget Impact Analysis** 311
Somen Saha, Kedar Mehta

Chapter 44: **Drawing up the Protocol for an Economic Evaluation Study** 314
Farah Naaz Fathima, Chandralekha Kona

SECTION 6 SYSTEMATIC REVIEW AND META-ANALYSIS

Chapter 45: **Systematic Review and Meta-analysis: Rationale** 323
Pankaj Bharadwaj, Sourav Basu, Ashwini Lonimath

Chapter 46: **Writing a Good SRMA Research Question** 327
Sourav Basu, Ashwini Lonimath, Pankaj Bharadwaj

Chapter 47:	**Protocol Writing in Systematic Review and Meta-analysis** *Manoj Kumar Gupta, Dewesh Kumar, Suthanthira Kannan*	330
Chapter 48:	**Search Strategy in Systematic Review and Meta-analysis** *Akhil Dhanesh Goel, Medha Mathur, Suthanthira Kannan*	333
Chapter 49:	**PRISMA Flowchart** *Padmavathi S, Suthanthira Kannan, Akhil Dhanesh Goel, Sourav Basu*	336
Chapter 50:	**Data Extraction** *Suthanthira Kannan S, Rashmi Kundapur*	346
Chapter 51:	**Introduction to RevMan in Systematic Review and Meta-analysis** *Mahalaqua Nazli Khatib, Dhanajayan, Rashmi Kundapur*	350
Chapter 52:	**Choosing the Measures of Effect in Systematic Review and Meta-analysis** *Jaykaran Charan, Deepthi R, Suthanthira Kannan*	353
Chapter 53:	**Principles of Meta-analysis in Systematic Review and Meta-analysis** *Vikas Yadav, Pentapati Siva Santosh Kumar, Suthanthira Kannan*	355
Chapter 54:	**Risk of Bias Assessment for Systematic Reviews** *Manya Prasad, Rivu Basu*	357
Chapter 55:	**The GRADE Tool for Rating Certainty in Evidence and Recommendations** *Manya Prasad, Rivu Basu*	363

Index   *371*

"Light up the Researcher in you"

To seek the unknown and more of already the known,
You are here on this field,
A field that has no boundaries,
A field of galaxies.

From ages it is known,
When basic needs are met,
Humans have grown beyond,
Not just in thinking but beyond their intellect,
For only then can one explore their true potential.
Beyond dreams shall you float,
And catch a glimpse of you.

A glimpse that shall show you,
That, you are beyond the wants of worldly materials,
That, you can do much more than you are doing now,
That, you can give much more than you are giving now.

An action driven in the right direction with a right intent,
With no attachments whatsoever,
Shall pave the way for enlightenment.

Hence in this journey,
Take many along with you,
As human possibilities are boundless.

Rashmi Kundapur, Deepthi R, Anusha Rashmi, Suthanthira Kannan

SECTION

Basics of Research Methodology

SECTION OUTLINE

- **Chapter 1:** Title and Abstract for a Research Paper
- **Chapter 2:** Formulation of a Research Question and Hypothesis
- **Chapter 3:** SMART Objectives
- **Chapter 4:** Review of Literature
- **Chapter 5:** Methodology and Quantitative Study Designs in Research
- **Chapter 6:** Protocol Writing
- **Chapter 7:** Manuscript Writing
- **Chapter 8:** Research to Health Policy

CHAPTER 1

Title and Abstract for a Research Paper

Deepthi R, Suhitha R Das, Nirmala CJ

A good title is the title of successful research. The most abstract statements or propositions in science are to be regarded as bundles of hypothetical maxims packed into a portable shape and size.
—William Kingdon Clifford

NEED OF THE TITLE AND ABSTRACT

Title and abstract are the "first line" and "face" of the paper that is read when a reader goes through a journal article. The initial aim of a title is to capture the reader's attention and draw their attention to the research problem being investigated. Often both of these are drafted after the full manuscript is ready. Very few readers will read the full paper and most readers read only the title and the abstract of a research paper. It helps editors to decide whether to process the paper for further review, help reviewers to get an initial impression of the paper and help readers to choose to read full paper, as these may be the only parts of the paper freely available. Keywords in the title and abstract are the ones searched widely by readers to retrieve a particular paper during a search. Title and abstract should be captivating, informative and will introduce the subject to the reader in a clear and concise manner.

Types of Titles

Descriptive, declarative or interrogative titles are the types of titles. They can also be classified as nominal, compound or full sentence titles.

Descriptive or Neutral Title

This title has the essential elements of the research theme, that is, the patients/subjects, design, interventions, comparisons/control, and outcome, but does not reveal the main result or the conclusion. These allow the reader to analyze the paper in an impartial way with an open mind. These types of titles are preferred as it increases visibility of an article.

For example: Effects of intermittent fasting on HbA1c of diabetics.

Declarative Title

The main finding of the study itself is mentioned in the title. This may reduce curiosity of the reader, may create bias in the mind of the reader and hence is best avoided.

For example: Intermittent fasting among diabetics reduced HbA1c levels.

Interrogative Title

This title states a query or the research question in the title. This may sensationalize the topic leading to more downloads. Such titles may be distracting to the reader, hence best avoided for research.
For example: Can intermittent fasting reduce HbA1c levels among diabetics?
From a sentence construct point of view:

Nominal Titles

Titles may just capture only the main theme of the study.
For example: Prevalence of hearing impairment among elderly

Compound Titles

To provide additional relevant information subtitles such as context, design, country, importance are included.
For example: Prevalence of hearing impairment among elderly of Bangalore—A cross sectional study.

Full Sentence Titles

They indicate an added degree of certainty of the results and are longer.
For example: Increased prevalence of hearing impairment among elderly of rural Bangalore—A cross sectional study.
Any of these constructs maybe used depending on the type of article, the key message and the author's preference or judgement.

Components of a Good Title

A good title should have following six key components, i.e., Setting, Population, Intervention, Condition, Endpoint, and Design **["SPICED"].**

Setting

The situation in which the research takes place is known as setting. It could be community-based, home-based, school-based, hospital-based, or laboratory-based. Within the hospital itself, it could be amongst out-patients or inpatients or in the emergency room. Likewise, it could be a rural or an urban setting. If results are not generalizable to other settings, or if the setting reflects the magnitude of the research it is important to mention the setting in the title.

Population

The target of the research work is the population and needs to be explicitly stated (age and/or sex, where necessary).

Intervention

Key element of any clinical trial is intervention.

Condition

Clinical condition of the subjects is referred to as condition.

Endpoint

Unless we wish to use a declarative title, outcome is sparingly used in the title. The change or type of change the condition undergoes after being subjected to intervention, is referred to as the endpoint.

Design

The study design in the title itself makes the title complete and it is usually placed after a colon or hyphen.

Dos and Do nots in Title Writing

- A good title should avoid technical language, easily searchable, substantiated by data and should spark curiosity among readers.
- Fanciful, amusing or clever titles, though look appealing, may be missed or misread by the busy reader and very short titles may miss the essential keywords used by the indexing agencies to catch and categorize the paper. Also, amusing or hilarious titles may be taken less seriously by the readers and may be cited less often.
- An excessively long or complicated title may put off the readers. Titles should be of optimal length not too long nor too short.
- Nonstandard abbreviations and technical jargons should be avoided.

Consider your audience before finalizing the title. Discussing the title with a colleague is a worthwhile option.

Table 1 has the checklist for drafting a good title for a research paper and **Box 1** reviews and comments on a few titles of IJCM.

Table 1: Some titles from IJCM publications and remark/comment on their appropriateness.

Title	Comment/remark on the contents of the title
Challenges in Detection of Adolescent Anemia: Validation of Point-of-Care Device (Mission® Plus) for Hemoglobin Measurement Among Tribal Residential School Children of Selected Districts of Odisha, India	Long title (28 words) capturing the main theme; site of study is mentioned
Cost-effectiveness of Universal Repeat Human Immunodeficiency → Virus → Screening → In Pregnancy: A Cross-sectional Study from Western India	Optimum number of words capturing the main theme; site, type of study is mentioned, no abbreviation used
To Study the Awareness About Universal Health Precautions Among Nursing Professionals in a Medical College Hospital of India	The words "to study" can be deleted, site of study can be mentioned
Accountability in Healthcare in India	Very short title may miss out on the essential keywords required for indexing
Maternal Health Status in tribal India: A 5-Year Intervention Program and its Outcome	Site and type of study not mentioned
Journey to Death: Are Health Systems Failing Mothers?	Whimsical title, declarative title, reader may be biased while studying
Devadasi and Their Intimate Partners: Dynamics of Relationship	Short title, Jargons used, maybe missed when searching for keywords, type of study and site not mentioned

> **Box 1:** Checklist/useful tips for formulating a good abstract for a research paper.
> - The abstract should have simple language and phrases (rather than sentences)
> - It should be informative, cohesive and adhering to the structure (subheadings) provided by the target journal. Structured abstracts are preferred over unstructured abstracts
> - It should be independent and stand-alone/complete
> - It should be concise, interesting, unbiased, honest, balanced and precise
> - It should not be misleading or misrepresentative; it should be consistent with the main text of the paper (especially after a revision is made)
> - It should utilize the full word capacity allowed by the journal so that most of the actual scientific facts of the main paper are represented in the abstract
> - It should include the key message prominently
> - It should adhere to the style and the word count specified by the target journal
> - It should avoid nonstandard abbreviations and (if possible) avoid a passive voice
> - Authors should list appropriate "keywords" below the abstract (keywords are used for indexing purpose)

Drafting a Suitable Title

Title is generally written after the main body of the text and the abstract are drafted. Following stepwise process can be followed to draft an appropriate title. The paper should be described by the author in about three sentences ensuring that these sentences contain important scientific words/keywords that describe the main contents and subject of the paper. Then the author should join the sentences to form a single sentence, shorten the length, and finally edit the title to make it more accurate, concise (about 10-15 words) and precise.

Many journals ask the authors to draft a "short title" or "running head" or "running title" for printing in the header or footer of the printed paper. This is an abridged version of the main title of up to 40-50 characters, may have standard abbreviations and helps the reader to navigate through the paper.

THE ABSTRACT

Importance of Abstract

An abstract is a summary or synopsis of the full research paper. It also needs to have similar characteristics like the title. It needs to be simple, direct, specific, functional, unbiased, concise, self sufficient, comprehensive, scholarly and should not be misleading. This is the second most commonly read part of the manuscript and therefore it should reflect the contents of the main text of the paper accurately and thus act as a "real trailer" of the full article.

The readers will go through the full paper only if they find the abstract interesting and relevant to their practice; else they may skip the paper if the abstract is unimpressive. The title and the abstract should be constructed using keywords from all the sections of the main text.

Abstracts are also used for submitting research papers to a conference for consideration for presentation as oral paper or poster. Grammatical and typographic errors reflect poorly on the quality of the abstract, may indicate carelessness/casual attitude on part of the author and hence should be avoided at all times.

Types of Abstracts

The abstracts can be structured or unstructured. ***Structured*** and ***unstructured abstracts:***

Structured Abstracts

These are followed by most journals, are more informative and include specific subheadings/subsections under which the abstract needs to be composed. These subheadings usually include context/background, objectives, design, setting, participants, interventions, main outcome measures, results and conclusions. Structured abstracts are more elaborate, informative, easy to read, recall and peer review and hence are preferred; however, they consume more space and can have same limitations as an unstructured abstract.

Unstructured Abstracts

It is also known as nonstructured abstracts, are free flowing and do not have predefined subheadings. They are commonly used for papers that usually do not describe original research. Though structured abstract is understood better, final format depends on the journal style.

The following elements need to be properly written under each subheading:

Introduction/Background and/or Objectives

These states why the work was undertaken and is usually written in just a couple of sentences. The hypothesis/study question and the major objectives are also stated under this subheading.

Methods

This subsection is the longest, states what was done and essential details of the study setting, design, participants, blinding, sample size, sampling method, intervention/s, duration and follow up, research instruments, main outcome measures, parameters evaluated and how the outcomes were assessed or analyzed are given.

Results/Observations/Findings

This subheading states what was found. It is longer and is difficult to draft and needs to mention important details including the number of study participants, results of analysis of primary and secondary objectives and include actual data of numbers, mean, median, standard deviation, "P" values, 95% confidence intervals, effect sizes, relative risks, odds ratio, etc.

Conclusions

The take home message which is the "so what" of the paper and other significant findings should be stated here, considering the interpretation of the research question/hypothesis and results put together without over interpreting the findings and may also include the author's views on the implications of the study.

Drafting a Suitable Abstract

It is important to follow the instructions to authors like format, word limit, font size/style, and subheadings provided by the journal for which the abstract and the paper are being written. Most journals allow 200-300 words for the abstract and it is wise to restrict oneself to this word limit. To maintain accuracy and conformity with the main text of the paper it is recommended to draft the abstract in the end thus maintaining an easy linkage/alignment with title, on one hand and the introduction section of the main text, on the other hand. Subheadings of the structured abstract permitted by the target journal should be checked, phrases should be used rather than sentences to draft the content of the abstract and passive voice should be avoided by the authors.

Next, the authors need to edit the abstract meticulously, remove redundant words to the correct word count permitted. It is important to ensure that the key message, focus and novelty of the paper are not compromised; the rationale of the study and the basis of the conclusions are clear; and that the abstract is consistent with the main text of the paper. Similar caution must be taken while revising the abstract too.

Nonstandard abbreviations need to be avoided and do not cite references, tables or figures in the abstract. It is always helpful in getting an opinion of a colleague on the content of the abstract. Suitable "keywords" preferably chosen from the Medical Subject Headings (MeSH) list of the U.S. National Library of Medicine (https://meshb.nlm.nih.gov/search) should be written as they are used for indexing purposes. These keywords need to be different/variant of the words from the main title as the title words are automatically used for indexing. Some formats like International Committee of Medical Journal Editors (ICMJE); http://www.icmje.org/ recommends publishing the clinical trial registration number at the end of the abstract.

Relevance of Title and Abstract During Publications

- ❖ The "title" and the "abstract" need to be drafted accurately, carefully, and meticulously since they are "initial impressions" of a research article. One should adhere to the instructions by the "target journal" regarding the style and number of words permitted for the title and the abstract.
- ❖ A novice author may have to browse through titles and abstracts of several prominent journals to learn more about the wording and styles of the titles and abstracts, as well as the aims and scope of the particular journal.
- ❖ The abstract should be consistent with the main text of the paper and should include the key message prominently. It is very important to include the "keywords" in the title and the abstract for appropriate indexing purposes and for retrieval from the search engines and scientific databases. Such keywords should be listed after the abstract.
- ❖ One must adhere to the instructions of the target journal with regard to the style and number of words permitted for the title and the abstract. Great titles and clearly-outlined abstracts speed up the editorial process and increase readership.

KEY POINTS

- Title and abstract are the "first line" and "face" of the paper that is read.
- Title and abstract should be captivating, informative and will introduce the subject to the reader in a clear and concise manner.
- Three types of titles: Descriptive, Declarative or Interrogative. Further classified into nominal, compound or full sentence.
- A good title should have following six key components, i.e., Setting, Population, Intervention, Condition, End-point, and Design ["SPICED"].
- The abstract is a summary or synopsis of the full research paper.
- Two types of abstracts: Structured and Unstructured.
- A checklist is of immense importance while constructing a title and an abstract.

BIBLIOGRAPHY

1. Andrade C. How to write a good abstract for a scientific paper or conference presentation. Indian J Psychiatry, 2011;53:172-5.
2. Andrade C. How to write a good abstract for a scientific paper or conference presentation. Indian J Psychiatry. 2011;53:172-5.
3. Bavdekar SB. Formulating the right title for a research article. J Assoc Physicians India. 2016;64:536.

4. Cals JWL, Kotz D. Effective writing and publishing scientific papers, part II: Title and abstract. J Clin Epidemiol. 2013;66:585.
5. Dewan P, Gupta P. Writing the title, abstract and introduction: Looks matter! Indian Pediatr. 2016;53:23541.
6. Gupta P. Framing a suitable title. In: Gupta P, Singh N (Eds). How to Write the Thesis and Thesis Protocol. A Primer for Medical, Dental and Nursing Courses. First Edition. New Delhi: Jaypee Brothers Medical Publishers; 2014. p. 45-9.
7. Hartley J. Current findings from research on structured abstracts: An update. J Med Lib Assoc. 2014;102:146-8.
8. Jamali HR, Nikzad M. Article title type and its relation with the number of downloads and citations. Scientometrics 2011;88:653-61.
9. Papanas N, Georgiadis GS, Maltezos E, Lazarides MK. Writing a research abstract: Eloquence in miniature. Int Angiol. 2012;31:297-302.
10. Tullu MS, Karande S. Writing a model research paper: A roadmap. J Postgrad Med. 2017;63:1436.

CHAPTER 2

Formulation of a Research Question and Hypothesis

Arvind Kasthuri, Suhitha R Das, Nirmala CJ

> *"He who does not know what he is looking for will not lay hold of what he has found when he gets it."*
> —Claude Bernard

INTRODUCTION

Research questions are the crux of systematic investigation. Recording accurate outcomes is solely dependent on asking accurate questions.

Asking the proper questions when conducting research can assist you in gathering pertinent and illuminating information. This eventually has a good impact on your work. The best research questions are often simple to comprehend, concise and interesting.

Defining a Research Question

A research question is a particular question to which the study is trying to find an answer. It is at the center of systematic study and it aids in defining a clear course for the research procedure.

For example: "What is the prevalence of diabetes mellitus in elderly residents of ward no 100 in Mumbai city?"

Any research project must begin with a well-defined research question that is then further refined. As Howie suggested, "To find the right question requires that we understand what we are asking about and know how to keep the question simple enough to be answerable, but challenging enough to be interesting".

Importance of a Research Question

According to Creswell, the primary importance of framing the research question is that it narrows down a broad topic of interest into a specific one. Along with hypotheses, research questions act as a foundation for direction. Additionally, these questions clearly define the study's parameters, establishing its bounds and preserving its coherence.

Additionally, the study as a whole is impacted by the research question. These issues have an impact on things like research technique, sample size, data collection and data analysis.

Characteristics of a Good Research Question

A query that is well-stated but only partially addressed. A question's wording is frequently more significant than its answer. A good question will possess certain traits. It frequently refers to recent experiences that the person asks about and ones that they are interested in. It shouldn't be excessively broad or little.

Table 1: FINER criteria for creating a strong research question.	
Feasible	• Adequate number of subjects
	• Adequate technical expertise
	• Affordable in time and money
	• Manageable in scope
Interesting	• Getting the answer intrigues investigator, peers and community
Novel	• Confirms, refutes or extends previous findings
Ethical	• Amenable to a study that institutional review board will approve
Relevant	• To scientific knowledge
	• To clinical and health policy
	• To future research

The FINER criteria **(Table 1)** should be used when creating a strong research topic, according to Hulley and colleagues. The FINER criteria highlight practical elements that might improve the likelihood of creating a fruitful research endeavor. A good research question should identify the target group, be relevant to the clinical setting, advance field knowledge and be of interest to both the scientific community and the general public.

By Richardson et al. in 1995, the PICOT framework was initially made public. It is possible to create research questions that cover key aspects of the study, such as the population being examined, the anticipated results, and the amount of time needed to attain the results, using the PICOT framework. Clinical research and evidence-based studies increasingly frequently use the framework with these components.

❖ P – population, patients, or problem
❖ I – intervention or indicator being studied
❖ C – comparison group
❖ O – outcome of interest
❖ T – timeframe of the study

How to Formulate a Strong Research Question

A good research question should, in general, be pertinent, determined and significant. There is a certain approach you can use to make the process of developing a research question easier. The following list of stages is for this approach:

Start with a Broad Topic

A large subject gives authors a lot of options to consider as they look for a strong research question. Using brainstorming and concept mapping, you can break down a topic into subtopics and possible research questions. These methods can help you structure your ideas so you can find connections and important topics within a big topic.

Do Preliminary Research to Learn About Topical Issues

After choosing a subject, you can begin your preliminary research. This first phase of research achieves two objectives. A preliminary analysis of the relevant literature will first help you identify the topics that academics and other researchers are currently debating. You acquire current, pertinent knowledge about your subject in this manner.

Second, a preliminary analysis of relevant literature enables you to identify any knowledge gaps or constraints in your field. You can later use these gaps as the subject of your research topic with a little bit of fine-tuning.

Narrow Down Your Topic and Determine Potential Research Questions

You can begin concentrating on a more specialized area of study once you have accumulated sufficient knowledge of the subject you wish to explore. Focusing on lacunae in current knowledge or recent publications is one possibility. Problematization is another strategy. Likewise, researchers can select study topics that build upon or supplement the results of prior literature. This entails developing research questions that cast doubt on your assumptions or expertise in the field of investigation.

Evaluate the Soundness of Your Research Question

Your preliminary investigation and analysis of the pertinent material should have led to several intriguing questions that seem worthwhile for further investigation. But not all intriguing queries are good choices for investigation. Remember that a research question is answered or drawn to a conclusion by an examination of the available data.

The "FINER" and "PICOT" criteria can be used to determine whether a research question is sound.

Types of Research Questions

Broadly there are three types of questions.

Descriptive Research Questions

The seek to measure the responses of a study's population to one or more variables or describe variables that the research will measure. Typically, these queries start with "what."

Comparative Research Questions

The focus is on identifying differences between two or more groups for an outcome variable. These queries may also be causal. For instance, the researcher might contrast two groups: one in which a particular variable is present, and the other in which it is not.

Relationship Research Questions

The looks for trends and interactions between two or more variables along with studying and describing them. These inquiries frequently use the terms "association" or "trends," as well as dependent and independent variables.

Good and Bad Research Question Examples

The following examples of good and bad research questions can help researchers craft a research question more effectively.

Example no. 1

- ❖ **Bad:** What impact does social media have on people's actions?
- ❖ **Good:** What impact does everyday YouTube use have on youngsters under the age of 16 in terms of their attention span?

The first research question is deemed inadequate due to the ambiguity of the term "social media" and the lack of precision in the query. A good research topic should be well defined and have a clear response that can be ascertained through data collection and analysis.

Example no. 2
- **Bad:** Has childhood obesity increased in the US during the past ten years?
- **Good:** How have parental education levels and school intervention initiatives impacted the prevalence of childhood obesity among kids in first through sixth grades?

In the above-given example, the first research question is not the best choice because it is too straightforward and can be answered with a simple "yes" or "no." The second research topic is more challenging; in order to respond to it, the researcher must gather information, conduct a thorough analysis of the information and develop an argument that encourages further discussion.

Hypothesis in Research

A hypothesis is a tentative answer to a problem, which implies that before discovering the outcomes based on a review of the literature, we will first construct a hypothesis based on the issue at hand. For instance, while defining a problem: According to this assertion, the notion is that the "urbanization problem is more prevalent in smaller cities than it is in larger ones." Based on this the investigator can state the hypothesis.

Concept of Hypothesis

A hypothesis is an assertion of the researcher's expectation or prediction about relationships among the study variables. The research question identifies the ideas under consideration and inquires about their potential relationships. A hypothesis is a prediction of a result.

Essentially, it is a statement that hints at a description, an association or an outcome. Scientific research can be used to test a good hypothesis. It outlines your expectations for the results of your investigation. The object of your study serves as the foundation for your research question.

Example:
"There is an association between smoking tobacco and lung cancer among persons aged 20 years and above in Bangalore city"

In this example,
- **INDEPENDENT** variable is "... smoking tobacco..."
- **DEPENDENT** variable is "... Lung cancer..."
- The **INDEPENDENT** variable is the cause and its value is independent of other variables.
- The **DEPENDENT** variable is the effect and its value is dependent on the changes in the independent variable.

Importance of Research Hypothesis
- It ensures that the research methodologies are scientific and valid.
- It aids to assume the probability of research failure and progress.
- It assists in the provision of links to the theory and research question.
- It helps to analyze the data and validity measurement of research.
- It aids as a basis to prove the validity of the research.
- It assists to describe research study in cemented terms rather than in a theoretical way.

Types of Research Hypothesis

Based on research, there are simple and complex types.

Simple Hypothesis

It predicts the relationship between the dependent and the independent variable.

For example: "There is an association between blood vitamin D levels and incidence of fractures among persons aged 60 years and above in Bangalore city."

Complex Hypothesis

It examines the relationship between two or more independent variables and two or more dependent variables.

For example: "There is an association between physical activity and vitamin D levels and the incidence of falls and fractures among persons aged 60 years and above in Bangalore city."

Based on a statistical standpoint, there are two types of hypotheses: Null and Alternate types:

Null Hypothesis

A null hypothesis is a general statement which states no relationship between two variables or two phenomena. It is usually denoted by H_0.

For example: "There **is NO association** between smoking tobacco and lung cancer among persons aged 20 years and above in Bangalore city."

Alternate Hypothesis

An alternative hypothesis is a statement which states some statistical significance between two phenomena. It is usually denoted by H_1 or H_A.

For example: "There **IS an association** between smoking tobacco and lung cancer among persons aged 20 years and above in Bangalore city."

An Example of Research Question V/S Research Hypothesis V/S Research Objective

Research Hypothesis

"**There is an association** between blood vitamin D levels and incidence of fractures among persons aged 60 years and above in Bangalore city."

Research Question

"**What is the association** between blood vitamin D levels and incidence of fractures among persons aged 60 years and above in Bangalore city?"

Research Objective

"**To study the association** between blood vitamin D levels and incidence of fractures among persons aged 60 years and above in Bangalore city."

KEY POINTS

- A research question is a particular question to which the study is trying to find an answer.
- The best research questions are often simple to comprehend, concise, and interesting.
- The feasible, interesting, novel, ethical and relevant (FINER) criteria highlight practical elements that might improve the likelihood of creating a fruitful research endeavor.
- Population, intervention, comparison group, outcome of interest and timeframe of study (PICOT) framework is increasingly frequently used by clinical research and evidence-based studies.
- To be borne in mind the four stages of framing a strong research question.
- A hypothesis is an assertion of the researcher's expectation or prediction about relationships among the study variables.

BIBLIOGRAPHY

1. Bhandari P. Independent vs. Dependent Variables|Definition & Examples Scribrr. [Online]. Available from: https://www.scribbr.com/methodology/independent-and-dependent-variables/ [Accessed 22 February 2022].
2. Bouchrika I, Researchcom. How to Write a Research Question: Types, Steps, and Examples. Weblog. [Online] Available from: https://research.com/research/how-to-write-a-research-question#:~:text=The%20primary%20importance%20of%20framing,study%20(Creswell%2C%202014).&text=These%20questions%20also%20specifically%20reveal,its%20limits%2C%20and%20ensuring%20cohesion. [Accessed 22 February 2022].
3. Creswell JW. Educational research: Planning, conducting and evaluating quantitative and qualitative research, 5th edition. Upper Saddle River, NJ: Pearson Education; 2014.
4. Dennis FP. Nursing Research: Generating and Assessing Evidence for Nursing Practice, 9th edition. New Delhi: Lippincott Williams and Wilkins; 2012:58-93.
5. Howie JGR. Refining questions and hypotheses. In: Norton PG, Stewart M, Tudiver F, Bass MJ, Dunn EV (eds). Primary Care Research: Vol 1. Traditional and Innovative Approaches. Newbury Park: Sage Publications; 1991:13-25.
6. Hulley S, Cummings S, Browner W, et al. Designing clinical research. 3rd edition. Philadelphia (PA): Lippincott Williams and Wilkins; 2007.
7. Khoo, Ee Ming. Research questions and research objectives. The Family Physician. 2005;13:25-6.
8. Lipowski EE. Developing great research questions. Am J Health Syst Pharm. 2008; 65(17):1667–70. https://doi.org/10.2146/ajhp070276
9. Nursing Research Society of India, Nursing research and statistics. 1st edition. India: Pearson Publication; 2013: 48–51
10. Stone, P. Deciding upon and refining a research question. Palliative Medicine. 2002;16:265–7. https://doi.org/10.1191/0269216302pm562xx

CHAPTER 3

SMART Objectives

Manish Rana, Nirmala CJ, Suhasini Kanyadi, Suhitha R Das

A goal properly set is half way reached. —Zig Ziglar

OBJECTIVES OF A STUDY

Research studies usually start with an idea; an idea or thought that you probably come across in your life and plan to execute it. However, prior to planning a research study, the following questions should come in your mind:

- ❖ **WHAT** are we going to do?
- ❖ **WHY** is it important for us to accomplish this activity?
- ❖ **WHO** is going to be responsible for the activities?
- ❖ **WHEN** do we want this to be completed?
- ❖ **HOW** are we going to do these activities?

It is very essential that we first answer these questions. Once you have answered the questions listed above you need to define your SMART objectives to move those ideas into action.

What are SMART Objectives?

S-Specific	What is the specific task? Who will perform it?	Concrete, detailed, and well defined so that you know where you are going and what to expect when you arrive at it Will this/these objectives lead to the desired results? Is the outcome specified? When you review the objective (preferably from others) it should be clear to them. Their understanding of objectives should be the same as yours
M-Measurable	What are the standards or parameters for measurement?	Numbers and quantities provide means of measurement and comparison How are we going to measure it (outcome) should be clear and shall be identified?
A-Achievable	Is the task feasible?	Feasible and easy to put into action Can this objective be achieved within a given time frame and with available resources? Are the limitations and constraints understood? We should know how we are going to achieve it?

Contd...

Contd...

R-Realistic/ Relevant	Are sufficient resources available?	Consider constraints such as resources, personnel, cost and time frame for achieving the objective. Whether the objectives are realistic in terms of achievement It should be relevant to scientific community and policy makers in decision making
T-Time Bound	What are the start and end dates?	A time frame helps to set boundaries around the objective and will enable you to achieve the objectives in the desired time period Deadline for achieving the objective should be set

Why Use SMART Objectives?

SMART objectives offer a structured approach to work plan development and design. They serve as a systematic framework for monitoring progress towards a target or ultimate goal, allowing for precise measurement of performance and the identification of improvement opportunities. Furthermore, SMART objectives enable the concise communication of intended impact and current progress to stakeholders. They provide a concrete roadmap for how goals will be achieved, enhancing clarity and accountability in the pursuit of organizational or project objectives. Devoting time and resources early on to intentionally writing SMART objectives is an investment in the future of a plan, program or service.

By starting out with SMART objectives, a research/health activity can systematically and meaningfully measure progress, show achievements and identify opportunities for improvement.

Steps in Framing SMART Objectives?

In order to understand how the parts of SMART objectives flow together, the order of the SMART components listed below will go out of order—**SMTRA**.

This is because the **Specific, Measurable and Time-Bound** parts are clearly visible in the standard written format for objectives. They are easy to comprehend and require less elaboration.

The **Relevant** and **Achievable** pieces are more abstract and require deliberation. Each of these parts will include an example objective that will be re-written to be SMART.

Specific

Objectives should be well-defined and clear to investigators, other team members as well as the stakeholders or funding organizations for them to understand the plan of study.

Consider these prompts:

What

- What exactly will you do?
- What is the plan of action?
- What do you intend to impact or what is the likely outcome?

Who

- Who is responsible for carrying out the action?
- What are you intending to impact or who is your target population?

It is important to consider that not all of these questions will be applicable to every objective.
Example: **Original objective:** Staff of the hospital shall be assessed for quality care.
Do we need to fix the objective?
What do we need to fix in this objective?
As mentioned above we need to address **WHAT** and **WHO**?
What - What quality care are we intending to assess?
We intend to assess high quality patient care during hospitalization
Who - Which staff shall provide quality care to patients?
It could be a particular staff in hospitals such as doctors, nurses or ward attendants or it could be all the health care staff.
SMART objective: *Nursing staff of hospital shall be assessed for high quality patient care.*

Measurable

It involves selecting what will be measured to show improvement, impact or success. There may be existing measures and targets that are required for a specific program or grant. Try to pick a measure that is meaningful as the easiest things to measure may not be the most meaningful.

Consider these prompts:
- **How much** and in **what** direction will the change occur?
- **What data** will be used to prove the **target** is met?
- **Where** will this data come from?
- Is there a **stand-in or proxy measure** to use, if, this objective cannot be directly measured, or is there **another measure** that would be more appropriate to use instead?
    Example: **Original objective:** Nursing staff of hospital shall be assessed for high quality patient care
    Do we need to fix the objective?
    We need to clarify how we are going to **MEASURE** and what is it that we are going to measure, i.e., **TARGET**
    We need a criteria to measure high quality patient care provided by nursing staff during hospitalization. What will be the target for the same, if any? Do we have a criteria or shall we use a standard criteria.
    We can use Quality Patient Care Scale **(QUALPACS)** a US based scale.
    We can also use **NABH** scale or other standardized scale considering regional or global comparison as our target.
    SMART objective: *Nursing staff of hospitals shall be assessed for high quality patient care using QUALPACS.*

Time Bound

Objectives should be achievable within a specific time frame. It should not be so soon as to prevent success, or so far away as to encourage procrastination.

Consider these prompts:
- **When** will this objective be achieved?
- Is this **time-frame realistic**?
- Should it be closer or further in the future?
    Original objective: Nursing staff of hospitals shall be assessed for high quality patient care using quality patient care scale (QUALPACS)

Do we need to fix the objective?
We need to clarify when will this objective be achieved; **a date or a month**?
This could be April–May 2022
Is April–May 2022 a realistic target or not. What do we need to consider for this?
We need to consider the number of nursing staff involved in patient care and whether we can achieve the objectives within the time frame.
It may be possible to assess 100–150 nursing staff in 2 months but it may not be feasible to assess 500–600 nursing staff even in 4 months.
The sample size, availability of nursing staff for assessment as well as assessors will also play an important role in deciding the time frame.
SMART objective: *Nursing staff of hospitals shall be assessed for high quality patient care using QUALPACS during April–May 2022.*
Note: We can elaborate the time frame in the methodology section of the proposal but it would be good to include it in the objectives of the proposal. It should also include the time required for data entry, data cleaning, analysis and report writing. We often fail to or refrain from incorporating it in objectives.

Realistic/Relevant

Objectives should align with a larger goal. One should review, if and how successfully completing an objective will be relevant to achieving the goal.

It is essential to consider if an objective relates to the larger program, a plan, an organization's mission or a vision.

It should also be considered whether an objective is relevant or important to the team as well as stakeholders or funding organizations. If the objectives are related to the organization's mission and guiding principles then they are more likely to be accepted and approved by the organizational leadership.

Similarly, if the objectives are the priority of stakeholders or funding organizations it will have a greater probability of being sanctioned.

Consider these prompts:
- Will this objective lead to **achieving the organization's goals?**
- Does it seem **worthwhile to measure this objective**? Does it seem **reasonable to measure this objective**?

Original objective: Nursing staff of hospitals shall be assessed for high quality patient care using QUALPACS during April–May 2022.
Do we need to fix the objective?
For relevance we need to consider how many staff are already providing high quality patient care.
If a high number of staff is already providing patient care, then it probably may not be useful to conduct the assessment or we need to realign our objective with a higher scale of assessment (If available).
If the nursing staff is poorly trained and is just providing basic patient care services then a training for the same can be organized first, followed by assessment.
If no existing data is available a pilot study shall be considered for assessment of level of nursing care and hence the relevance of study.

Achievable

Objectives should be within reach for your team or program, considering available resources, knowledge, time and capacities.

Consider these prompts:
- ❖ **How can this objective** be accomplished?
- ❖ **Given the current time frame or environment,** can this objective be achieved? Should we scale it up or down?
- ❖ **What resources** will help us achieve this objective? What limitations or constraints stand in our way?

Original objective: Nursing staff of hospitals shall be assessed for high quality patient care using QUALPACS during April–May 2022.

Do we need to fix the objective?

It is important to review and understand whether the team is competent and has capacities for assessment. One should consider if the method of assessment is feasible to the team.

If there are other priorities (for organization or stakeholders) such as COVID-19 surge of cases and objectives are not achievable; one should consider submitting proposals at a later stage.

Are there enough resources to meet the objectives of study (availability of budget, logistics, reagents, human resources, etc). If adequate resources are not available then the objectives shall be realigned accordingly.

Other Examples of SMART Objectives

Original Objective

Assessment of weekly IFA supplementation on hemoglobin levels among females.

Do we need to fix this objective? For this we shall use the SMART (SMTRA) criteria to determine it. Whether it is specific, Measurable, Time Bound, Relevant & Achievable.

SMART Objective

Assessment of weekly IFA Supplementation on hemoglobin levels among school going adolescent females in Mehsana district of Gujarat using automated hemoglobinometer during October–December 2022.

Original Objective

Prevalence of hypertension in Bidar district of Karnataka.

Do we need to fix this objective? We shall use the SMART (SMTRA) criteria to determine it. Whether it is specific, Measurable, Time Bound, Relevant & Achievable.

SMART Objective

Prevalence of hypertension among adults above 30 years of age in rural areas of Bidar district of Karnataka using digital sphygmomanometer during August–September 2022.

KEY POINTS
▪ After planning a research study you need to define your SMART objectives to move those ideas into action.
▪ Smart - Specific, measurable, achievable, relevant and time-bound.
▪ The order of the SMART components listed below will go out of order—SMTRA.
▪ Specific, measurable and time-bound parts are easy to comprehend and require less elaboration.
▪ The Relevant and achievable pieces are more abstract and require deliberation.

BIBLIOGRAPHY

1. Bjerke MB, Renger R. Being smart about writing SMART objectives. Eval Program Plann. 2017;61:125-7. doi: 10.1016/j.evalprogplan.2016.12.009. Epub 2016 Dec 23. PMID: 28056403.
2. Chatterjee D, Corral J. How to Write Well-Defined Learning Objectives. J Educ Perioper Med. 2017;19(4): E610. Available from: https://www.ncbi.nlm.nih.gov/pmc/articles/PMC5944406/pdf/i2333-0406-19-4-1a.pdf
3. Jung LA. Writing SMART Objectives and Strategies That Fit the ROUTINE. TEACHING Exceptional Children. 2007;39(4):54–8. https://doi.org/10.1177/004005990703900406
4. Ogbeiwi O. Why written objectives need to be really SMART? Br J Health Care Manag. 2017;23(7): 324-36.
5. Wolf A, Akkaraju S. Teaching Evolution: From SMART Objectives to Threshold Experience. The Journal of Effective Teaching. 2014;14(2):35-48.

Review of Literature

Farah Naaz Fathima, Suhitha R Das, Suhasini Kanyadi

> *Literature always anticipates life. It does not copy it but moulds it to its purpose.*
> —Oscar Wilde

WHAT IS REVIEW OF LITERATURE?

Review of literature is a "survey of scholarly sources of academic value on a specific topic." It is a search that gives us an overview of the current knowledge on the topic, outlines the relevant theories on the subject, describes the methods used to study the topic and helps us to identify gaps in the existing research thereby giving us pointers on how to design our study. There is no need to search, read and include every source that has been ever published on the topic, but it is important to include all key sources.

Traditional sources of literature include articles published in peer reviewed journals, books and reports by international, national or regional organizations. In addition to these, other sources of literature include conference proceedings, empirical studies, theses/dissertations, blogs, newspaper reports and websites. These are called "grey literature" because they may not have gone through the process of rigorous peer review. Journals, books and reports are the preferred sources of literature for a review. If information is not available on the topic in traditional literature, then information from grey literature can be included.

Need for Review of Literature

A good review of the literature helps us answer three critical questions about the research topic of interest.
1. What do we know about the topic?
2. What open questions and knowledge do we not yet know?
3. Why is this information important?

Reading previously published work provides a background to the research topic of interest. Summarizing this into different categories helps to demonstrate the change in knowledge over time. It helps to clarify areas of controversy and agreement and identifies dominant viewpoints. In the process, the researcher will be able to identify gaps, unexplored areas and unanswered questions that will highlight the need for new research.

When Should Review of Literature be Done?

Review of literature is a continuous and iterative process. It is often the first task undertaken while initiating research and one of the last to be completed. It is intricately linked to every stage of a research study.

While writing the introduction section of a research protocol or a manuscript, review of literature helps to familiarize yourself with the language, common terminologies, standard abbreviations, current knowledge and the gaps in knowledge.

The methods section of a research protocol draws from existing literature to identify the research design that is best suited to answering the research question of interest. It is critical for the estimation of the sample size required for the current research. It helps in identifying variables that need to be studied and the most appropriate way of measuring them. It also helps in finding validated questionnaires and other standardized tools that can be used for current research.

Review of literature provides inputs to write the discussion section of a study. Results from other studies will help to provide context for the current study and to explain the reasons for similarities or differences between previous findings and current research. It can be used to explain the public health implications and significance of the findings of the current research and the ways in which these results could be translated into changes in existing policy or clinical practice. Review of literature also helps to explain the reasons for the limitations of the current research and the external validity of the findings.

Steps in Review of Literature

The following are the three key steps in conducting a good review of literature:
1. **Search** for relevant literature
2. **Analysis and synthesis**—evaluate sources and identify themes, debates and gaps
3. **Organize and write** your literature review

Step 1: Search for Relevant Literature

This can be done by identifying the "keywords" related to the topic of research. A simple search by entering the keywords on a generic search engine like Google will result in millions of hits. The output will include everything on the topic like news, announcements, advertisements in addition to journal articles and books. Browsing through all of these is unnecessary and time consuming. This can be refined by doing a smart search. Some ways of doing smart search are as follows:

Use Inverted Commas

For example, when you type diabetes mellitus into any search engine, the output will contain all sites that contain the terms either diabetes or mellitus. When you use inverted commas (E.g., "diabetes mellitus") at the beginning and end of the term, the output will contain only those sites where both the terms appear as one.

Use Boolean Operators

There are three Boolean operators—**AND, OR, NOT**
1. AND gives only outputs that contain both the keywords. For example, the keywords diabetes AND India will give articles that contain both the terms diabetes and India. Thus, the Boolean operator AND helps in narrowing down the search.
2. OR gives outputs that contain either one of the keywords. For example, the keywords, diabetes OR hypertension will give all articles that contain either diabetes or hypertension. Thus, OR helps in broadening the search.
3. NOT is used to specifically exclude certain articles from your search. For example, the keywords, diabetes NOT type 1 will exclude all articles on type 1 diabetes.

Therefore, the use of Boolean operators helps in refining the search for literature on the research topic of interest.

Table 1: Creating search strategy in PubMed.				
Concept (what do you want to search)	Keyword (your keywords)	Mesh term (corresponding terms from mesh data base)	Search inputs (Combination of terms using boolean operators)	Number of articles

PubMed Search (Table 1)

PubMed is a search engine maintained by the National Library of Medicine (NLM) at the National Institutes of Health, USA for its MEDLINE database. It is available free of cost for use by researchers all over the world. Medical subject headings (MeSH) terms are controlled vocabulary terms in PubMed.

Researchers should check the MeSH database to identify the MeSH terms for the "keywords" for their current topic of research. The MeSH terms may or may not be the same as the keywords. For example, the MeSH term for cancer is neoplasm. MeSH terms can be combined with Boolean operators to develop a search strategy. Prepare a summary **Table 1** like the one depicted below for your search.

Step 2: Analysis and Synthesis

Analysis and synthesis are complementary processes while doing a review of the literature. Analysis is the systematic breakdown of relevant literature into its constituent parts. It is similar to zooming in to get to see the individual components. In practical terms, this involves identifying articles related to different sub-topics under the main research topic. For example, a researcher could search the articles on different aspects of diabetes like complications, prevalence, control rates, adherence, rural and urban differences, quality of life, etc. Each of these components would have a separate search strategy.

Synthesis, on the other hand involves making connections between the different components identified during analysis. It is similar to zooming out to see the bigger picture. In this process, the researcher can examine the connections between the different articles and to identify trends and patterns, recurring themes, areas of debates, conflicts and contradictions and pivotal publications on the topic. During synthesis, the researcher will be able to identify areas where lots of literature is available and also areas where there are literature gaps.

Analysis and synthesis are twin processes that happen simultaneously during the literature review process. At the end of this step, the researcher should be able to produce a working "literature review matrix". This matrix will help the researcher to get a good grip on the situation at a glance and appreciate the change in findings based on the sample size and the setting. The researcher needs to break down the main research topic into subheadings and prepare a matrix for each subheading.

Table 2: Literature review matrix template.

Author	Year	Location	Target population	Study design	Sample size	Findings	Comments

The literature review matrix is a table that depicts the name of the author, year of publication, location, target population, study design, sample size, main findings and the researcher's own comments on the study. Summarizing the information in this format will help the researcher in getting a bird's eye view of the available literature which will help in designing the current study and in writing the discussion section of the final manuscript. A sample literature review matrix is depicted below in **Table 2**.

Step 3: Organization and Writing

A structure is essential while writing the review of literature section. This structure consists of an introduction, a body and a conclusion.

The introduction should establish the focus and purpose of the review. This should be aligned with the objectives of the study.

It is preferable to divide the body of the review into subsections. The classification of the subsections may be chronological or thematic or methodological. Chronological subdivisions help us to trace the evolution of the evidence on the topic over time. Thematic subdivisions depend on the identification of the main threads under which the topic can be discussed. Methodological subdivision is a classification based on the study designs generating the evidence in the review.

The conclusion section provides a summary and the main take home messages from the review.

Plagiarism

Plagiarism refers to representing another author's work as one's own original work. This may include use of language, thoughts, ideas or expressions and is done without giving due credit to the original source. Plagiarism is a moral, ethical and a legal issue that authors must be aware of.

There are many plagiarism detection software that is available. All researchers should run their manuscripts through one of these before final submission. Commonly used plagiarism detection software includes ithenticate, Turnitin and plagiarism detector.

Some Tips for Good Writing

- ❖ Plan the outline of the review before beginning. This can be done by outlining the main themes and then adding subthemes for each point to be discussed.
- ❖ Construct well-structured paragraphs. Begin each paragraph with a topic sentence that captures the overall essence of what you want to convey. Use transition words to connect your thoughts.

- Use standard abbreviations and consistent terminology throughout the manuscript.
- Add your own interpretations and explanations in your own words to explain findings.
- Write short simple sentences. Avoid long, complicated and difficult to understand sentences.
- Check grammar, punctuation, spelling and meanings. Install software (E.g., grammarly) if English is not your native language.

KEY POINTS

- Review of literature is a continuous and iterative process which shapes all stages of research.
- Learn skills to do a smart PubMed search using MeSH terms and Boolean operators.
- Prepare a literature review matrix.
- Technology has made our lives easier. Use software for plagiarism check, reference management and grammar.
- Strive to improve with every paper that you write.

BIBLIOGRAPHY

1. Creating a Search Strategy in PubMed-Public Health - Research Guides at Dartmouth College [Internet]. [cited 2021 Dec 29]. Available from: https://researchguides.dartmouth.edu/TDI- MPH/search-pubmed
2. Karas L. LibGuides: Literature Review: Purpose of a Literature Review. [cited 2021 Dec 30]; Available from: https://uscupstate.libguides.com/c.php?g=627058andp=4389968
3. Lai P. Academic Guides: Common Assignments: Literature Review Matrix. [cited 2021 Dec 30]; Available from: https://academicguides.waldenu.edu/writingcenter/assignments/literaturereview/matrix
4. Learn how to write a review of literature – The Writing Center – UW–Madison [Internet]. [cited 2021 Dec 30]. Available from: https://writing.wisc.edu/handbook/assignments/reviewofliterature/
5. McCombes S. The Literature Review|A Complete Step-by-Step Guide [Internet]. Scribbr. 2019 [cited 2021 Dec 28]. Available from: https://www.scribbr.com/dissertation/literature-review/
6. Seven Steps to Writing a Literature Review-Write a Literature Review-Guides at University of Guelph [Internet]. [cited 2021 Dec 30]. Available from: https://guides.lib.uoguelph.ca/c.php?g=130964andp=5000948
7. Sydney University Library Study Smart W. Library Study Smart Literature review purpose. 2017 [cited 2021 Dec 30]; Available from: http://services.unimelb.edu.au/academicskills/all_resources/writing-resources
8. VanLeer L. Academic Guides: Keyword Searching: Finding Articles on Your Topic: Select Keywords. [cited 2021 Dec 30]; Available from: https://academicguides.waldenu.edu/library/keyword/search-strategy
9. Westrick J. LibGuides: Guide to the Basics: AND, OR, NOT-Which to Choose? Boolean searches explained. [cited 2021 Dec 30]; Available from: https://rushu.libguides.com/basics/booleanBasics
10. What is grey literature?|Grey literature|Library|University of Leeds [Internet]. [cited 2021 Dec 30]. Available from: https://library.leeds.ac.uk/info/1110/resource_guides/7/grey_literature

CHAPTER 5

Methodology and Quantitative Study Designs in Research

Pradeep Kumar, Ipsa Mohapatra, Nirmala CJ, Meely Panda, Suhitha R Das

Who, what, when, where, how, and why: the ingredients in the recipe for a successful methods section.
—*Thomas M Annesley*

INTRODUCTION

The methods section is the most important aspect of a research paper because it provides the information by which the validity of a study is ultimately judged. Changes that have been brought about in the last decades have led to an amalgamated structure and style of scientific writing, that is the Introduction, Materials and Methods, Results, and Discussion (IMRAD) structure. As per IMRAD, methodology describes what and how the proposed study is to be done. It must be written in the future tense for a study proposal which is yet to be done and the past tense for the study already done.

The research design is an overall strategy, a blueprint of the analytical approach that a researcher chooses in order to integrate, in a coherent and logical way, the different components of the study, thus ensuring that the research problem will be thoroughly investigated. It constitutes a plan of action to collect, measure and interpret the information and data collected to answer the research question. The study design, being the skeleton of any research, needs to be chosen properly. The decisions regarding—what, where, when, how much, by what means—constitute a research design.

It must be written with enough information so that the experiment could be repeated by others to evaluate whether the results are reproducible and the audience can judge whether the results and conclusions are valid. The methods section ties the introduction to the results section to create a clear story line. It should present the obvious approach to answering the research question and define the structure in which the results will be presented later.

A well-written "material and methods" section helps the peer review process, enhancing the chances of acceptance of the manuscript. It also increases the chance of inclusion of study findings in secondary analysis of existing data, in systematic reviews and meta-analyses.

Essentials Steps of Methodology

1. Overall study design should be mentioned
2. Setting where the study will be done or done
3. Study subjects
4. Sample size and sampling method
5. Data collection/measurements
6. Intervention (if any)

7. Data analysis and interpretation
8. Ethical considerations

Study Design

The study design of a scientific paper is the guide leading to an accurate approach to collection of data and helps the reader to interpret the results properly. The authors should mention the specific design of the study, as to whether they are planning an observational study or an experimental study with further details on whether it is a cross-sectional study or a cohort study (prospective/retrospective) or a randomized controlled trial and also describe its key components (interventional vs. observational study, longitudinal vs. cross-sectional design).

Study designs can be descriptive, cross-sectional, observational study, prevalence study in population or its sub groups, correlational study between determinants and outcomes, Knowledge, Attitude, Practice (KAP) type studies, qualitative studies, mixed methods, operational research or interventional studies.

Classification of Study Designs in Epidemiology (Flowchart 1)

Case Report

It describes a patient with an unusual disease or with the simultaneous occurrence of more than one condition.

Case Series

It is an aggregation of multiple (often only a few) similar cases. It may report an unrecognized disease and hence plays an important role in advancing medical knowledge and science.

Cross-sectional Study

It is also called a *snapshot study,* as it captures a moment in time. It requires a sampling frame for selecting study participants. It measures the exposure and outcome status of the study participants at the same time; the health outcome is based on prevalence (hence also called a *prevalence study*). The limitation is its inability to prove cause-effect relationship. Its advantages are: relatively easy, quick and inexpensive; can measure multiple exposures and outcomes; estimates prevalence of disease and exposures; good for hypothesis generation; and often an

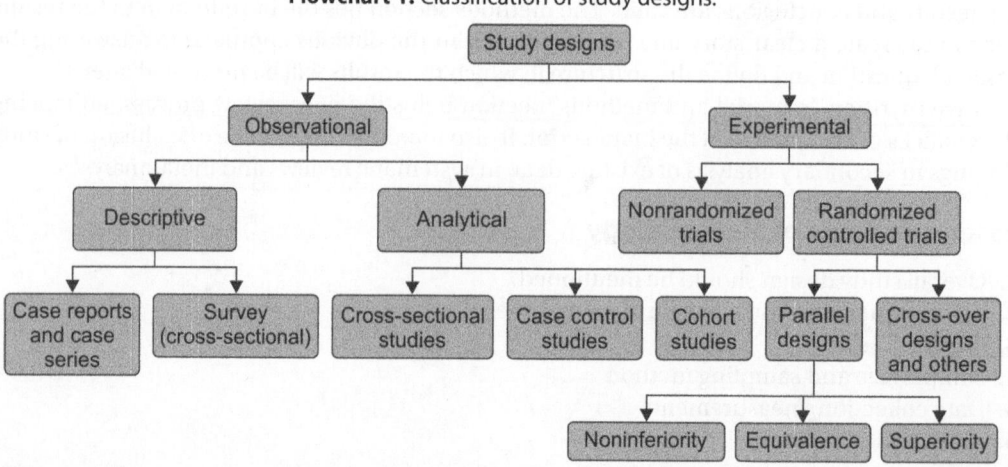

Flowchart 1: Classification of study designs.

early study design in a line of investigation. The disadvantages are: it cannot infer causality, may miss latent disease and may be subject to recall bias.

Case-control Study

These are studies of disease etiology, in which the researchers begin by selecting a group of patients (cases) with a particular disease and a similar group without the disease (controls). The cases and controls are selected by a criterion called matching; with a ratio of cases to controls varying from 1:1 to a maximum of 1:4. Prior exposure status and risk factors are assessed for both cases and controls. The major challenges lie in selecting cases, when the investigator is not sure whether these are incident or prevalent ones and in matching controls (group or individual). The advantages are: it is inexpensive and efficient (especially for rare diseases) and is useful for studying diseases with long latencies. The disadvantages are the difficulty in selecting an appropriate comparison group and the potential bias in measuring exposure (recall bias due to disease).

Cohort Study

It starts with identification and selecting the study population, then classifying the study population according to exposure status and other risk factors and following up the cohort members over time to determine the occurrence of health outcomes by exposure status subgroups. The advantages are: establishes causality, can determine incidence rates and risk and can be efficient for studying rare exposures. The disadvantages are: expensive, a rare exposure will require a large sample size, results may not be available for a long time and bias due to attrition and loss of follow-up.

Interventional Studies

The researcher actively interferes to determine the effect of the intervention on the natural course of events. They are always prospective. Based on the effect of the intervention being measured, they are divided into:
1. **Superiority trial:** To assess if one intervention is different compared with the existing intervention or placebo, in terms of showing that the "new intervention is better" than the standard one.
2. **Equivalence trial:** To show that the "new intervention is equivalent" to the existing one; however, the new intervention may be cost-effective or less toxic compared with the existing one.
3. **Noninferiority trial:** To show that "new intervention is not worse" compared with the existing one; the new intervention may be less harmful or toxic.

Types of Study Design Based on Time or Direction of the Study (Fig. 1)

Based on time or direction of the study, i.e., whether we are looking into the past, doing it in the present moment or continuing it to the future, study design can be of the following types:

Choice of study design based on the type of research question, as given in following **Table 1**, whereas appropriate study is based on type of question **(Table 2)**

Settings

The author should explain when and where the study was conducted, how the sample was recruited or selected. The study setting can be
- Community or hospital (institution) based
- Rural health training center (RHTC)/urban health training center (UHTC) areas

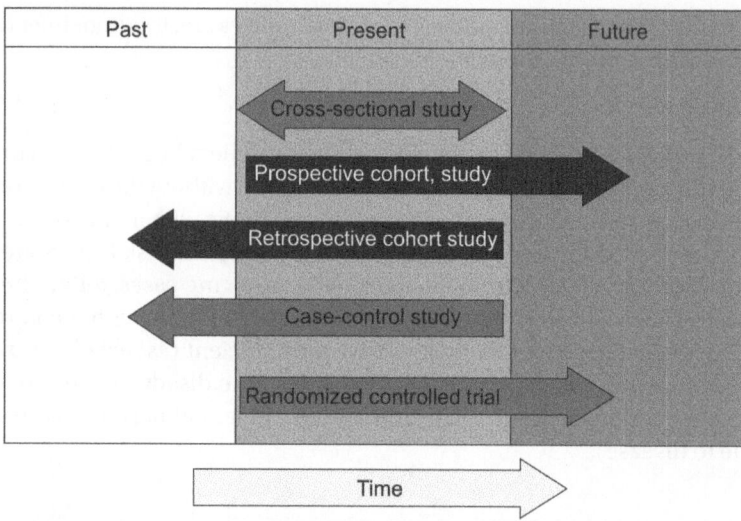

Fig. 1: Types of study design based on time or direction of the study.

Table 1: Choice of study design based on the type of research question.	
Type of question	*Study design to adopt*
Diagnosis	Prospective, blind comparison to a gold standard
Therapy	RCT > cohort > case-control > case series
Prognosis	Cohort > case-control > case series
Harm/etiology	RCT > cohort > case-control > case series
Prevention	RCT > cohort > case-control > case series

Table 2: Appropriate study is based on type of question.	
Type of question	*Appropriate study*
Burden of illness	Cross-sectional study
Prevalence	Cross-sectional survey
Causation, risk and prognosis	Case control study
Treatment efficacy	Randomized controlled study
Diagnostic test evaluation	Randomized controlled
Cost effectiveness	Randomized controlled study

Study Subjects

Judging the external validity of a study involving human subjects requires that descriptive data be provided regarding the basic demographic profile of the sample population, including age, gender and possibly the racial composition of the sample.

For human observational studies, the eligibility criteria, the sources and methods of selection of participants and methods of follow-up (in cohort studies) should be described. For case-control studies, the sources and methods of sampling of the control group and the rationale for the choice of cases and controls must be described.

Clinical trials, it is expected to inform about the details of target population, sample size and sampling method, sample representativeness, method of recruitment of the participants and how the randomization process is implemented. Socio-demographic profile of the study population is to be mentioned and as for any other study the inclusion and exclusion criteria should be clearly defined. Such information is needed to evaluate both the internal and external validity of the study.

When animals are the subjects of a study, the details of the animal including the species and strain, gender, age at the time of experiment are to be mentioned. The study subjects in the context of the research question must be clearly described. The inclusion and exclusion criteria including the justification for keeping those criteria must be stated.

Sample Size and Sampling Techniques: (Details in Chapter 12 and 13)

- Provide a sample size calculation for studies set up to statistically test a specific hypothesis.
- Sample—representative of universe—sufficiently large and randomly selected.
- Avoid purposively or conveniently selected population.
- Sampling method has to be mentioned.

Data Collection and Measurements

The research protocol is the series of steps to be followed systematically in a sequential manner with appropriate manipulations and accurate measurement. Typically, this first involves a description of baseline conditions and any associated baseline measurements, followed by the sequence of manipulations of the independent variable and the subsequent measurement of changes in the dependent variable.

Researchers need various data gathering tools and techniques which vary in complexity, design, administration and interpretation. They help to collect the right responses of a sample/population under study. Each tool is appropriate for certain kinds of evidence or information. Tools are decided at planning/design stage of a research study but can be refined during piloting.

Study Tool

Questionnaire or proforma can be self-administered or through online, may be open or close ended or both, checklist for responses might be given. A short but comprehensive data collection form with the help of experienced researchers should be designed. While inserting each variable, it should be thought whether it will be analyzed and temptation for more variables should be avoided.

With regard to the data collection, define precisely what **exposure** (e.g., stressful life events) or **intervention** (e.g., cognitive behavioral therapy) you investigated, what outcomes you measured (e.g., depression), how were the outcomes measured/quantified (e.g., using a self-reported depression scale) and when exactly were the measurements done/documented(e.g., during the screening visit and after 12 months of follow-up). Original research on existing measurement tools used in the present study should be appropriately cited and also mention if a specific tool has been designed for the study. Provide details of measurement properties (reproducibility, validity, and responsiveness) if these are crucial for the interpretation of the main results.

Any laboratory method used to collect data should be elaborately explained under this section with appropriate references. Describe what variables were measured and how those measurements were made. The description of measurement instruments should include specifics about the manufacturer and the specific model used in the present study, calibration procedures carried out to ensure the accuracy of the equipment and procedure/steps followed during measurement. Details of measurement characteristics (i.e., reproducibility, validity, and responsiveness) that influence the interpretation of the main results should also be described, validity and reliability, key indicators of the quality of measurement instruments (e.g., equipment and questionnaires) used for data collection or measurement should be appropriately reported. It also may be necessary to justify why and how certain variables were measured.

List of tools or instruments for data collection
- Observation checklist
- Interview guide for in-depth interviews
- Interview schedule
- Questionnaires
- Rating scales
- Laboratory based tests
- Physical instruments/equipment for various investigations

Intervention

It can range from various treatments to strategies that are directly proportional to the outcome of the experiment, e.g. Cognitive behavioral skill, a new drug regimen or vaccine, etc.

Analyze and Interpret Data

To describe how the data will be presented in the results section (e.g., mean vs median), which statistical tests will be used for the inferential data and what p value is deemed to indicate a statistically significant difference.

The basic requirement of writing the statistical section is providing description and justification for the statistical approaches and selection of statistical tests. Mention in detail regarding general considerations for analyses (preliminary, primary, and supplementary) derived from statistical reporting guidelines.

Data collection and entry in database (data cleaning):
- Formulate dummy tables
- Identify statistical tests beforehand based on type of data/objectives of study—Statistical software SPSS or MS Excel?
- Keep an open mind and let data reveal the truth. Uni-variate analysis "characterized or depending upon only one random variable"—distributions of variables were evaluated using means, SD, median, range and proportions

Multivariate analysis—carried out using multiple independent mathematical or statistical variables—differences in proportions evaluated using X^2 tests, difference in means using t-test. OR with 95% CI using logistic regression.

Ethical Considerations

When working with human or animal subjects, there must be a declaration that the medical center's institutional review board governing research on living matter has determined that the study protocol adheres to ethical principles. Without such approval, no research project can be conducted nor can it be published in a reputable, peer review science journal.

Approval by Institutional review boards or Institutional Ethics Committee is a must and prerequisite for publication.

All human studies need a clarity regarding informed consent/assent which needs to be a written consent in a language that the study subjects can understand and the same to be mentioned in the ethics approval section. Briefly, informed consent is a process by which an adult human subject confirms his/her willingness to participate in a research after being properly informed of the research protocol.

In case of clinical trials, the registration number of study protocols obtained from the clinical trials' registries should be mentioned. According to the Declaration of Helsinki-2008, "every clinical trial must be registered in an easily accessible database for the public before recruitment of the first participant". This approach is vital in making clinical trials more transparent and also decreases the publication bias.

Important Considerations in Methodology

Pilot Study

Pilot study is a minireplica of study to test all aspects of design. It is essential to pretest all tools/measurements/instruments on small scale.

This helps in finding population and its variability, quality of sampling frame, to evaluate validity and reliability in procedures, to identify mechanical (in equipment) and field problems, to estimate time, cost and staff requirements, to detect ambiguities/weaknesses and evaluate for inconsistencies, nonresponse/refusals,—to change questions/rephrase, to decide on limitations, for data analysis like coding, statistical tests, expertise required, etc., and to adapt questionnaire for local setting.

Address Problems of Bias

Bias: A systematic error (versus random error) introduced into sampling/testing by selecting or encouraging one outcome or answer over others.

Various Types of Bias Include

- **Selection bias:** To avoid selection bias—choose a random sample from a stable population
- **Response bias:** Tespondents differ systematically from nonrespondents.
- **Information or measurement or observer's bias:** Systematic difference among the measurements recorded in different study groups do standardization and frequent calibration of equipment, training of investigators (if > 1) and blinding of subjects (single) or observers (double)

KEY POINTS

- Study design is crucial in research, guiding data collection, measurement and analysis, is influenced by the research question, goals, resources and time.
- It varies between quantitative and qualitative research and is central in addressing the research problem and reviewing relevant literature.
- The methods section, pivotal in a research paper, details the experimental procedures, measurements, and statistical analyses, ensuring reproducibility and aiding peer review by linking the introduction and results with a coherent narrative.
- Study design in research is a blueprint used for collection, measurement and analysis of data, it should be properly chosen.
- The choice of any study design is determined by the research question, goals of the research, availability of resources and time.
- It must be written with enough information so that the experiment could be repeated by others to evaluate whether the results are reproducible.

BIBLIOGRAPHY

1. Marta MM. A brief history of the evolution of the medical research article. Clujul Med. 2015;88(4):567–70
2. Kotz D, Cals JW. Effective writing and publishing scientific papers, part IV: Methods. J Clin Epidemiol. 2013;66(8):817. doi:10.1016/j.jclinepi.2013.01.003.
3. Erdemir F. How to write a materials and methods section of a scientific article? Turk J Urol. 2013;39(Suppl 1):10–5. doi: 10.5152/tud.2013.047.
4. Stroup DF, Smith CK, Truman BI. Reporting the methods used in public health research and practice. J Public Health Emerg. 2017;1. doi:10.21037/jphe.2017.12.01.
5. Knight KL. Study/experimental/research design: Much more than statistics. J Athl Train. 2010;45(1):98–100. doi: 10.4085/1062-6050-45.1.98.
6. Kimberlin CL, Winterstein AG. Validity and reliability of measurement instruments used in research. Am J Health Syst Pharm. 2008;65(23):2276–84. doi: 10.2146/ajhp070364.
7. Lang TA, Altman DG. Basic statistical reporting for articles published in biomedical journals: The "statistical analyses and methods in the published literature" or the SAMPL Guidelines. Int J Nurs Stud. 2015;52(1):5–9. doi: 10.1016/j.ijnurstu.2014.09.006.
8. Yip C, Han N-LR, Sng BL. Legal and ethical issues in research. Indian J Anaesth. 2016;60(9):684–8. doi: 10.4103/0019-5049.190627.
9. Borovecki A, Mlinaric A, Horvat M, Supak SV. Informed consent and ethics committee approval in laboratory medicine. Biochem Med (Zagreb). 2018;28(3):30201. doi: 10.11613/BM.2018.030201.
10. Ann LK. Study design III: Cross-sectional study. Evidences Based Dentistry. 2006,7:24-5.
11. Gordis L. Epidemiology. 5th edition. Canada: Elsevier Saunders; 2014.
12. Rothman KJ, Greenland S, Lash TL. Modern epidemiology. 3rd edition. Philadelphia, PA: Wolters Kluwer Health/Lippincott Williams and Wilkins; 2012.

CHAPTER 6

Protocol Writing

Anil Purty, Raghavendra R Huchchannavar, Suhitha R Das, Sridevi Kulkarni

"By failing to prepare, you are preparing to fail." —Benjamin Franklin

INTRODUCTION

All new inventions and discoveries in the world right from the stone age to the present era were just a thought process in someone's mind. There were many novel ideas but only few worked on it and did not stop until they reached a satisfying end point. All medical personnel's irrespective of the field they are working in need to have a keen interest in their work and the ways and means to improve the modalities of treatment, ease of administration of therapeutic agents, prevent occurrence of diseases and overall improvement in the quality of life of the patients. In the present era of evidence-based medicine and the very dynamic nature of the medical field makes the life of a doctor as well as a patient a very challenging one. It is quintessential to stay up-to-date with the ongoing research in our field, which is not only for the day-to-day teaching, learning and treating but also helps us in asking the right questions regarding the future steps that need to be taken in terms of research.

Benefits of Writing Research Protocol

Writing a research protocol is the very first step of conducting research. This forms the basement on which the research you are planning to conduct stands, hence needs to be well thought through with appropriate scientific backing. To form a strong research protocol the basic requirement is the current and up-to-date knowledge regarding the topic of interest. One needs to review and critically evaluate the published literature on the topic, thereby assisting in developing novel ideas and asking research questions that are relevant to the present medical scenario. Since writing a research proposal requires in-depth knowledge and comprehensive assessment of the present situation, it will help in convincing not only yourself but also others regarding the importance of your study. This will also aid in keeping oneself focused on research and gaining the expertise on the subject.

Components of a Research Protocol

Understanding of the research methodology helps in preparing a good research protocol and this protocol when implemented appropriately will result in capturing of ground reality. This combined with a well thought analysis and interpretation of results will bring out the best in the field of medical research. A list of components that make a protocol wholesome are mentioned

Table 1: Components of a research protocol.	
Title	Data collection—methods and tools
Background including justification/rationale	Ethical issues and approval
Study objectives	Plan for analysis of collected data
Generating hypothesis that can be tested	Plan of reporting the results
Study design	Budgeting
Study population and sampling technique	Timeline
Sample size	References

in **Table 1**. The first and the foremost of these components is the title of the study. The title of the research proposal is the face of the whole protocol. It gives an impression to the reader regarding the type of research activity that is being planned, study population, location of the study and also a curiosity towards the research topic. Too short or too long title doesn't give a good impression as either there is too little information or too much information which is not actually required in a title. Therefore, the title of the research proposal must be precise, but also covey the gist of the study conducted with due mention of study design, study setting, study population and information regarding study hypothesis.

Background and Significance

The introduction/background part of the protocol must be brief, precise and must set induction for what the study is being conducted. This section should begin with points relevant to the topic proper and only those details that are required to understand the current situation. Avoid unnecessary details that may be remotely related to the topic but are not of importance to the present study. For example, if you are planning to study two different treatment approaches and want to give history/origin story regarding these approaches, it is better to do the same in few lines or maximum a paragraph rather than going on for pages regarding the same.

Before heading into the research topic proper, critical evaluation of the existing knowledge is essential. Taking an example of a communicable disease/any disease of interest, first we need to understand the general situation and the disease trend. Next step is to understand the situation if the condition remains unchecked and the possible complications/disease progression. Identification of the gaps in the knowledge and understanding of the disease and filling up of the specific gaps by the study being planned provides the basis for the rationale of the study. Another important factor considered in selection of the study for research grant is the novelty of the study with clear and concise statements regarding importance of the study. Significance of your research can be further clarified under following points:

- ❖ Scientific contribution
- ❖ Improvement in public health
- ❖ Change in health policies
- ❖ Change in patient care

The Study Objectives in the Protocol

The aims and objectives of the study need to be stated explicitly in the protocol after writing up the introduction and the need for the research. The study aims and objectives arise from the knowledge gap identified during the literature review. They must be logical, relevant, coherent, feasible, concise, realistic and consider the local conditions.

Key points of any protocol are:
- ❖ What is your research question explained by "hypothesis"?
- ❖ How is your study going to contribute to the scientific knowledge, i.e., significance of the study?
- ❖ How are we going to achieve our objectives and find the truth or reality of the hypothesis stated?

Study Designs

The type of study design selected depends on the research hypothesis/objectives. Selection of the study design must also consider the sample size, time limit, feasibility in terms of resources available-manpower, funding, etc. Study designs follow the hierarchy of evidence in research protocol.

Study Population and Method of Recruitment

One of the most important tasks during the protocol stage is deciding on the study area and the study population. Study area should be chosen wisely, you need to have an adequate number of individuals for the study, should be accessible for conducting the study and if the study requires follow up then the issue of monitoring of study participants must be thought of at the protocol stage itself. Study population is one wherein the disease/event of interest can be observed and from this pool the study participants will be selected (sample size should be fulfilled). Method of recruitment is a vital part of the study protocol as the sampling technique has an influence on the external validity of the study. If you are planning to recruit the study participants by any of the probability sampling techniques (simple random sampling, stratified sampling, etc.), it is essential to have the line-listing of the population in the study area. The issue of nonresponders also needs to be addressed at this stage itself. Once the details of the study area and study population are obtained, the next step is identifying the potential study participants. This can be done by clearly defining the inclusion/exclusion criteria for the study and the known confounding factors have to be considered while setting up these criteria. Role of the researchers at every step must be properly defined to avoid any confusion at the time of implementation. All studies that involve interaction of the researcher/research team with the study participants, it is mandatory to mention informed consent in the patient's vernacular language.

Sample Size

Sample size of the study should be adequately large to capture the outcome/exposure of interest. However, a very large sample will overshoot the estimated budget. Decision on choosing the formula for sample size calculation will depend on the type of study being conducted. The primary objectives of the study are to be considered for calculation of sample size. The previous study used and the data used for calculation of sample size must be mentioned in the protocol with proper referencing. In case no appropriate previous study is available for calculation of sample size, a pilot study needs to be carried out and the results of the pilot study should be used for calculation of sample size.

Data Collection—Methods and Tools

Next step in writing a research protocol is identifying the appropriate collection method. This depends on the type of study being carried out and the type of data that needs to be collected. It is necessary to quantify the variables of interest as accurately as possible. Units of measurement of quantitative data have to be mentioned in the protocol. Another important aspect of data collection is data triangulation. This helps in increasing the accuracy of the data being collected.

Ensuring the quality of data being collected is of utmost importance. If the data is collected by the researcher/subject expert as per the laid down guidelines then the quality of data collected is ensured. But many a times this may not be possible and an additional workforce might be required for collection of data. In such situations, it is necessary to adequately train these personnels to ensure the accuracy and quality of data being collected. If any equipment is being used for collection of data, then it has to be calibrated and validated before the start of data collection. The data collection tool also needs to be selected carefully; it must capture all the essential data required for proving/disproving the research hypothesis. Pretesting of the study tool is a good practice to identify any potential issues related to the study tool and if necessary amendments can be made or a particular question can be added or omitted. The study tool as far as possible is to be in the local language—linguistic validation of the tool should be done by first translating it into local language and then back translation from local language. Construct and content validity of the tool has to be done with the help of subject experts before utilizing the tool in the study.

Plan of Analysis

Data analysis is vital for any research and without efficient analysis important findings in the study might be missed. It is essential to identify and list out all possible statistical tests that can be applied in the proposed study with a proper plan of how the results will be presented. This further provides the funding agency clarity about the researcher's expertise on the proposed study.

Budget Details

The budget required for execution of the study must be prepared as per the guidelines provided by the concerned funding agency. The overall budget and cost of individual manpower/material requirements should be within the limits announced by the funding agency. Hence, it is quintessential to go through the details of the budgeting requirements of the agency. The fund required is usually divided year-wise with separate sections for recurring and nonrecurring expenditure. Further break-up of the budget (manpower, consumables, equipment, reagents, transport, etc.) with due justification of each must be provided.

Timeline

A well-planned study needs to have a proper timeline for proper execution of the study as well as to keep a check on the progress of the study. Most of the funding agencies ask for timeline of the proposed study. It is also necessary that the targets be achieved in the planned timeline. In case we underestimate the study duration, the results may not be reflected in our study and over-estimation of study duration may lead to exhaustion, loss of interest or over-shooting of the budget. Gantt chart is one of the effective means of representing. An example of timeline of a study requiring follow-up is shown below in **Figure 1**.

Referencing

All literatures mentioned should duly be recognized by referencing it in the protocol and the same listed by a standard referencing style (Vancouver, Harvard, APA, etc.) at the end of the

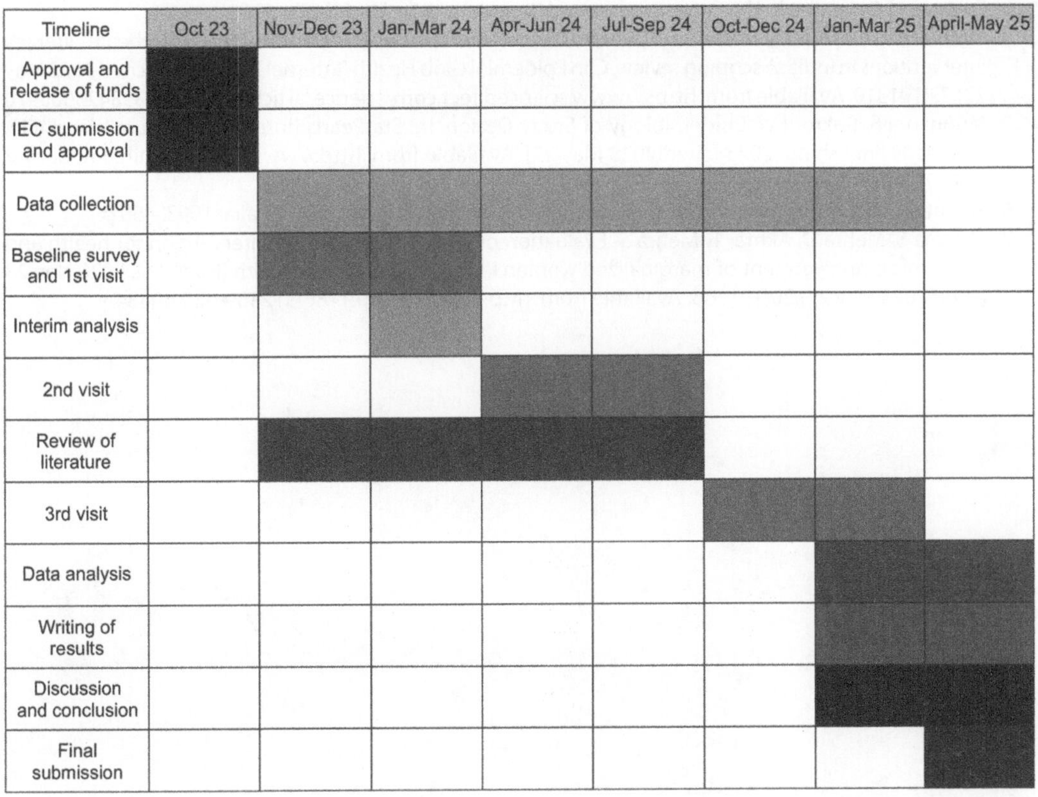

Timeline	Oct 23	Nov-Dec 23	Jan-Mar 24	Apr-Jun 24	Jul-Sep 24	Oct-Dec 24	Jan-Mar 25	April-May 25
Approval and release of funds								
IEC submission and approval								
Data collection								
Baseline survey and 1st visit								
Interim analysis								
2nd visit								
Review of literature								
3rd visit								
Data analysis								
Writing of results								
Discussion and conclusion								
Final submission								

Fig. 1: Gantt chart for presentation of timeline with achievable targets for a study requiring follow-up.

document as per the guidelines of the funding agency. Referencing is of paramount importance as without proper referencing the write-up will be considered as an act of plagiarism.

KEY POINTS

- Protocol writing is the bird eye view of the intended research and details the process of carrying out the study.
- It is an essential document for getting the grant approval and ethical clearance post which the study can be initiated.
- Study protocol includes—Introduction, need for the study, objectives, methodology, funding requirement, consent form, ethical clearance, references.
- Results, discussion, conclusion and recommendations are not a part of protocol writing.

BIBLIOGRAPHY

1. Al-Jundi A, Sakka S. Protocol Writing in Clinical Research. J Clin Diagn Res JCDR [Internet]. 2016 Nov [cited 2023 May 25];10(11): ZE10. Available from: https://www.ncbi.nlm.nih.gov/pmc/articles/PMC5198475/
2. Belbasis L, Bellou V. Introduction to Epidemiological Studies. Methods Mol Biol Clifton NJ. 2018;1793:1-6.

3. Dayanand Anupama K. Hypothesis Types and Research. 2018 Jan 1;2455–6351.
4. Mathias EG, Dhyani VS, Krishnan JB, Rani U, Gudi N, Pattanshetty S. Community based health literacy interventions in India: A scoping review. Clin Epidemiol Glob Health [Internet]. 2023 Jul 1 [cited 2023 May 27];22:101310. Available from: https://www.sciencedirect.com/science/article/pii/S2213398423000970
5. Munnangi S, Boktor SW. Epidemiology of Study Design. In: StatPearls [Internet]. Treasure Island (FL): StatPearls Publishing; 2023 [cited 2023 May 27]. Available from: http://www.ncbi.nlm.nih.gov/books/NBK470342/
6. Sarantakos S. Social research. South Melbourne: Macmillan Education Australia; 1993. 459 p.
7. Sharma S, Mehra D, Akhtar F, Mehra S. Evaluation of a community-based intervention for health and economic empowerment of marginalized women in India. BMC Public Health [Internet]. 2020 Nov 23 [cited 2023 May 27];20(1):1766. Available from: https://doi.org/10.1186/s12889-020-09884-y

CHAPTER 7

Manuscript Writing

Sanjay Zodpey, Raghavendra R Huchchannavar, Aditi Mohta, Suhitha R Das, Manjula R

> "Writing is thinking. To write well is to think clearly. That's why it's so hard."
> —David McCullough

INTRODUCTION

The pinnacle of research and possibly one of its most crucial steps is the publication of a scientific manuscript. Your knowledge and experience become citable science through the publication of a scientific manuscript, providing new knowledge to medical professionals and scientists for both the present and the future.

Publication of your findings is most valuable when your coworkers can locate your article in the medical literature, comprehend your paper and believe the results, understand the ramifications of the results along with the positive impact of your research and incorporate your data into their own knowledge base and quote or cite your article in their own publications.

One of the few effective strategies available to scholars for persuading their colleagues of their academic progress is regular publication. Successful research publications draw attention to academics and their institutions. This could result in the institute receiving more money and ensuring a person's advancement in their field. The quantity of publications a person has to their credit is frequently used by academic institutions and universities as a gauge of competence. This is becoming a more important criterion for the hiring process.

The quality of a manuscript's preparation determines whether it will make a decent publication. Each journal has a distinct method for providing guidelines for manuscript preparation. A well-written paper can easily find its way to publication in a reputable journal.

There are three types of manuscripts according to Borja,
1. **Full article or original article:** This refers to a large completed piece of research.
2. **Letter/rapid communications/short communications:** They are very brief according to the type of journals.
3. **Review papers or perspectives:** These might be critical or noncritical summaries of a trending subject or previously published data.

The algorithm that O'Connor and Holmquist published is helpful for writing scientific manuscripts. The creation of figures and tables, according to these authors, should come first, followed by summary statements (conclusions that summarize the main contributions of the manuscript to the scientific community), audience identification, materials and methods, results, discussion, references and introduction, title and conclusion. This method is intended to help scientists who struggle with writer's block and non-native English speakers by providing the manuscript's structural backbone.

"Like every well-written story, a scientific manuscript should have a beginning (introduction), middle (materials and methods), and an end (results). The discussion (the moral of the story) puts the study in perspective. The abstract is an opening summary of the story and the title gives the story a name".

Title, Keywords and Abstract

The article's title determines how it will be indexed and significantly increases the paper's visibility. It ought to capture the heart of the piece, as well as its uniqueness and applicability to the biological sector it addresses. It should represent the goal of the study and indicate the issue(s) addressed rather than the results. It should be concise, straightforward and detailed, without jargon or unusual or confusing acronyms.

The keywords should be given in accordance with the guidelines for authors as they enable database searches for the paper. The likelihood that a publication will be retrieved and cited by other writers increases dramatically with careful selection from the Medical Subject Headings (MeSH) in the National Library of Medicine (NLM) controlled vocabulary thesaurus used to index articles in PubMed.

The abstract is the last piece to be prepared, but it is the most crucial because readers typically read it first and use the information in it to decide whether or not to continue reading the entire work. It should be a brief synopsis of the manuscript that doesn't go above the length allowed by the guidelines for authors. Typically, references, acronyms and abbreviations are not usually permitted. If necessary, it must be formatted in the manner prescribed.

Introduction

It is advised that the introductory section be brief, avoiding lengthy reviews regarding the contents of the article, even though the requirements for the length of the introduction vary among scientific fields (for instance, they are longer in psychology publications). It has been suggested that the introduction section should be organized like a cone or funnel, beginning with the key points of the general topic, highlighting the knowledge gap, the article's hypothesis or major question and concluding with a brief summary of the methodology used in the current work.

Another suggestion is to keep it short and concise, with three main paragraphs: the first one describing what is known, the second describing what is unknown and the third describing the objective of the study and how it would advance scientific understanding.

When stating what is known, it should not be a comprehensive analysis of the literature but rather the key details required to comprehend the context. The discussion and the introduction shouldn't use the same information. The reader should be given as much information as possible in the paragraph outlining what is unknown to better grasp the purpose of the investigation. The research hypothesis or question should be stated in the final paragraph.

Materials and Methods

This part is crucial and should be written in a way that will make it easy for other researchers to repeat the study. This section has been equated to a recipe because it lists all the elements and how to combine them. Important information about the methods used, including the study's overall design, inclusion and exclusion criteria, sample sizes and statistical power, should be presented. It can also be divided into sections using subheadings, such as "study design," "setting," "subjects," "data collection," and "data analysis".

Results

The orderly presentation of the data that was gathered makes up the results section. In the results section, all measurements that the authors mentioned in the materials and methods section must be recorded and organized in the same manner. Because the results were collected in the past, the write up should be in the past tense.

Tables and figures can be used to report results for primary and secondary outcomes to provide more clarity. It is necessary to justify the choice of endpoint and the lack of data collection on significant unmeasured factors.

Discussion

The major goal of the debate is to interpret the significance of the findings. This part should be organized as though it were a natural progression of ideas, and it should begin with a concise summary of the major findings and a determination of whether or not they are consistent with the research goals stated in the final sentence of the introduction. The research's advantages, drawbacks and contributions to existing knowledge should next be discussed.

Reference

The vancouver style is widely used in medical publications, while each journal often has its own citation format. Numerous tools, both free and paid for, are available that make it easier to cite sources and create bibliographies, complete with information about various citation styles. *For examples*, include EndNote, Zotero and Mendeley.

A significant remark should always be cited in its original form, so be sure the reference you cite isn't just quoting another source. Consider the strength of the evidence, the year of publication, and the caliber of the work when making a decision between several references.

Acknowledgments

The acknowledgments section must include all contributors, even if they don't match the requirements for authorship. Therefore, the authors must include a statement about the kind of assistance, if any, they received from the sponsor or the sponsor's representative, as well as the names of any individuals who helped with the manuscript's technical or writing aspects, provided editorial support or otherwise contributed in any way.

Accepting and Rejecting a Manuscript

According to '8 reasons I accepted your article' which is a small study conducted among 5 editors of Scopus indexed journals by Elsevier's company and reported by Zwaff, the following are the 8 reasons for accepting the manuscript:
1. It provides insights into an important issue.
2. The insight is useful to people who makes decisions.
3. The insight is used to develop a framework or theory.
4. The insight stimulates new important questions.
5. The methods used to explore the issues are appropriate.
6. The methods used are applied rigorously and explain why and how the data support conclusions.
7. Connections to prior works in the field or from other fields are made.
8. The article tells a good story.

According to Thrower,
The 8 reasons for rejection of a manuscript are the follows:
1. It fails in technical screening.
2. It does not fall within the aims and scope of the Journal.
3. It is incomplete.
4. The procedures and/or analysis of data is seen to be defective.
5. The conclusion cannot be justified on the basis of the rest of the paper.
6. It is simply a small extension of a different paper, often from the same authors.
7. It is incomprehensible.
8. It is boring.

How to Select a Journal?

The writers should consider a number of factors when choosing a journal, including regional publication norms, the journals' visibility or influence and their affinities with the manuscripts' topics. Verifying journal indexing in important databases like PubMed, Scopus/SCimago (quartiles) and Journal Citation Reports (impact factor) is strongly advised.

Viewing the list of references in your study can help you decide which publication is best. Make sure the journal's scope and preferred editors fit your manuscript before choosing it. Read all the requirements. List 3–5 journals and prioritize them before selecting the appropriate one.

The results, whether positive or negative, should not impact the study. Every article has to reach the public, as it is knowledge to be gained. If a journal rejects the article, one should not be disheartened rather, it can be a learning curve. Rewriting the manuscript till it reaches a fineness plays a very important role. Years of hard work and dedication are needed to make a strong and concrete impact in the world of research publication. Therefore, it is necessary to structure the work and strive for the positive best.

KEY POINTS

- Publishing scientific papers is key in research, transforming knowledge into valuable resources for future medical and scientific work.
- Manuscript quality is crucial for publication success, with different types (full articles, short communications, reviews) and guidelines for writing.
- The title, keywords, and abstract of a paper determine its visibility and help readers decide whether to read the full content.
- A paper's structure (introduction, methods, results, discussion) is essential, with each section serving a specific purpose.
- Choosing the right journal depends on various factors and manuscripts may be accepted for their insights or rejected due to technical flaws or lack of originality.

BIBLIOGRAPHY

1. Annesley TM. Who, what, when, where, how, and why: The ingredients in the recipe for a successful Methods section. Clin Chem. 2010b;56:897–901.
2. Balch et al. Steps to Getting Your Manuscript Published in a High-Quality Medical Journal. Ann Surg Oncol. 2018;25(4):850-5.
3. Borja, Angel. Six things to do before writing your manuscript. Elsevier Connect. (2014). Available at https://www.elsevier.com/connect/six-things-to-do-before-writing-your-manuscript. Accessed on 02/08/2022.
4. Cals JW, Kotz D. Effective writing and publishing scientific papers, part III: introduction. J Clin Epidemiol. 2013a;66:702.

5. Cals JW, Kotz D. Effective writing and publishing scientific papers, part VIII: references. J Clin Epidemiol. 2013c;66:1198.
6. Falagas ME, Pitsouni EI, Malietzis GA, Pappas G. Comparison of PubMed, Scopus, Web of Science, and Google Scholar: Strengths and weaknesses. FASEB J. 2008;22:338–42.
7. International Committee of Medical Journal Editors. Uniform Requirements for Manuscripts Submitted to Biomedical Journals. Updated April 2010. Available at: http://www.icmje. org/urm_full.pdf. Last accessed on 02/08/2022.
8. Kotz D, Cals JW, Tugwell P, Knottnerus JA. Introducing a new series on effective writing and publishing of scientific papers. J Clin Epidemiol. 2013;66:359–60.
9. Martín-Martín A, Orduna-Malea E, Thelwall M, López-Cózar ED. Google Scholar, Web of Science, and Scopus: A systematic comparison of citations in 252 subject categories. JOI. 2018;12:1160–77.
10. Thrower Peter. Eight reasons I rejected your article. Elsevier Connect. (2012). Available at https://www.elsevier.com/connect/8-reasons-i-rejected-your-article. Accessed on 02/08/2022.
11. Zwaff Elizabeth. 8 reasons I accepted your article. Elsevier Connect. (2013). Available at https://www.elsevier.com/connect/8-reasons-i-accepted-your-article. Accessed on 02/08/2022.

Research to Health Policy

AM Kadri, Somen Saha, Chandana H, Sudha Sharma, Nishanth Krishna K, Sivaram Kiraseni

"The best public policy is made when you are listening to people who are going to be impacted."
—Elizabeth Dole

HEALTH TECHNOLOGY ASSESSMENT

Health Technology Assessment (HTA) is the systematic evaluation of the properties, effects, and impacts of health technologies and interventions, covering both their direct and indirect consequences. It is a multidisciplinary process that aims to determine the value of a health technology and to inform decision-making in the health sector by providing evidence about the given technology. It also considers the social, ethical, economic and organizational implications of technology and its use.

HTA is a tool for evidence-based decision making to achieve health care benefits. Health technologies are broadly defined as any intervention that may be used to promote health, prevent, diagnose, or treat disease, or improve rehabilitation or long-term care. They include drugs, devices, procedures, programs, and systems. Health interventions are the application of health technologies in a specific context, such as a clinical setting, a health program, or a health policy.

Health Technology Assessment in India (HTAIn) is a sub-scheme under the Department of Health Research (DHR), Ministry of Health & Family Welfare (MoHFW), Government of India to facilitate the process of transparent and evidence-informed decision making in the field of healthcare. HTAIn was established in 2017 as an institutional arrangement for evaluation of the appropriateness and cost effectiveness of available and new health technologies in the country as part of the research governance mandate of the DHR.

Objectives and Significance of HTAIn

- ❖ To undertake HTA studies aiming at maximizing health in the population, reducing out of pocket expenditure (OOP) and reducing inequity.
- ❖ To support the process of decision-making in health care at the central and state policy level by providing reliable information based on scientific evidence.
- ❖ Develop systems and mechanisms to assess new and existing health technologies by a transparent and inclusive process.
- ❖ To appraise health interventions and technologies based on available data on resource use, cost, clinical effectiveness, and safety.
- ❖ To collect and analyze evidence in a systematic and reproducible way and ensure its accessibility and usefulness to inform health policy.

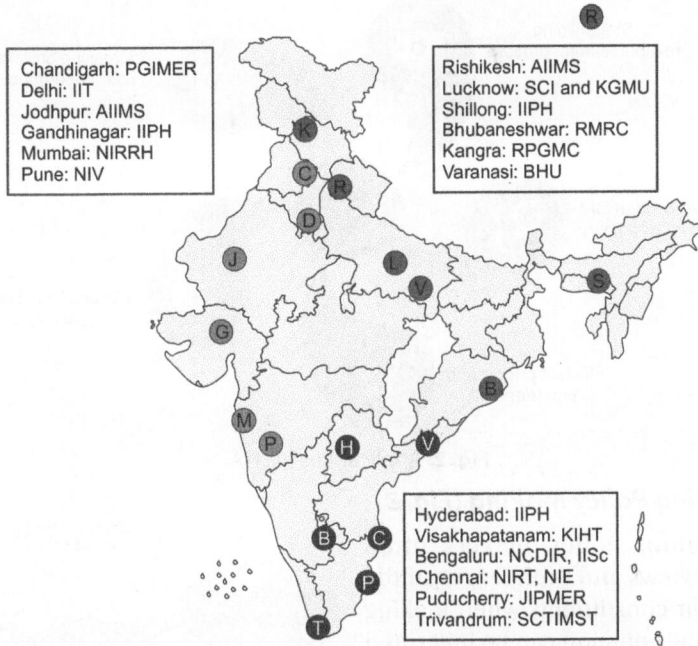

Fig. 1: Health technology assessment India Resource Centres.

❖ Disseminate research findings and resulting policy decisions to educate and empower the public to make better informed decisions about health.

Structure of HTAIn

HTAIn consists of an in-house HTAIn Secretariat, Board, Technical Appraisal Committee (TAC) and Regional Resource Centres (RRCs) **(Fig. 1)**.

Applications of Health Technology Assessment

HTA can be applied for various purposes and at different levels of the health system, such as:
1. Selection and prioritization of health technologies and interventions for research, development, adoption, or disinvestment.
2. Regulation and approval of health technologies and interventions for safety, quality, and efficacy.
3. Pricing and reimbursement of health technologies and interventions for affordability and cost-effectiveness.
4. Coverage and access of health technologies and interventions for equity and appropriateness.
5. Implementation and delivery of health technologies and interventions for effectiveness and efficiency.
6. Evaluation and monitoring of health technologies and interventions for performance and impact. Application of HTA represents in **Fig. 2.**

Policy Making

Policy making is the process of creating and implementing rules, regulations, laws, or programs that affect the public or a specific group of people.

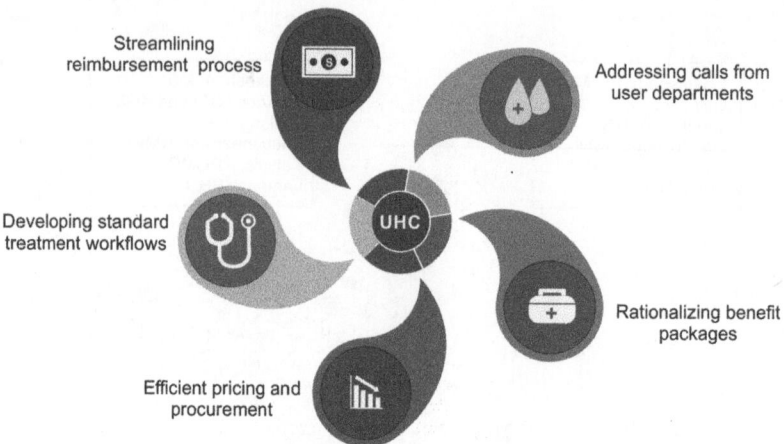

Fig. 2: Applications of HTA.

Factors Affecting Policy Making (Fig. 3)

- **Public opinion:** Policy makers often consider the views and preferences of the public or their constituents when making decisions. Public opinion can be measured through polls, surveys, letters, emails, phone calls, or social media. Public opinion can also be influenced by the media, education, culture, and personal experiences.
- **Economic conditions:** Policy makers must balance the costs and benefits of different policy options, considering the available

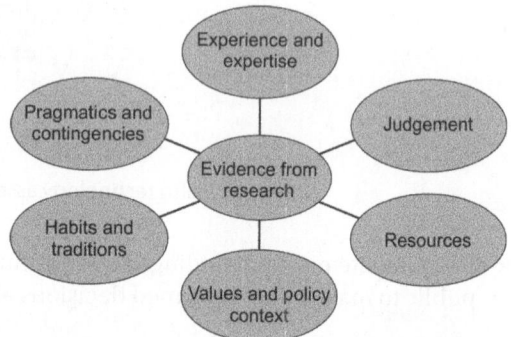

Fig. 3: Factors influencing policy-making.

resources, the budget constraints, the economic impacts, and the opportunity costs. Economic conditions can also affect the demand and supply of certain goods and services, the income and wealth distribution, inflation and unemployment rates, and the trade and investment flows.
- **Scientific discoveries:** Policy makers may use scientific evidence and data to support or challenge their policy choices. Scientific discoveries can also create new opportunities or challenges for policy making, such as new health technologies, environmental issues, or security threats.
- **Technological changes:** Policy makers must adapt to the rapid and constant changes in technology, which can affect the production, distribution, and consumption of goods and services, the communication and information systems, innovation and competitiveness, and the social and ethical norms.
- **Interest groups:** Policy makers may be influenced by the pressure and persuasion of various groups that have a stake or interest in a particular policy issue, such as businesses, unions, NGOs, professional associations, or social movements. Interest groups can use various tactics to advance their interests, such as lobbying, advocacy, education, mobilization, or litigation.
- **Political activities:** Policy making is also shaped by the political system and institutions, such as the constitution, the laws, the courts, the parties, the elections, the coalitions, the bureaucracy, and the international organizations. Political activities can also include the agendas, ideologies, strategies, and behaviors of the political actors, such as the leaders, the candidates, the legislators, the officials, the diplomats, or the voters.

These can be assessed by conducting PEST analysis. PEST focuses on **political, economic, social, and technological factors** affect the feasibility of a policy.

Writing a Policy Brief

A policy brief is a short description of a particular issue, the policy options for solving it, and some recommendations for the best solution. They serve as a vehicle for providing evidence-based policy recommendations to assist readers in making well-informed decisions. A policy brief fulfills one of the most important goals of public health, which is to convey suggestions to policymakers in a clear and succinct manner so that they can act on them.

A policy brief distills or synthesizes a large amount of complex detail to bring the reader closer to the issue's heart, its background, the players ("stakeholders"), and any recommendations or even educated forecasts about the future of the issue. Research findings must be transformed into understandable, accessible, and relevant information that decision-makers may utilize to mobilize resources, formulate policy, implement programs, and evaluate impact. The purpose of the policy brief is to persuade the intended audience of the urgency of the current problem and the need to implement the chosen alternative or course of action outlined, and so function as a catalyst for action. Planning a policy brief involves a knowledge of its vital elements namely its **purpose, audience, content, and structure.**

The purpose is to give readers a clear background of a particular issue, suggest possible policy options, and make recommendations supported by evidence from research. It is important to keep that one issue in focus, communicate its urgency and the benefits of following the recommendations.

Policy briefs should be accessible and targeted at a specific audience. It should be framed keeping in mind the prospective readers, their interest in and level of knowledge of the subject, the information they will need to make a decision and their openness to the recommendations made.

A policy brief should be clear, succinct, and focused on a single topic. It should use plain language, should not describe the methodology in detail, should be drafted afresh, not cut down an existing report and should not exceed 1,500 words or two pages in length.

The structure should lead the reader from problem to solution. The policy recommendations should be clear, supported by evidence and reflect the audience's interests. A policy brief should relate to the big picture: The policy brief may build on context-specific findings, but it should draw conclusions that are more generally applicable.

Objectives of a Policy Brief

- ❖ Convince a specific audience that a problem is important.
- ❖ Present a list of available and feasible choices for resolving the issue.
- ❖ Assistance in making evidence-based, well-informed decisions.
- ❖ Make specific recommendations to motivate action to solve the problem.

Attributes of an Effective Policy Brief

- ❖ An identified audience
- ❖ Language and format suitable to that audience
- ❖ Helpful signposts and orienting information
- ❖ The balance between length and breadth
- ❖ Logically organized, persuasive arguments
- ❖ Evidence-based, value-driven arguments
- ❖ Practical, feasible, and culturally appropriate recommendations

Some Initial Considerations before Writing a Policy Brief

Determine who your Audience is!

- Who am I writing this brief for?
- How knowledgeable are they about the topic?
- How open are they to the message?
- What questions need answers?
- What are their interests, concerns?
- What does it take to reach a specific audience?

Use the Power of Persuasion

- Answer the question, "How valuable is this to me?"
- Describe the situation's urgency.
- Speak in terms of advantages and benefits.
- Concentrate on a single subject.
- Define your goal.
- Determine the most important points that support the goal.
- Reduce the number of points to the most important information.
- Set a word count limit of 1,500 words.

Cover Following Points

- What is the extent of the issue? What are the health ramifications?
- What is the problem with public health or the global health challenge?
- What are the elements that put you at risk? Who is the most impacted?
- Are there any nonhealth consequences to this condition (e.g., economic, societal, or political)?
- What is the relationship between this issue and other global health issues?
- What initiatives, strategies, and policies are available to address this issue?

Steps of Effectively Writing a Policy Brief

Front-loaded

The conclusions of policy briefs are placed on the first page.

An executive summary should be included on the top page, offering a brief (1–2 paragraphs) outline of the brief's goal and main suggestions.

Policy Brief Template

- Title
- Executive summary
- Introduction
- Approach/policy options critique
- Implications and recommendations
- Sometimes, addenda such as references or recommended reading

Policy Brief Title

It needs to be **Descriptive, Punchy, and Relevant.**

Policy Brief Executive Summary

The executive summary is intended to persuade the reader that the brief is worthy of further consideration. A time-pressed audience needs to recognize the brief's relevance and importance when reading the summary.

As a result, a one- to two-paragraph executive summary often includes:
- A description of the problem being addressed.
- A statement explaining why the present approach/policy option needs to be altered.
- Your recommendations for action.

Policy Brief Introduction
- Provides an answer to the question "why?"
- Explains the issue's importance/urgency and describes the research goal.
- Provides an outline of the findings and conclusions.
- Curiosity is piqued for the remainder of the short.

Critique of Policy Options/Approaches

The goal of this section is to highlight the flaws in the present strategy or options in use, demonstrating the need for change as well as the areas where change should be focused. The following are typically included in policy options critiques:
- A brief overview of the policy option(s) under consideration.
- An explanation of why and how the present or proposed method is ineffective.
- Recognize all points of view in the debate on the problem for credibility.
- Provides a synopsis of the information.
- It describes the problem and background, as well as the study and analysis that went into it.
- Explains how the research was carried out and those who were involved in the research.
- Should not be very technical.
- Identifies the method utilized to acquire data.
- Highlights issues, rewards, and opportunities.

Policy Implications or Recommendations

Implications (what could happen):
- Describe what the researcher believes the effects will be.
- Advice is less straightforward than suggestions.
- When you don't want to give counsel, this is a good tool to have.
- A gentler approach that is still persuasive.

Recommendations (what should happen):
- Clearly state what should happen next.
- Describe the steps in detail.
- An outline of the specific practical tasks or measures that must be taken.
- A final paragraph that re-emphasizes the necessity of action is sometimes included as well.

Appendices

Although the brief is a short and focused document, authors may decide that their position requires more evidence and include an appendix.
Appendices should only be used if necessary.

Conclusion

This final section should detail the actions recommended by research findings.* Persuasive language can be used to present the recommendations. Conclusion should be kept short

---

*In case of competing data and perspectives, PEST analysis, which focuses on political, economic, social, and technological factors, which affect the feasibility of a policy, can help one to form recommendations.

but should include **Implications** (the effects that the research could have in the future) and the recommendations (the effects it will have, as evident from the research). Beyond being descriptive, the recommendations should act as a call to action by stating precise, relevant, credible, and feasible next steps.

Sources and References

- Many writers of the policy brief decide not to include any sourcing of their evidence, as their focus is not on an academic audience.
- Many authors choose to direct their readers to more reading by including a section on suggested readings.
- Include a brief bibliography at the end of the paper.
- Names, positions, institution, and email address for correspondence.

Acknowledgments

Who made significant contributions to the content of the policy brief.

A policy brief should be convincing and interesting to read. Compelling titles and headings, sidebars featuring interesting details, bulleted lists to summarize important points, and graphics such as charts and images can help make it interesting.

Limitations

The policy brief lacks an in-depth analysis of the textual features of each structural element and the use of parts of sample papers to illustrate the elements.

KEY POINTS

- HTA evaluates health technologies and their broader impacts, with India's HTAIn guiding healthcare decisions based on evidence.
- HTA helps choose, approve, price, and monitor health technologies, ensuring they are safe, effective, and beneficial to health systems.
- Policy briefs summarize key issues and recommend actions based on research, aiming to clearly communicate solutions and influence decision-making.
- A policy brief can bridge the gap between research and the implementation of its findings by communicating possible solutions to the policy makers and key stake holders thus ensuring that the benefit of the research reaches the population.

BIBLIOGRAPHY

1. "An essential guide to writing policy briefs.pdf [Internet]. [cited 2023 Nov 15]. Available from: https://www.icpolicyadvocacy.org/sites/icpa/files/downloads/icpa_policy_briefs_essential_guide.pdf
2. How to Write a Policy Brief (Step by Step) [Internet]. 2021 [cited 2023 Nov 15]. Available from: https://fiscalnote.com/blog/guide-writing-policy-brief
3. The double burden of malnutrition: policy brief [Internet]. [cited 2023 Nov 15]. Available from: https://www.who.int/publications-detail-redirect/WHO-NMH-NHD-17.3.

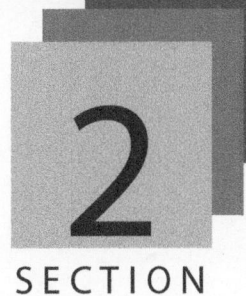

Quantitative Research Methodology

SECTION OUTLINE

- **Chapter 9:** Descriptive Studies
- **Chapter 10:** Analytical Study Designs
- **Chapter 11:** Cross-sectional Study Design
- **Chapter 12:** Case-control Study Design
- **Chapter 13:** Cohort Study Design
- **Chapter 14:** Experimental Study Designs
- **Chapter 15:** Sample Size Estimation
- **Chapter 16:** Sampling Methods and Errors
- **Chapter 17:** Basic Statistics
- **Chapter 18:** Test of Significance
- **Chapter 19:** Advanced Statistics
- **Chapter 20:** Referencing and Discussion

9 CHAPTER

Descriptive Studies

Deepthi R, Raghavendra Huchchannavar, Suhitha R Das, Manjula R

"In the world of research, detail is not a luxury, but a necessity. The devil is in the details, but so is salvation."
—*Hyman G Rickover*

INTRODUCTION

In the realm of scientific research, descriptive studies serve as a foundational pillar for understanding various phenomena, behaviors and patterns in a systematic and organized manner. These studies are essential for building the initial framework of knowledge before delving into more complex investigations. It is rightly named as "The first scientific inquiry". It is concerned with and designed only to describe the existing distribution of variables related to population characteristics, without regard to causal hypotheses. This is the most frequently encountered epidemiologic design strategy in the medical literature as it is less expensive and less time consuming than analytical studies.

Types of Descriptive Studies (Flowchart 1)

Case Studies

Case studies are a type of descriptive study that involves an in-depth examination of a single individual, group, event or phenomenon. Researchers gather detailed information through multiple sources, such as interviews, observations and historical records, to construct a

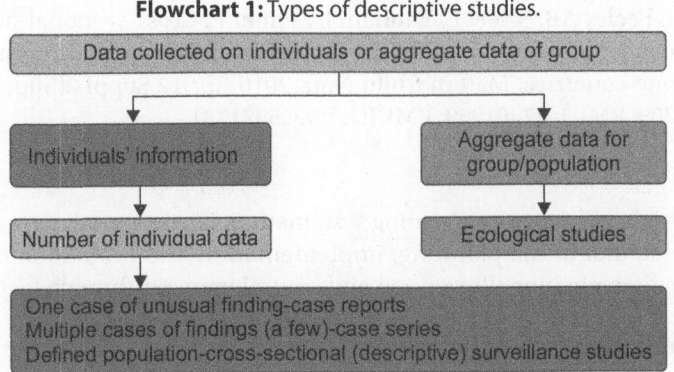

Flowchart 1: Types of descriptive studies.

comprehensive narrative. Case studies are often used in psychology, medicine and social sciences to explore unique or rare cases and generate hypotheses for further research. Examples include previous undescribed disease, unexpected link between diseases, unexpected new therapeutic effect and adverse events.

For example: Gottlieb GJ, Ragaz A, Vogel JV, Friedman-Kien A, Rywlin AM, Weiner EA, Ackerman AB. A preliminary communication on extensively disseminated Kaposi's sarcoma in young homosexual men. Am J Dermatopathol. 1981 Summer;3(2):111-4. doi: 10.1097/00000372-198100320-00002. PMID: 7270808.

Andrews MA, Areekal B, Rajesh KR, Krishnan J, Suryakala R, Krishnan B, Muraly CP, Santhosh PV. First confirmed case of COVID-19 infection in India: A case report. Indian J Med Res. 2020 May;151(5):490-492. doi: 10.4103/ijmr.IJMR_2131_20. PMID: 32611918; PMCID: PMC7530459.

Case Series

Case series expand upon the concept of case studies by examining a collection of similar cases or a series of events with common characteristics. These studies aim to identify patterns and trends within a specific group of cases, often in a clinical or medical context. Case series can provide valuable insights into the natural history of diseases or the effects of interventions. Cases may be identified from a single or multiple sources and generally report on new/unique condition. Hence may be only realistic design for rare disorders.

For example: Freise NF, Kivel M, Grebe O, Meyer C, Wafaisade B, Peiper M, et al. Acute cardiac side effects after COVID-19 mRNA vaccination: A case series. Eur J Med Res. 2022 Jun 2;27(1):80. doi: 10.1186/s40001-022-00695-y. PMID: 35655235; PMCID: PMC9160507.

Descriptive Cross-sectional Studies

Descriptive cross-sectional studies, also known as 'prevalence studies' or 'disease frequency studies', involve the simultaneous collection of data from a representative sample of a population at a single point in time. These studies are designed to provide a 'snapshot' of a population's characteristics, behavior or attitudes. They are widely used in public health, sociology and market research to assess prevalence, make comparisons, and identify associations. Data collected on individual characteristics (presence or level of variable of interest), including exposure to risk factors, alongside information about the outcome. The distribution/descriptive triad—or pentad (Five "W" questions) time, place and person or agent, host and environment explaining who, what, when, where, why and 'so what'.

For example:
Pereira C, Ford R, Feeley AB, Sweet L, Badham J, Zehner E. Cross-sectional survey shows that follow-up formula and growing-up milks are labeled similarly to infant formula in four low and middle income countries. Matern Child Nutr. 2016 Apr;12 Suppl 2(Suppl 2):91-105. doi: 10.1111/mcn.12269. PMID: 27061959; PMCID: PMC5071731.

Surveillance

Watchfulness over a community: Ongoing systematic collection, analysis and interpretation of health data essential to the planning, implementation and evaluation of public health practice—timely dissemination. Prevention and control happens through feedback loop.

Ecological Studies or Correlational Studies

These examine population (records/registry/database). It studies the association between exposure and an outcome across population rather than individuals. It is convenient if the data are available in reliable source. It studies if the difference in exposure within group is smaller than the difference between groups.

The limitations of ecological studies are:
- Ecological fallacy—association at group level may not be true at individual level.
- Confounding—association may be related to third factor.
- Error—due to migration of people with varied exposure between regions.
- Variations in definition or criteria in different populations.

Steps in Development of a Protocol for Descriptive Studies
- **Research question:** Descriptive triad—or pentad (Five "W" questions)
- **Aims and objective:** To describe or to estimate
- **Study design:** Cross-sectional descriptive
- **Etting**: General and specific (Hospital/description of study area)
- **Study population**: Describe or define the population (denominator)
- **Inclusion and exclusion criteria:** Whom to include and exclude after inclusion
- **Sample size:** Depending on what do you want to describe or estimate
- Sampling technique
- **Ethical consideration:** Informed consent, mention the risk involved
- Data collection procedure and tools
- Plan of analysis.

Reporting Guidelines for Descriptive Studies
- **CARE Checklist** of information to include when writing a case report.
- **STROBE Statement**—Checklist of items that should be included in reports of cross-sectional studies.

Uses of Descriptive Studies
- **Understanding burden of disease:** There studies measure or quantify the burden of disease or risk factors which is crucial for having a baseline data. It provides distribution of attribute with respect to time, place and person.
- **Source of ideas:** It helps us in planning and set priorities in designing of a preventive strategy or to implement a new public health program.
- **Trend analysis:** It helps in understanding trends of the disease which in turn assists in prevention of disease and prepare for the expected outcome.
- **Evaluation of services:** Descriptive studies helps in evaluating services by service documentation, assessing service processes, utilization, quality assessment, service costs and resources.
- **Generating hypotheses:** Descriptive studies often serve as a starting point for scientific research. Through detailed observations and data collection, researchers can generate hypotheses and research questions that can be further explored through experimental or analytical studies. It stimulates the initiation of a more detailed study.
- **Clinical insights:** In medicine and healthcare, case studies and case series can offer valuable insights into rare diseases, unusual presentations or unexpected treatment outcomes. They can guide clinical decision-making and suggest areas for further investigation.
- **Public health surveillance:** Descriptive cross-sectional studies play a crucial role in public health by monitoring disease prevalence, risk factors and health behaviors within a population. This information informs public health policies, interventions and resource allocation.

- **Social science research:** In sociology and anthropology, descriptive studies help researchers understand social phenomena, cultural practices and human behavior by providing a detailed account of specific cases or groups within a society.

Advantages of Descriptive Studies

- **Exploratory nature:** Descriptive studies allow researchers to explore new areas of interest and generate hypotheses for future research because of its diverse nature of data.
- **In-depth understanding:** Case studies and case series provide rich, detailed information about individual cases or small groups, offering insights that quantitative research may miss.
- **Practicality:** Descriptive cross-sectional studies are often cost-effective and can be conducted relatively quickly, less severe ethical issues making them suitable for assessing population-level data.
- **Real-world applicability:** Findings from descriptive studies often have direct relevance to real-world situations and can inform decision-making.

Disadvantages of Descriptive Studies

- **Limited generalizability:** The findings of descriptive studies may not be applicable to broader populations due to their focus on specific cases or groups.
- **Bias:** Selection bias, information bias, and confounding variables can affect the validity of results in descriptive studies, especially in observational research.
- **Lack of causality:** Descriptive studies cannot identify associations or establish causation because of its descriptive design.
- **Subjectivity:** Interpretation of data in descriptive studies can be subjective, potentially leading to researcher bias.
- **Lack of validity:** Validity of the study depends on representativeness of the sample and standardization of the tools.

KEY POINTS

- Descriptive studies are an essential component of the research landscape, providing valuable insights, generating hypotheses and laying the groundwork for more rigorous investigations.
- Researchers must carefully design and conduct descriptive studies while acknowledging their limitations to ensure the reliability and validity of their findings.
- These studies are indispensable tools for advancing knowledge across various fields of study.

BIBLIOGRAPHY

1. Aggarwal R, Ranganathan P. Study designs: Part 2—Descriptive studies. Perspect Clin Res. 2019 Jan-Mar;10(1):34-36. doi: 10.4103/picr.PICR_154_18. PMID: 30834206; PMCID: PMC6371702.
2. Catherine R Lesko, Matthew P Fox, Jessie K Edwards. A Framework for Descriptive Epidemiology. Am J Epidemiol. 2022;191(12):2063-2070. https://doi.org/10.1093/aje/kwac115
3. Dulock HL. Research Design: Descriptive Research. J Pediatr Oncol Nurs. 1993;10(4):154-157. doi:10.1177/104345429301000406
4. Grimes DA, Schulz KF. Descriptive studies: what they can and cannot do. Lancet. 2002 Jan 12;359(9301):145-9. doi: 10.1016/S0140-6736(02)07373-7. PMID: 11809274.
5. Omair A. Selecting the appropriate study design for your research: Descriptive study designs. J Health Spec. 2015;3:153-6.
6. Siedlecki, Sandra L. PhD, RN, APRN-CNS, FAAN. Understanding Descriptive Research Designs and Methods. Clinical Nurse Specialist 34(1):p 8-12, 1/2 2020. | DOI: 10.1097/NUR.0000000000000493

CHAPTER 10

Analytical Study Designs

Tulika Goswami, Nirmala CJ, Sweta Balappa Athani, Baidurjya Mahanta, Mridushman Saikia, Manjula R

Beautiful Evidence is about the theory and practice of analytical design. —Edward Tufte

INTRODUCTION

Analytical study design is an observational study design where from generation of hypothesis to testing of hypothesis for better evidence generation to know the burden of different conditions, its distribution in different communities and determinants and its strength of association can be assessed. Analytical study design is subjected to less ethical issues compared to intervention studies and it is also useful for planning and implementation of different programs.

Analytical studies are intended to test hypotheses on the relationship between exposure and outcome to address why certain populations or individuals get affected by a health situation and others do not. Thus, the objective of analytical studies is to establish a causal inference answering the question: Are exposure and disease linked?

In real life situations however, such clear demarcation may not be available and data generated from a descriptive study may be used to analyze variables of subgroups within the study sample.

This accentuates the importance of specific and clear objectives mentioned a-priori to initiation of the study. Furthermore, analytical study design uses a control (or comparator) group to analyze the hypothesis whereas, the sole purpose of a descriptive study is to describe the target population only. This chapter will be pivoted around analytical study design.

Classification of Analytical Studies

Based on the three main aspects of any study design, viz.
1. Directionality
2. Sample selection
3. Timing, analytical studies are subdivided into:
   * Cross-sectional study
   * Case control study
   * Cohort study

Details of each study is explained in detail in further chapters. **Table 1** explains how to choose a analytical study design.

Table 1: Choice of study.

Basis	Cohort	Case-control	Cross-sectional
Rare condition	Not practical	Bias	Not appropriate
To determine a precise risk	Best	Only estimate possible	Gives prevalence
To determine whether exposure preceded disease	Best	Not appropriate	Not appropriate
For administrative purposes	Not appropriate	Not appropriate	Best
If attrition is a serious problem	Not appropriate	Attrition is usually minimal	Attrition may have occurred before the study
If selective survival is problem	Best	Not appropriate	Not appropriate
If all factors are not known	Best	Not appropriate	Less appropriate
Time and money	Most expensive	Least expensive	In between

KEY POINTS

- Analytical study designs are observational methods used to explore associations between variables, assess disease burdens, and determine their distribution and determinants in communities.
- These studies do not manipulate variables but observe natural settings to generate hypotheses.
- While they offer valuable insights into potential relationships, they cannot establish causality and may be affected by biases like selection and confounding.
- Despite these limitations, analytical observational studies are vital in informing decisions in medicine, public health and social sciences.

BIBILIOGRAPHY

1. Bonita R, Beaglehole R, Kjellström T, Organization WH. Basic epidemiology [Internet]. World Health Organization; 2006.
2. Celentano Dd. Gordis Epidemiology 6th (Indian Edition). Elsevier; 2019.
3. Kramer MS. Clinical Epidemiology and Biostatistics [Internet]. Berlin, Heidelberg: Springer; 1988.
4. Rao PSS, Richard J. Introduction to Biostatistics and Research Methods. PHI Learning Pvt. Ltd.; 2012.
5. Rothman KJ. Epidemiology: An Introduction. 2nd ed. New York: Oxford University Press; 2012.

CHAPTER 11

Cross-sectional Study Design

Pradeep Aggarwal, Darshan BB, Sudip Bhattacharya, Rubina Saha, Meely Panda

"One must credit a hypothesis with all that has had to be discovered in order to demolish It."
—Jean Rostand

INTRODUCTION

Cross-sectional studies are a type of observational studies, commonly used in epidemiology and social studies. They involve collection of data at a specific point of time and taking a snapshot of a population or a subset of it. The primary goal of cross-sectional study is to examine the relationship between different variables within the population and determine the prevalence or distribution of specific characteristics or conditions. It examines the relationship between diseases (or other health-related characteristics) and other variables of interest as they exist in defined population at one point of time.

In a cross-sectional study, data is collected from a sample of individuals or units within a population and information is gathered regarding the variables of interest. These variables can include demographic information, behaviors, attitudes, disease prevalence or other relevant factors. Data is obtained on both exposure and outcome at a single point of time and analyzed to identify associations between variables. The study does not follow individuals over time, prospectively or retrospectively. Therefore, it is also known as *snapshot study*.

Prevalence refers to the proportion of persons, in a population, with a particular disease or attribute at given point of time, irrespective of the onset of disease. Since cross-sectional studies have been mainly used to estimate the prevalence of a disease, they are referred to as *prevalence study*, also.

A cross-sectional study measures the prevalence of health outcomes or determinants of health or both, in a population at a point in time or over a short period. Such information can be used to explore etiology—for example, the relation between cataract and vitamin status has been examined in cross-sectional surveys.

Steps in Cross-sectional Study

The following are the general steps followed in conducting a cross-sectional study:
- **Define the research objectives:** Define the research objective, identify the variables and population or subset which needs to be studied.
- **Sampling:** Determine the appropriate sampling strategy to select participants or units for the study. It involves defining the target population, selecting a representative sample and deciding on the sample size.

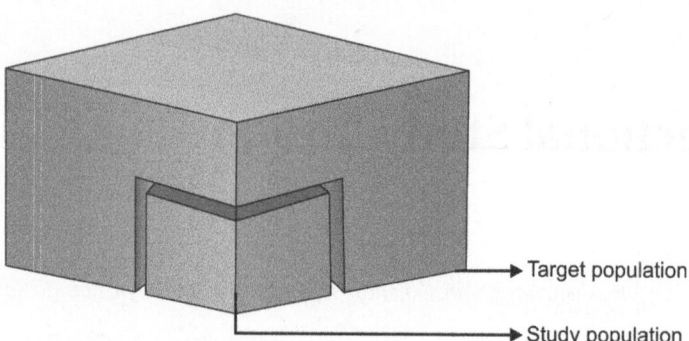

Fig. 1: Selection of study population in analytical studies.

- **Data collection:** Develop a data collection plan and choose the appropriate methods and tools to gather the required information. This can include questionnaire, survey interviews, physical measurement or other relevant techniques. The data collection method should be reliable and valid.
- **Ethics and consent:** Ensure that ethical considerations are addressed and informed consent are obtained from the participants. Protect the privacy and confidentiality of the individuals involved.
- **Data analysis:** Clean and organize the collected data and perform appropriate statistical analyses to explore the relationships between variables. Descriptive statistics, such as frequencies and percentages, can be used to summarize the data. Inferential statistics, such as chi square tests or regression analyses, may be employed to examine associations between variables.
- **Interpretation of findings:** Analyze the results of the data analysis and interpret the findings in the light of the research objectives. Identify patterns, trends or significant associations between variables.
- **Reporting and communication:** Prepare a report and clearly communicate the results in a way that is understandable to the intended audience.
- It is important to note that the specific steps and procedures may vary depending on the nature of the study, the research field and the variables being investigated. Consulting relevant literature and seeking guidance from experienced researchers can provide further insights into conducting a cross-sectional study effectively.

The study is conducted by selecting the study population in a target population who represent the whole population, which is done by using appropriate sampling method **(Fig. 1)**.

Types of Cross-sectional Study

Descriptive

They characterize the prevalence of one or multiple health outcomes in a specified population.

For example: A cross-sectional study was conducted in a village to find out the prevalence of diabetes mellitus. It was found that out of 1,000 population surveyed, 200 had diabetes mellitus, amounting to 20% prevalence of diabetes mellitus. In other words, one out of five people had diabetes mellitus.

Analytical

While collecting the data, the investigator collects information on both exposure as well as outcome. Then they compare outcome results on both exposure group and nonexposure group.

For example: A cross-sectional study was conducted in a village to investigate the association between alcoholism and diabetes mellitus. The village harbored 1,000 persons. The data collected was as follows:

	Disease or outcome (Diabetes mellitus)		
	+	−	Total
Alcoholism +	a (400)	b (200)	a + b (600)
Alcoholism −	c (160)	d (240)	c + d (400)

- Alcoholic with DM [exposed and outcome +]
- Alcoholic without DM [exposed and outcome −]
- Nonalcoholic with DM [not exposed and outcome +]
- Nonalcoholic without DM [not exposed and outcome −]
  So, we analyze the data as follows:
  - Prevalence of DM in alcoholic = $\dfrac{a}{a+b} = \dfrac{400}{600} = 66\%$
  - Prevalence of DM in nonalcoholic = $\dfrac{c}{c+d} = \dfrac{160}{400} = 40\%$

We conclude that the prevalence of DM is more in alcoholics compared to nonalcoholics.

Advantages

- Quick and cost-effective
- Less ethical issues
- Multiple outcomes
- Health-related variables apart from disease can also be studied
- Easy for generating hypothesis.

Disadvantages

- Temporal relation cannot be proved, so we rely on case-control and cohort study.
- We identify prevalent cases, but not new (incident) cases.
- We exclude cases who died because of the disease. So, results reflect association with survival with/after the disease rather than association with developing a disease.

Limitations

Cross-sectional studies are liable for many biases that can impact the validity and generalizability of the research study. The common biases encountered in cross-sectional studies are:
- **Selection bias:** It occurs when there is a systematic difference in the characteristics between those who participate and those who do not participate in the study. It can lead to a sample which is not representative of the target population and lead to bias.
- **Information bias:** It occurs when there are errors or inaccuracies in measurement or collection of data.
- **Reverse causality bias:** To illustrate reverse causality bias let us take a suitable example of decreased levels of Vit D in patients suffering from depression. Without being aware that lower levels of Vit D may lead to depression, a parallelly opposite inference could be that depression may lead to lower levels of Vit D, as depressed people are less likely to go outside and often so less exposed to sunlight. We are uncertain as to which has occurred first to cause the outcome. For the same reason such bias is also called "cart before horse bias."

Important Considerations

Cross-sectional studies can also be repeated over time to examine trends over time, helping us identify surge of any outcome to take preventive or curative steps in future.

Pseudo-cohort study: Pseudo cohort studies are actually cross-sectional studies carried out at regular intervals for a protracted period of time. Different age groups are studied cross-sectionally rather than following one group over time. Thus, making such a study seem longitudinal as the outcome data is based on the age of different participants rather than on the same subject over time. The advantage of such studies is that it is not always feasible to follow the same individual over time, confidentiality being one major deterrent.

KEY POINTS

- Cross-sectional study is a type of observational study that examines the relationship between diseases (or other health-related characteristics) and other variables of interest as they exist in defined population at one point of time.
- Cross-sectional study allows us to calculate the prevalence rate.
- Cross-sectional study does not require follow up.
- Cross-sectional study is susceptible to information bias and selection bias.

BIBLIOGRAPHY

1. Ann LK. Study design III: Cross-sectional study. Evidences Based Dentistry. 2006;7:24-5.
2. Gordis L. Epidemiology. 5th edition. Canada: Elsevier Saunders; 2014. p. 210-2.
3. Last JM. A dictionary of epidemiology. 4th edition. New York: Oxford University Press; 2001. p. 44.
4. Wang X, Cheng Z. Cross-sectional studies strengths, weakness and recommendations. CHEST 2020;158(1S):S65-S71.

12
CHAPTER

Case-control Study Design

Amir Maroof Khan, Chandralekha Kona, Aditi Mohta, Ekta Gupta, Meely Panda

"Its methods may be scientific, but its objectives are often thoroughly human."
—Alex Broadbent

INTRODUCTION

Case-control studies are observational type of studies, which are conducted to explore the association between a disease or a health condition and their hypothesized risk factors. These are suited to explore the association of multiple risk factors with the disease. Herein, we select a group of cases, i.e., those with the disease or health condition in question, and a group of controls, i.e., those without the disease or health condition in question, and compare the risk factor exposure in both these groups. Traditionally, a case-control study begins once the cases have already occurred and therefore, all case-control studies are retrospective. However, it is possible that a researcher, in their study, waits for a case to occur and on its occurrence, they find an appropriate control for this case and so on. This makes a case-control study, prospective in nature. We will learn about variations of traditional case-control studies, such as nested case-control studies and case-cohort studies, later in this chapter.

Selection of Cases and Controls in a Case-control Study

- Define the cases as specifically as possible.
- Exposure should be measured similarly in both cases and controls.
- Measurement of exposure must be done using valid and reliable techniques.
- Diagnostic criteria for identifying cases should be valid and reliable.
- Controls should preferably be selected from the source population from where the cases have come.
- Controls should be selected in a manner which is independent of exposure.
- Controls may be selected from neighborhood, among their friends, or other patients within the hospital. However, hospital-based controls can lead to certain biases, the most well-known being the **Berkson's bias**, which is also known as *hospital admission rate bias*. This occurs while attempting to find out the association between two diseases, where one disease condition is considered as a risk factor for another disease. Hence cases and controls are selected from admitted patients, leading to risk of overestimation of the odds ratio. This is because the chances of hospital admission may be higher for those with two diseases in the same person in contrast to a person who has any one of these two diseases.

* The number of cases and controls should be equal, i.e., 1:1, to ensure comparability. If it is not possible to get the required number of cases for a 1:1 case-control study, the researcher may opt for two controls per case, with a maximum of four controls per case. As number of controls per case increases, the number of cases required for the same amount of power decreases. Hence there is no meaningful gain beyond four controls per case.

Confounding Factors

Confounding variables are those variables which are associated both with the disease and with the risk factor, but do not lie in the causal pathway. They can distort the true association between the disease and the risk factor. For example, in a case-control study of smoking and lung cancer, age can confound the results by modifying the actual odds ratio (OR), since age is associated with smoking as well as lung cancer.

Confounding can be adjusted by either matching or by using certain statistical techniques during analysis. ***Matching*** means selecting controls which are similar to cases in terms of certain characteristics which can be the potential confounders such as age, sex etc. For example, if a case is a 45-year-old female, then the control selected should also be a female of around 45 years. A margin of a few years on either side should be allowed for, as it would not be possible to find cases and controls with the exact same age. We should avoid matching too many variables *(overmatching)*, since it may lead to similar exposure rates in both the groups and underestimate the odds ratio. Matching should preferably be done for those variables which are already known to be confounders.

To control for a confounder during analysis, stratified analysis can be done, with one stratum consisting of subjects with the confounding variable and another stratum consisting of those without the confounding variable. If the OR in these two strata is different from the crude OR, it indicates the presence of confounding. In such cases, either odds ratios can be given separately for each stratum, and/or pooled odds ratio, known as Mantel-Haenszel odds ratio, can be given. Another statistical technique to adjust for confounders is regression analysis, which gives an adjusted odds ratio (AOR) by adjusting for the confounding effect of the other variables.

Outcome Measure in Case-control Studies

Let us understand about odds ratio, which is the outcome measure of a case-control study using a 2 × 2 table **(Table 1)** given below.

Table 1 depicts the relationship between disease and risk factor. This type of 2 × 2 table can be constructed for case-control study as well as cohort study. The difference between the two is that in case-control study we begin the study by selecting cases and controls, i.e., the disease has already occurred; whereas in the cohort study, we select the groups based on their exposure to a particular risk factor. It is therefore imperative to clearly identify the disease or the health outcome and the risk factor before designing an observational study to explore association between them.

Table 1: A 2 × 2 table depicting the relationship between disease and risk factor			
	Cases	*Controls*	*Total*
Exposed	a	b	a + b
Nonexposed	c	d	c + d
Total	a + c	b + d	a + b + c + d

Odds ratio (OR) tells us about the odds of exposure in cases with respect to the odds of exposure in controls. First, let us understand what is meant by odds. Odds is the probability of the occurrence of an event divided by the probability of nonoccurrence of that event.

From **Table 1**, we derive that:
- Odds that a case was exposed are $[a/(a + c)] \div [c/(a + c)] = a/c$
- Odds that a control was exposed are $[b/(b + d)] \div [d/(b + d)] = b/d$
- Odds ratio, i.e., odds that a case was exposed to odds that a control was exposed = $[a/c] \div [b/d] = ad/bc$.

The odds ratio can be a reasonable estimate of the relative risk (RR), in case of rare diseases, i.e., when the prevalence of the disease is less than 5%. This is known as the *rare disease assumption*.

The relative risk, if calculated from **Table 1** will be as follows:
- Relative risk (RR) = Risk of disease among exposed/Risk of disease among nonexposed

$$= [a/(a + b)] \div [c/(c + d)]$$

- In case of rare disease assumption, a and c will be very less. Hence,

$$(a + b) \approx b \text{ and } (c + d) \approx d$$

- Implying, RR $\approx (a/b) \div (c/d) = (ad/bc)$ which is the same as the odds ratio given above.

Advantages of Case-control Studies

- Quick and inexpensive, since they do not require long-term follow-up of large groups of people.
- Well-suited for studying rare diseases or outcomes: For rare diseases, researchers would have to follow very large number of participants and wait for a long time to be able to get adequate number of cases to draw inference from cohort studies. In contrast, case-control studies can be conducted with a relatively small number of cases and controls, and therefore they are more suited for rare diseases or outcomes.
- Can be used to explore the association of multiple risk factors with the disease or outcome.

Limitations of Case-control Studies

- **Can not prove causal relationship:** As temporality is not established in case-control studies, we can only infer association from these studies. For causation, cohort or trials are appropriate study designs.
- **Recall bias:** People with a disease may be more likely to remember an exposure by a risk factor than those without the disease. This introduces recall bias in case-control studies. For example, those involved in accidents may remember not wearing seatbelts more than those not involved in accidents.
- **Survivorship bias:** The case-control study includes only the surviving cases. It is possible that exposure among diseased persons who died due to the disease is different from exposure among diseased persons who are surviving. This may lead to biased odds ratio.

So far, we have discussed about traditional case-control study design wherein the cases have already occurred by the time we are conducting the study. It is possible to conduct case-control studies wherein the participants are followed up for a sufficiently long period of time to arrive at adequate number of incident cases who can be recruited in the study. These studies can only be conducted within a cohort which is being studied and from which data is being collected at regular intervals. Case-cohort and nested case-control are two such study designs.

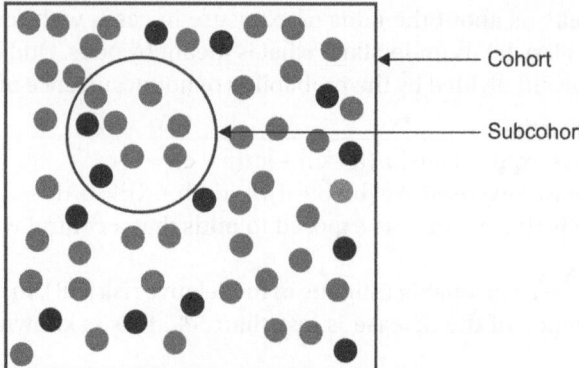

Fig. 1: Schematic diagram of a case-cohort study design. All the black dots whether inside the circle (subcohort) or outside the circle (cohort) are the cases. Grey dots inside the circle (subcohort) are the controls.

Case-cohort Study Design (Fig. 1)

This variation of case-control study is built within an existing cohort being followed up. Baseline data of all the participants of the cohort is available. A subcohort of the participants enrolled in the cohort acts as a control group, irrespective of whether any of its participants develops the disease and becomes a case later. This method of selection of controls is called *case-base sampling* or *inclusive sampling*. As the whole cohort is being followed up which includes the subcohort too, the participants who develop the disease in the whole cohort are considered as cases. The risk factor under study is compared between the cases (incident cases) and the control (subcohort) group.

The advantage of case-cohort study design is that the odds ratio approximates relative risk, and is represented as the number of diseased among exposed with respect to the number of diseased among the nonexposed. The rare disease assumption is not applicable here. Multiple risk factors can be studied in one study. Analysis is done using weighted Cox's regression.

Nested Case-control Study Design (Fig. 2)

This is also built within an existing cohort being followed up and those participants who develop the disease in the follow up period are designated as cases. At the time point at which an incident case is detected, the control for that case is also selected from the remaining participants who have not developed the disease. Thus, cases and controls are time-matched. This method of sampling is called *risk-set sampling*, as the control is being selected from all those participants who have not yet developed the disease and so are the 'at-risk' group. It is also known as *density sampling* or *concurrent sampling*.

This type of study design also produces odds ratio which is similar to relative risk and the rare disease assumption is not applicable. Nested case-control study design can also be developed within an existing randomized controlled trial. A limitation is that multiple risk factors cannot be studied in a single nested case-control study design. Analysis is done using stratified Cox's regression and conditional logistic regression.

Case-crossover Study Design

Let us see one more variation of the case-control study design. The case-crossover study design may be used to study fleeting exposures on acute disease. Only cases are selected, i.e., those who suffered an event. Each participant serves as their own control. The study is used to determine

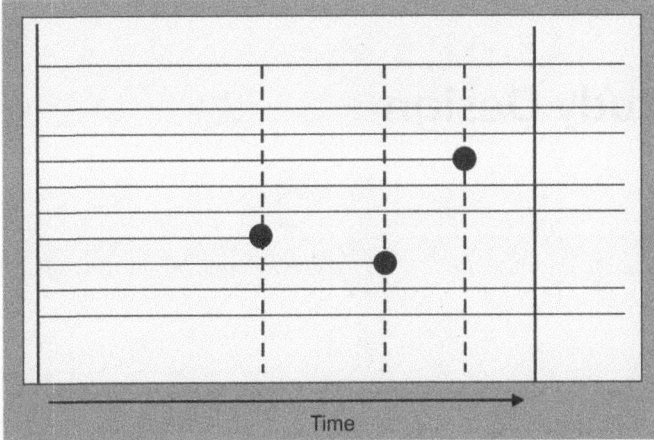

Fig. 2: Schematic diagram of a nested case-control study. The horizontal lines indicate the participants in the cohort study followed for a time duration which is represented by two vertical lines at two time points. The black colored dots represent the participants who turned into cases. The dashed lines indicate the time point at which the incident cases emerge and that the control/s for that incident case will be selected from the participants free of the disease at that point in time.

whether the exposure times are associated with the outcome times. The probability of exposure during the outcome time, i.e., the time period just before the event occurred (case window), is compared with exposure frequency during the exposure time, i.e., the time period relatively earlier than outcome time (control window). It is a matched study design and analysis must also be done using appropriate techniques such as conditional logistic regression.

KEY POINTS
▪ Case-control studies are common observational study designs in medical literature, used to explore the association of exposure to a risk factor with the disease or outcome. ▪ Care must be taken to select controls from the source population. ▪ Traditionally it was believed that all case-control studies are retrospective and rare disease assumption is a necessary criterion for the odds ratio to be approximately equal to the relative risk. ▪ There are newer variations to the traditional study design in the form of case-cohort study, nested case-control study design and case-crossover design.

BIBLIOGRAPHY

1. Abramson JH, Abramson ZH. Research methods in community medicine: surveys, epidemiological research, programme evaluation, clinical trials. 6th ed. England: John Wiley & Sons; 2008.
2. Gordis L. Epidemiology. 5th ed. Canada: Elsevier Saunders; 2014.
3. Kartsonaki C. Nested case-control and case-subcohort studies Oxford, United Kingdom: Nuffield Department of Population Health; 2017.
4. Lombardi DA. The Case-Crossover Study: A Novel Design in Evaluating Transient Fatigue as a Risk Factor for Road Traffic Accidents. Sleep. 2010;33:283-4.
5. Mann CJ. Observational research methods. Research design II: cohort, cross sectional, and case-control studies. Emerg Med J. 2003;20:54-60.
6. O'Brien KM, Lawrence KG, Keil AP. The Case for Case–Cohort: An Applied Epidemiologist's Guide to Reframing Case–Cohort Studies to Improve Usability and Flexibility. Epidemiology. 2022;33:354-61.
7. Partlett C, Hall NJ, Leaf A, Juszczak E, Linsell L. Application of the matched nested case-control design to the secondary analysis of trial data. BMC Medical Research Methodology. 2020;20:1-8.

CHAPTER 13

Cohort Study Design

Prem Mony, Bhushan Kamble, Chandralekha Kona

> *"Research is formalized curiosity. It is poking and prying with a purpose."*
> —*Zora Neale Hurston*

INTRODUCTION

Cohort studies are a type of analytical studies. The term "cohort" is derived from the Latin word "Cohors" – originally referring to a "division of Roman Legion". One legion is equal to 10 cohorts. It refers to a group of warriors marching forward together in time. It is a type of nonexperimental or observational study design. The terms "prospective", and "longitudinal" study (contrasted with "retrospective" for case-control study) are used synonymously for cohort studies, but the term "cohort study" is preferable. The term "cohort" refers to a group of people who have been included in a study by an event that is based on the definition decided by the researcher. For example, a cohort of people born in Mumbai in the year 1980, will be called a "birth cohort". Another example of a cohort will be people who smoke.

Design of Cohort Study

Cohort study design shown in **Flowchart 1**:

Flowchart 1: Cohort study design.

Steps of Cohort Study

Approach to studying risk factors and disease incidence:
1. Start with a population at risk
2. Estimate sample size
3. Measure exposures (and covariates) at baseline
4. Follow up the cohort over time with: (a) Surveillance for events or (b) re-examination
5. Keep track of attrition/withdrawals/dropouts
6. Compare event rates in people with and without exposures of interest
7. Incidence is the appropriate measure of effect or event or outcome
8. Adjust for confounders and compute adjusted Incidence
9. Compute relative risk, attributable risk, and population attributable risk.

Types of Cohort

Closed Cohort

It has fixed membership. Once the cohort is defined by enrolling subjects and follow up begins, no one can be added. The number of subjects may decline because of death or loss to follow up, but no additional subjects are added. As a result, closed cohorts always get smaller over time.

For example, Birth cohort: group of people born on the same day, etc.

Open Cohort

It is dynamic, meaning that members can leave or be added over time. Rothman gives the example of a state cancer registry. Subjects are continually added when they are diagnosed with cancer, so cohort size increase over the time. Subjects can also leave the cohort by moving to a new state or dying.

For example, cohort: people exposed to an infection or drug, etc.

The great majority of cohort studies are conducted in closed (or fixed) cohorts, because it is more difficult to establish eligibility and track people in an open cohort, since they can enter and leave at any time. This problem becomes greater as the size of the cohort gets larger and/or the study continues for a longer period of time.

Types of Cohort Study

Cohort studies are also designated by the timing of the data collection (retrospectively or prospectively):

Historical or Retrospective

Collect data on events that have already occurred.

Prospective

Most widespread use is to refer to studies in which the investigators observe occurrence of events.

Ambidirectional

Retrospective and prospective combined

Examples of Prospective and Retrospective Cohort Studies

Example 1: Our objective is to estimate the incidence of cardiovascular events in patients with psoriasis. We have decided to conduct a 10-year study. All the individuals who are diagnosed with psoriasis are eligible for being included in this cohort study. However, one has to ensure that none of them have cardiovascular events at baseline. Thus, they should be thoroughly investigated for the presence of these events at baseline before including them in the study. For this, we have to define all the events we are interested in the study (such as angina or myocardial infarction). The criteria for identifying psoriasis and cardiovascular outcomes should be decided before initiating the study. All those who do not have cardiovascular outcomes should be followed at regular intervals (predefined by the researcher and as required for clinical management). This will be a prospective cohort study.

Example 2: Our objective is to assess the survival in HIV-infected individuals and the factors associated with survival. We have clinical data from about 430 HIV-infected individuals in the center. The Follow up period ranges from 3 months to 4 years, and we know that 33 individuals have died in this group. We decide to perform the survival analysis in this group of individuals. We prepare a clinical record form and abstract data from these clinical forms. This design will be a retrospective cohort study.

Special Types of Cohort Study

Nested Case-control Study

This study is conducted within the methodology of a prospective cohort design that has a large source of cohort participant lab samples and risk factors at baseline. The case-control study is "nested" within the prospective cohort in that participants are derived from the cohort and analyzed. Case participants are compared to control participants on lab samples and risk factors related to an outcome of interest.

Case-cohort Study

This design was proposed by Prentice as a cost-effective alternative to the nested case-control design. In a case-cohort design, a sub cohort is randomly drawn from the full cohort and the case-cohort sample consists of the sub cohort plus those subjects from the entire cohort whose outcome occurred during the study period.

How is 'Exposure' Measured?

- History, e.g., smoking
- Validation in a subset
- Physical examination
- Choice of robust equipment/calibration of equipment/training manual/lead anthropometrist/standardization training and certification of fieldworkers
- Biological markers
- Blood sampling/test/laboratory issues

How is 'Outcome' Measured?

- Cause-of-death by 'hospital diagnosis' or by 'verbal autopsy'
- Myocardial infarction definitions—definite/probable/possible (depending on certainty of diagnosis)
- Case definition predefined by researcher

Analysis of Cohort Studies

	Disease		
	+	−	Total
Exposure +	a	b	a + b
Exposure −	c	d	c + d

Measure of association: ***Relative risk*** or ***risk ratio (RR)***
= incidence among exposed (I_e)/incidence among unexposed (I_u)
= [a/ (a+b)] ÷ [c/(c+d)]
Values can be on either side of 1; interpretation = risk or protection
Interpretation of RR: Incidence of lung disease among exposed is so many times higher as compared to that among nonexposed
If RR = 1, it implies no association
If RR > 1, it implies positive association
If RR < 1, it implies negative association (protective)

Strength of association in a cohort study is also evaluated by:
- ❖ **Attributable risk (AR)** = (Incidence among exposed − Incidence among nonexposed)/ Incidence among exposed × 100
  i.e., $AR = [(I_e - I_{ne})/I_e] \times 100$
  Interpretation of AR: It tells about the amount of disease that can be attributed to exposure
- ❖ **Population attributable risk (PAR)** = (Incidence among total—Incidence among nonexposed)/Incidence among total × 100
  i.e., $PAR = [(I_t - I_{ne})/I_t] \times 100$
  Interpretation of PAR: If risk factor is modified or eliminated, the value calculated shall represent the annual reduction in incidence of the disease in the given population.

Advantages

Clarity of Temporal Sequence (Did the Exposure Precede the Outcome?)

Cohort studies more clearly indicate the temporal sequence between exposure and outcome, because subjects are known to be disease-free at the beginning of the observation period when their exposure status is established. In case-control studies, one begins with diseased and nondiseased people and then ascertains their prior exposures, which may lead to diminished recall and thus bring in recall bias.

Allow Calculation of Incidence

Cohort studies allow for calculation of incidence of disease in exposure groups, so we can calculate:
- ❖ Absolute risk (incidence)
- ❖ Relative risk (risk ratio or rate ratio)
- ❖ Risk difference
- ❖ Attributable proportion (attributable risk %)

Facilitate study of Rare Exposures

While a cohort design can be used to investigate common exposures (e.g., risk factors for cardiovascular disease and cancer in the nurses health study), they are particularly useful for evaluating the effects of rare or unusual exposures, because the investigators can make it a point to identify an adequate number of subjects who have an unusual exposure, e.g., unusual occupational exposures (e.g., asbestos, or solvents in tire manufacturing).

Allow Examination of Multiple Effects of a Single Exposure

When we follow up a cohort, multiple outcomes of single exposure can be studied at different timeline. Even the combined effect of multiple exposures on the outcome can be determined.

Avoid Selection Bias at Enrolment

Cohort studies, especially prospective cohort studies, reduce the possibility that the results will be biased by selecting subjects for the comparison group who may be more or less likely to have the outcome of interest, because in a cohort study the outcome is not known at baseline when exposure status is established. Nevertheless, selection bias can occur in retrospective cohort studies (since the outcomes have already occurred at the time of selection) and it can occur in prospective cohort studies as a result of differential loss to follow up.

Results from Cohort Studies May be More Generalizable in Clinical Practice

Researcher may obtain large samples and reach greater power in statistical analysis relative to a randomized controlled trial. Furthermore, cohort studies often have broader inclusion and fewer exclusion criteria compared with randomized controlled trials.

Provide Insight Into the Dynamic Relation Between Exposure and Outcome

The longitudinal nature of cohort studies means that changes in levels of exposure over time and changes in outcome, can be measured to provide insight into complex relation between exposure and outcome over the period.

Disadvantages of Prospective Cohort Studies

- You may have to follow large numbers of subjects for a long time.
- They can be very expensive and time consuming.
- They are not good for rare diseases.
- They are not good for diseases with a long latency.
- Differential loss to follow up can introduce bias.

Disadvantages of Retrospective Cohort Studies

- As with prospective cohort studies, they are not good for very rare diseases.
- If one uses records that were not designed for the study, the available data may be of poor quality.
- There is frequently an absence of data on potential confounding factors if the data was recorded in the past.
- It may be difficult to identify an appropriate exposed cohort and an appropriate comparison group.
- Differential losses to follow up can also cause bias in retrospective cohort studies.

Examples

Framingham Cohort Study

This cohort study was initiated in 1948 in Framingham, USA. Framingham, at the time of initiation of the cohort, was an industrial town 21 miles west of Boston with a population of 28,000. This Framingham Heart Study recruited 5,209 men and women (30-62-year-old) in the study to assess the factors associated with cardiovascular disease (CVD). The researchers also recruited second generation participants (children of original participants) in 1971 and the third general participants in 2002. This has been one of the landmark cohort studies and has contributed immensely to our knowledge of some of the important risk factors for CVD. The investigators have published nearly 3,064 publications using the Framingham Heart Study data.

The Danish Cohort Study of Psoriasis and Depression

This is another large cohort study that evaluated the association between psoriasis and onset of depression. The participants in the cohort were enrolled from national registries in Denmark. None of the included participants had psoriasis or depression at baseline. The outcome of interest was the initiation of antidepressants or hospitalization for depression. The authors compared the incidence rates of hospitalization for depression in psoriasis and reference population. The psoriasis group was further classified as mild and moderate psoriasis. The authors found that psoriasis was an independent risk factor for new-onset depression in young people. However, in the elderly, it was mediated through comorbid conditions.

Limitations

Loss to follow up: Retention of study participants till end is an important issue in conducting the cohort study. Loss to follow up usually occurs due to dropouts or death of study participants, which often occurs in studies with long Follow up duration and is a major source of potential bias. A general rule of thumb requires that the loss to Follow up rate does not exceed 20% of the sample.

Confounding: It often occurs in cohort studies. Confounding could result in a distortion of the effects; it may lead to overestimation or underestimation of an effect or even reverse the direction of an effect. Many statistical methods can be applied to control for confounding factors, both at the design stage and in the data analysis stage such as restriction, stratification, multivariable regression and propensity score.

KEY POINTS

- Cohort studies track a group with shared characteristics over time to measure outcomes and are key for understanding incidence and natural history of conditions.
- They enable calculation of incidence rate, cumulative incidence, relative risk and hazard ratio, offering generalizable results for general practice.
- However, they are prone to loss to Follow up, making them less reliable than cross-sectional studies in this aspect.
- Prospective cohort studies, while providing valuable insights, are costly and time-intensive.
- Retrospective cohort studies face challenges with information and recall biases.

BIBLIOGRAPHY

1. Conato J, Shah N, Horwitz RI. Randomized, controlled trials, observational studies, and the hierarchy of research design. N Engl J Med. 2000;342:1887-92.
2. Ernster VI. Nested case-control studies. Prev Med. 1994;23(5):587-90.
3. Euser AM, Zoccali C, Jager KJ, Dekker FW. Cohort studies: prospective versus retrospective. Nephron Clin Pract. 2009;113(3):c214-7.
4. Merrill RM. Introduction to epidemiology. 7th edition. Burlington, MA: Jones & Bartlett Publishers; 2015.
5. Prentice RL. A case-cohort design for epidemiologic cohort studies and disease prevention trial. Biometrika. 1986;73(1):1-11.
6. Rothman KJ, Greenland S, Lash TL. Modern epidemiology. 3rd edition. Philadelphia, PA: Wolters Kluwer Health/Lippincott Williams & Wilkins; 2012.
7. Setia MS. Methodology Series Module 1: Cohort Studies. Indian J Dermatol. 2016;61(1):21-5. doi:10.4103/0019-5154.174011

CHAPTER 14

Experimental Study Designs

NR Ramesh Masthi, Ashwath Narayan, Ravish H, Shivram, Ramesh Holla,
Suhasini R Kanyadi, Sweta Balappa Athani

"No research without action, no action without research." —Kurt Lewin

INTRODUCTION

Experimental epidemiology is a type of study design where we seek evidence of the effects of an intervention/procedure/therapy, etc. The objective both in clinical practice and public health is to modify the natural history of a disease so as to prevent/delay death or disability and to improve the health of the patient/population. Randomized control trial is observed to be an ideal study design for evaluating both the adverse events and efficacy of new forms of interventions. Experimental studies are also known as interventional studies in epidemiology. Experimentation involves small groups, block level or community. Effects of interventions are measured in two groups, which are, experimental and control group.

Experimental study designs involve application or withdrawal of a variable in the study group while no changes are made in the control group. The study and control groups are then observed for the outcomes of the investigation.

Historically, In the 1900s, Webster in the USA and Topley, Wilson and Greenwood in England, pioneered experimental studies on epidemics and herd immunity in animals, mainly mice. The earliest documented studies in humans are from James Lind, Scottish Physician on his experimental study on scurvy among sailors in the 17th century and Ignaz Semmelweis, Hungarian Physician in the 18th century pioneering randomized study on maternal mortality and hygiene.

Types of Experimental Studies

Clinical Trials or Randomized Controlled Trials

These are the most common type of experimental studies. They are done for interventional, diagnostic, therapeutic, prophylactic purposes, for devices, procedures, regimens, protocols, etc. The unit of study is "patient suffering from a disease".

Field Trials or Preventive Trials

They take place at community level, for preventive procedures or personal protective measures, etc. Healthy individuals are the study participants in field trials. *For example,* pulse polio program in the community.

Community Intervention Trials

Randomization is done at community level, but outcome assessment is done at individual level.

For example, health Health education at community level, such as steps in hand hygiene practices and diet modification for patients suffering from noncommunicable diseases.

Health System Evaluation Trials

They are used to measure cost-effectiveness of the intervention in the study.

For example, evaluation of reduction in incidence of diarrheal diseases following health education on personal hygiene practices.

Trials to Identify Etiologic Agents

They are done for identifying or detecting the causative organism of the diseases.

For example, RTPCR for COVID-19 and pulmonary infections.

Risk Factors Trials

The risk factor is the "'intervention,' e.g., studying the effect of risk factor (consumption of junk food) on lifestyle-related diseases (diabetes mellitus and hypertension).

Cessation Experiment Trials

A harmful factor is removed from the intervention group.

For example, people leading a sedentary lifestyle are divided into two groups, wherein one group is asked to perform physical activity for at least 30 minutes every day, while the other group is not asked.

The Quasi-experimental Design

It involves manipulation of an independent variable but typically lacks random assignment, making it useful when randomization is challenging or unethical. Quasi-experiments are often employed in real-world settings to study cause-and-effect relationships while accounting for practical constraints. e.g. study to assess the impact of electric vehicles (EVs) on air pollution.

Nonrandomized "Concurrent" Trial

A nonrandomized concurrent trial is a research design where participants are assigned to different treatment groups without randomization, typically based on practical or ethical considerations.

For example, comparing the effectiveness of two different exercise programs for improving cardiovascular health who enrolled voluntarily into different programs.

Natural Experiments

They leverage naturally occurring events or conditions as sources of variation in order to investigate cause-and-effect relationships. These studies provide valuable insights into real-world phenomena without direct manipulation of variables, making them especially useful for ethical or logistical reasons, e.g., study of the impact of a sudden increase in cigarette taxes on smoking rates.

Before and After Trial Using "Historical Controls"

This is a study design that compares outcomes from a group exposed to an intervention before and after its implementation with a separate group that serves as a historical reference, e.g., studying the effectiveness of a new traffic safety law.

Introduction to Randomized Controlled Trial

Introduction to randomized controlled trial (RCT) is an epidemiological experiment in which subjects in a population are randomly allocated into groups, usually called study and control groups, to receive and not receive an experimental preventive/therapeutic intervention or procedure. It is a prospective, comparative, quantitative study performed under controlled conditions with random allocation of interventions to different comparison groups. It is the most rigorous and robust research practical method of determining whether a cause-effect relation exists between an intervention and an outcome. It generates high-quality evidence when evaluating the effectiveness and safety of an intervention. Thereby, evidence-based clinical practice improves patient safety and outcomes. Designing and conducting an RCT, analyzing data, interpreting findings and disseminating results can be challenging as there are several practicalities to be considered.

RCT can also be an experimental form of impact evaluation in which the population receiving the program/policy (intervention) is chosen at random from the eligible population and a control group also at random from same eligible population (e.g., people, schools, villages, etc.). It tests the extent to which specific, planned objectives are being achieved, as measured by a predetermined set of indicators.

Research Question Formulation

A hypothesis must be formed for a research question to be answered using an RCT. The hypothesis should be precise. The key components of a sound research question should include:
* P (population of interest),
* I (intervention to be studied),
* C (comparator intervention),
* O (outcomes to be evaluated) and
* T (is there a time duration for intervention/outcome ascertainment time).

Adequate time and expertise is needed for converting a "free flowing" question arising from clinical context to convert into a properly answerable question. For example, to address the free-flowing research question, "Is the new antirabies vaccine safe and immunogenic to prevent rabies?", investigators need to convert it into a well-defined, feasible, specific, measurable, ethical and clinically important question: Is the new antirabies vaccine given by Essen regimen as a part of PEP in animal bites, safe and immunogenic as compared to the WHO prequalified vaccine among all age groups?

Points to Remember While Conducting an RCT

* Once a research question is generated, the next step is to clearly define the target population, inclusion and exclusion criteria, process of randomization, allocation, blinding of intervention, treatment and control delivery, outcomes assessment, definitions of outcomes, sample size required, ethical requirements, consent process and finally, data management.
* These topics should be written as a well-defined protocol. The protocol should be reviewed and approved by an independent ethics committee before starting the trial.
* For clinical trials registry (CTRI), it is now obligatory that protocols are registered with a publicly available trial registry before recruiting any participants. Apart from promoting transparency, most journals have this as a mandatory requirement and would not publish the results of an RCT unless trial registration details are provided.
* An RCT can be conducted at a single site or at multiple sites. RCTs conducted according to a single protocol but at more than one site are referred to as a multi-center trial. Including

several sites has the advantage of reaching the required sample size within a shorter time and may also improve generalizability of findings.
- ❖ The main premise of conducting an RCT is that the participants should be treated the same way in both arms, except for the intervention/control treatment.
- ❖ All other procedures of treatment, diagnosis, investigations, alterations, etc., should follow the routine process and *no undue advantage/testing should be performed on patients in the trial.*

Steps to Conduct RCT

1. Preparation of study protocol
2. Selection of reference and experimental populations
3. Randomization
4. Intervention
5. Follow up
6. Assessment

These steps have been described in detail in the upcoming sections.

Preparation of Study Protocol (Flowchart 1)

It is the blueprint of an RCT and specifies the following:
- ❖ Title of the study and registration number; DCGI approval
- ❖ Background information, rationale, aims and objectives of the study
- ❖ Selecting suitable population and reference population including sample size
- ❖ Duration of the study and roles and responsibilities of the study group
- ❖ Criteria for selection of study and control group (eligibility criteria) and description of study vaccines; their supplies and storage.

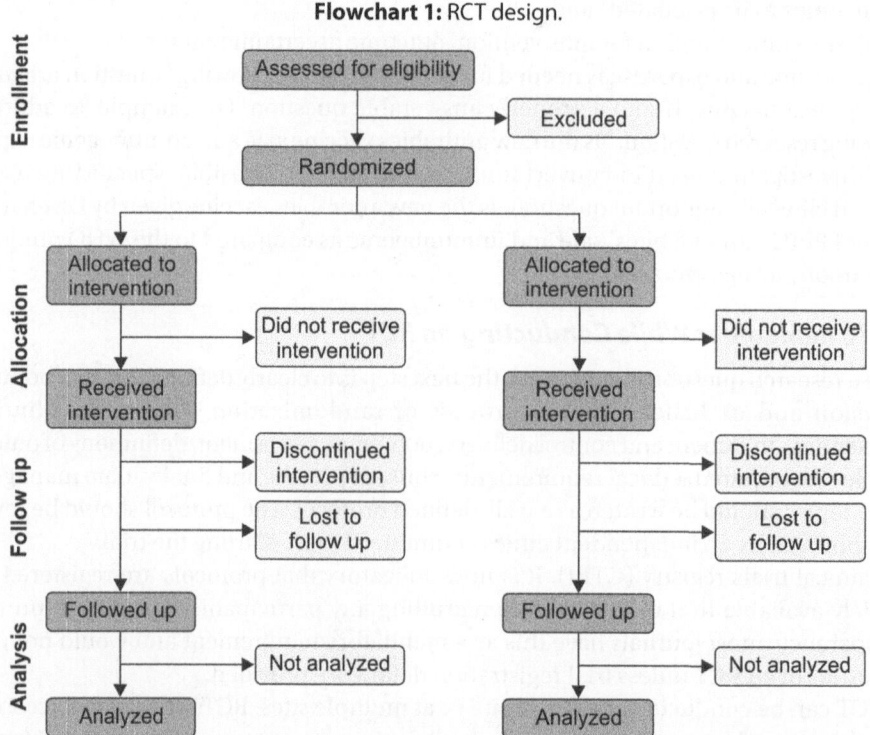

Flowchart 1: RCT design.

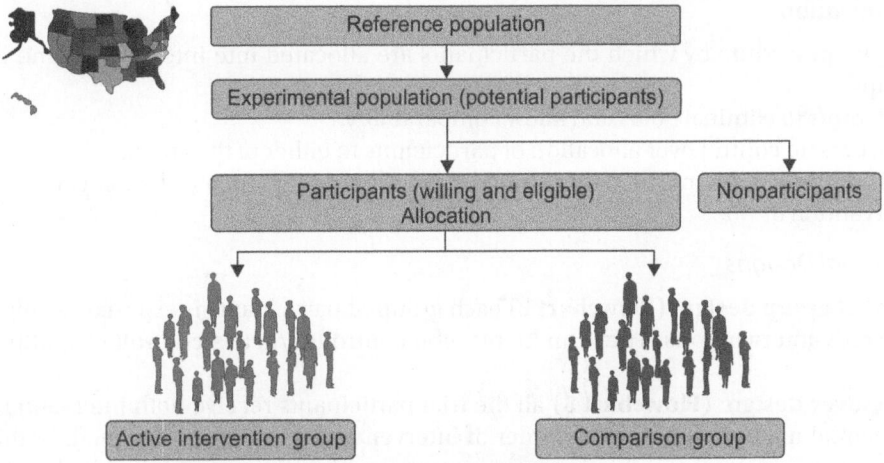

Fig. 1: Selection of reference and experimental populations.

- Informed consent process and randomization
- Intervention procedure and assessment of the intervention
- Follow up, end-points, evaluation, reporting, closure and archiving
- Statistical considerations and quality control and quality assurance (monitoring and audits)

Selection of Reference and Experimental Populations (Fig. 1)

Reference/Target Population

Population to which the findings of the trial, if found successful, are expected to be applicable, e.g., animal bite victims, children, workers, etc.

Experimental/Study Population

Derived from the reference population, that participates in the trial. It should ideally be randomly chosen from the reference population, so that it has the same characteristics to represent reference population. It is important to choose a stable population, whose cooperation is assured to avoid dropouts.

Reference population may be as **broad as mankind** or it may be **geographically limited** or **limited to persons** in specific age, gender, occupational or social groups, e.g., COVID 19 vaccine—applicable to the whole population shown in below:

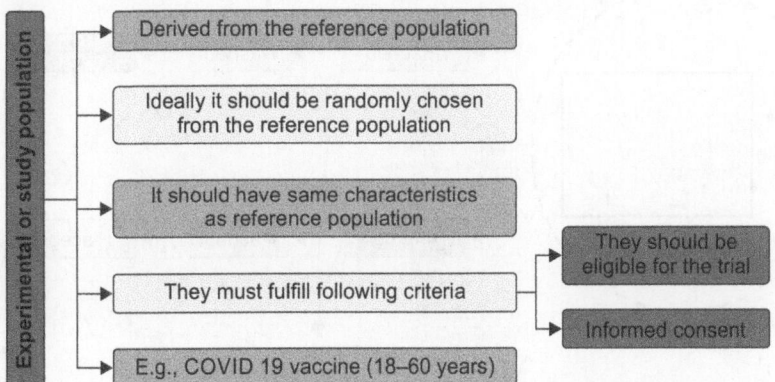

Randomization

- It is the procedure by which the participants are allocated into intervention and control groups.
- It attempts to eliminate bias and allow comparability.
- It ensures no control over allocation of participants to either of the group.
- Each of the eligible participants should have an equal chance to be allocated into the intervention or not.

Clinical Trial Designs

- **Parallel group design: (Flowchart 2)** each group of participants is exposed to only one of the study interventions. They can be placebo controlled/active controlled/multiple arm RCT.
- **Crossover design: (Flowchart 3)** all the trial participants receive both interventions in a sequential manner and only the order of intervention is randomly assigned. In this way, each participant serves as his/her own control, thereby eliminating individual participant differences.
- **Factorial design: (Flowchart 4)** commonly used as experiment plans to study the impact of several factors on a process.

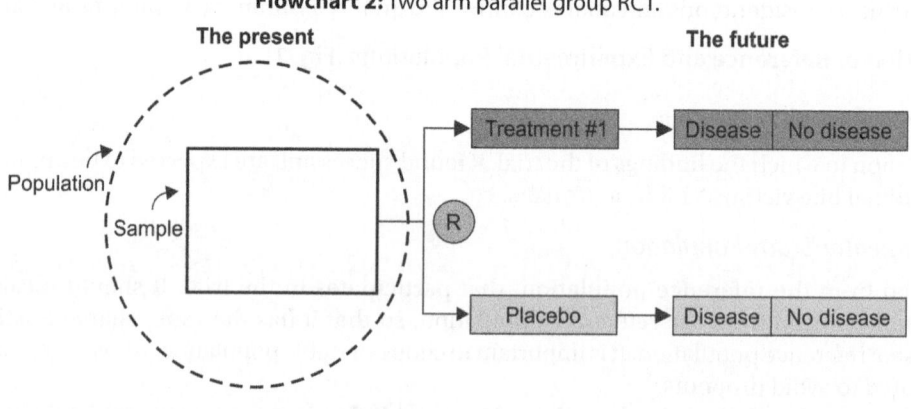

Flowchart 2: Two arm parallel group RCT.

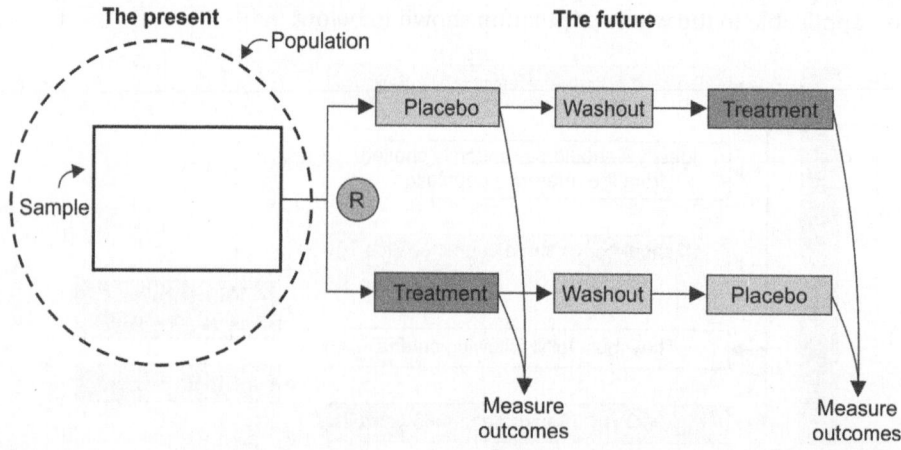

Flowchart 3: Crossover design of RCT.

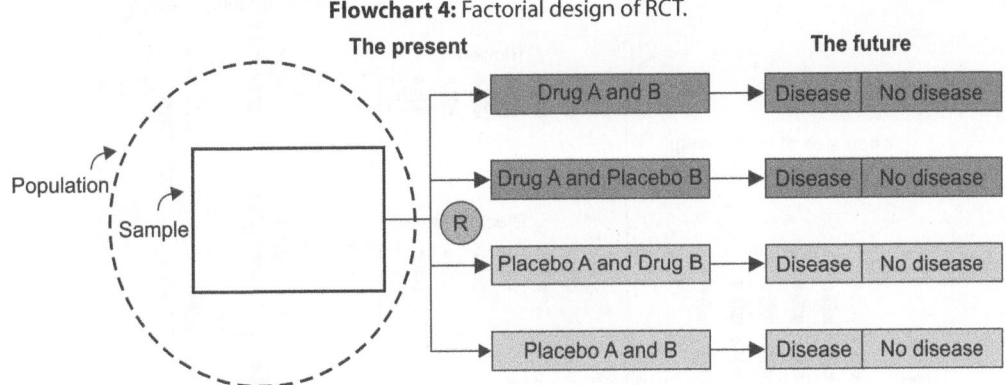

Flowchart 4: Factorial design of RCT.

Random Sequence Generation and Allocation Concealment

- **Random sequence generation:** An unpredictable allocation sequence must be generated based on a random procedure, such as random number table **(Table 1)**.
- **Allocation concealment:** It shields those involved in a trial from knowing upcoming assignments.

Generation of random sequence should be done by independent personnel, usually a statistician, who is not going to be involved in conduct of the RCT. The access to this sequence should be restricted to only a few individuals who absolutely need it (such as the pharmacist

Table 1: Random number table.									
07048	52841	54969	87057	30570	50494	29936	93967	1 0641	79871
09165	56926	17294	03803	31755	11321	33681	12997	17625	25954
35654	69761	83791	6337'1	28189	19944	04514	56533	89108	27861
79065	63956	39443	30373	55571	00919	1 5377	36851	28318	40846
27969	74368	77782	88616	06368	07345	00725	81221	78417	37992
47528	70548	25078	80729	27806	42877	80287	21759	61980	52447
65694	95760	64031	24046	77606	91 163	51492	20958	18384	49840
24253	39427	80642	36718	921 64	77732	69754	01 291	53704	33054
34302	60309	27186	22418	59962	13934	67591	17476	21 559	73437
76809	84341	74012	50947	83214	19967	44219	75929	13182	34858
85183	35958	04301	49628	91493	66103	65699	04241	82441	38112
27541	79187	99777	22894	83283	56218	86183	74497	21070	78935
74188	09083	54938	79920	27158	24864	31116	33173	43032	52000
13270	57457	30968	65978	67679	91216	47969	39204	46030	93954
891 50	53922	40537	23169	4-6948	05519	721 71	85417	31580	98102
49980	44551	99908	46115	92508	77184	44556	69725	42878	60298
26810	40280	15387	30976	15478	77703	341 09	02682	52877	36755
35056	23942	42645	67063	441 18	46433	83172	95689	60923	32769
09873	65959	7791 2	70059	07704	16015	57527	09818	84379	35903
40806	30051	54251	73489	4721 5	90651	90083	21019	63860	41369

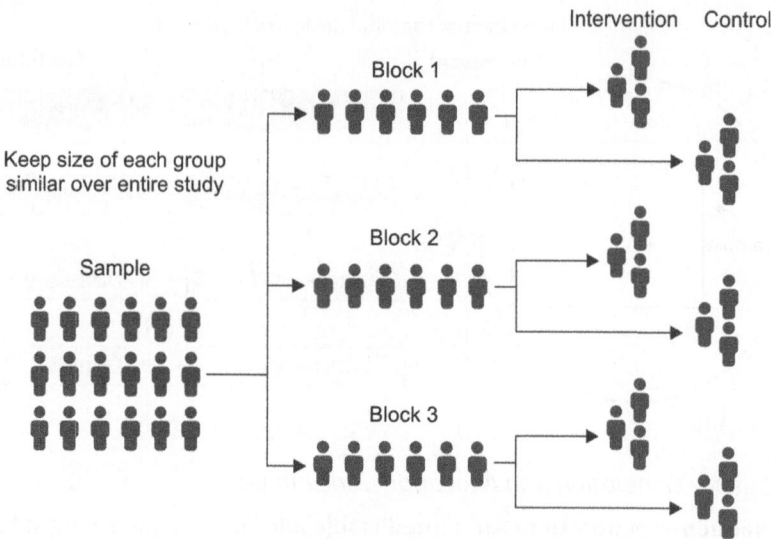

Fig. 2: Block randomization.

who will be preparing the medication) and not the investigators or personnel involved in ascertaining outcome.

Randomization Schemes

Randomization (Fig. 2)

It is used to maintain a balance between intervention group and control, so that the numbers are not too dissimilar, which could rarely happen by chance.

Group/Cluster Randomization

This type can be used when randomization of individual participants is not feasible/practical, in which case, hospitals, clinics, geographic areas, etc., can be used as units for the allocation of intervention.

For example, if an intervention seeks to change eating patterns by altering supermarket environments, since the treatment cannot be delivered to individuals separately, group randomization of communities utilizing those supermarkets would be appropriate for such a study.

Intervention

It is the deliberate application of the study drug/vaccine as laid down in the protocol.

The manipulation creates an independent variable (e.g., providing vaccine), whose effect is then determined by measurement of the final outcome, which constitutes the dependent variable (e.g., incidence of disease). Comparison of efficacy and effectiveness depict in **Fig. 3.**

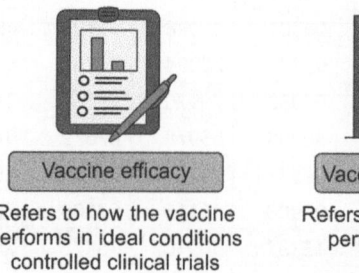
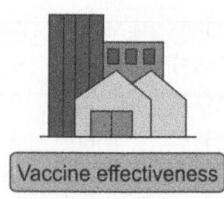

Vaccine efficacy — Refers to how the vaccine performs in ideal conditions controlled clinical trials

Vaccine effectiveness — Refers to how the vaccine performs in the wide populations

Fig 3: Comparison of efficacy and effectiveness.

Follow up

It comprises examination of the experimental and control groups at defined interval of time in a standard manner, with equal intensity, under the same circumstances, in the same time frame till final assessment of outcome. The duration of follow up depends upon the objectives laid under the protocol of the study and details about adverse drug events (ADEs). There may be some dropout because of various reasons such as migration, unwillingness to continue, etc., which is known as "attrition". If the attrition is substantial, it may be difficult to generalize the results of the study to the reference population. Therefore, every effort should be made to minimize the dropouts/attrition.

Outcome Assessment

The prespecified primary and secondary outcomes should be collected by independent observers who are unaware of the allocation and treatment arms of participants. As far as possible, it is advisable that objective measures are used for ascertaining outcome so that, bias on the part of the collector does not come into play. It is also important that the outcome is collected in all randomized patients. The number of patients with missing outcome data should be minimized as far as possible. A high rate of attrition will lead to reduced confidence in the results and may lead to biased estimates.

Interim Analysis

Randomized controlled trials are designed with an anticipated incidence of the primary outcome in the control arm. The observed incidence may be lower, making the trial underpowered or higher, making the trial unnecessarily prolonged. Interim analysis is a useful way to make sure that the observed incidence is not too different from the expected incidence. However, interim analyses should be preplanned and stated in the protocol. Analysis should be performed by an independent statistician blinded to the identity of either group. An independent data monitoring committee oversees the interim analysis.

Interim analysis may sometimes show that differences in the two groups are large and show a clear advantage of the intervention. In this case, continuing the trial is unethical because the control group will be denied the clearly superior alternative. On the other hand, early discontinuation may be advisable if the incidence of primary outcome in the control is far too low. When event rates are lower than anticipated or variability is larger than expected, methods for sample size re-estimation are available without unblinding.

Interpretation of RCTs

Interpretation of any trial should depend not only on the primary outcome, but on the totality of the evidence (i.e., primary, secondary, and safety outcomes). However, in most RCTs, if the difference in the primary outcome is significant at the customary level of $p < 0.05$, chances are that the observed difference is real.

The magnitude of the observed difference is also important. Instances where this magnitude may be small, but still statistically significant, the clinical significance is most often limited. When the magnitude is large, but statistically insignificant, the study remains underpowered. Appropriate sample size calculations before embarking on the study should prevent this situation. In many cases, the observed difference is small and is not statistically significant. When a trial is too small to detect modest treatment effects, it is appropriate to describe the findings as inconclusive rather than negative.

Bias and Confounding in Clinical Trials

Bias is systematic error which acts to make observed results nonrepresentative of true effects of an intervention. Biases in clinical trials can be broadly classified into:
- **Selection bias:** Study population does not reflect a representative sample of the target population.
- **Measurement/Information bias:** Improper, inadequate or ambiguous recording of individual factors—either exposure or outcome variables.

Confounding: Spurious association made between the outcome and a factor that is not itself causally related to the outcome and occurs if the factor is associated with a range of other characteristics that do increase the outcome risk.

Blinding (Masking)

The focus of conducting an RCT is elimination of bias. All these potential problems can be avoided if everyone involved in the study is blinded to the actual treatment the patient is receiving.

Blinding is intended to avoid bias caused by subjective judgment in reporting, evaluation, data processing and analysis due to knowledge of treatment.

The procedure of blinding the participants (***single blinding***) or both investigators and participants (***double blinding***) or including data analyzers (***triple blinding***) helps to eliminate this unconscious information bias.

It is not always possible to blind either the participants or investigators due to the nature of the RCT.

Advantages

- Scientifically ideal method.
- Gold standard for evaluating the efficacy of therapeutic, preventive and other risk interventions in both clinical medicine and public health.
- Assess new programs for screening and early detection or new ways of organizing and delivering health services.
- Confirming cause effect associations.
- Remove bias related to selection and measurement.
- Build up "faith" in the findings of the study.

Disadvantages

- Subjects are sometimes difficult to get or large numbers may be needed, e.g., Newer COVID 19 vaccine—difficult to get subjects who are yet to have received a covid vaccine.
- Ethical issues.
- High financial costs.
- Study of "risk factors" or "prognostic factors", one cannot randomly allocate human beings into two groups.
- A long period of time is often required to reach a conclusion.

Real life Examples

A clinical evaluation on **safety and immunogenicity** of purified chick embryo cell vaccine (**PCECV, Rabipur**) and purified vero cell rabies vaccine (**PVRV, Verorab**) administered as simulated postexposure prophylaxis using one week intradermal regimen (4-4-4-0-0) on healthy volunteers was conducted in Preventive Medicine Unit, Kempegowda Institute of Medical Sciences Hospital and Research Centre, Bangalore, depicts in Flowchart-5 below:

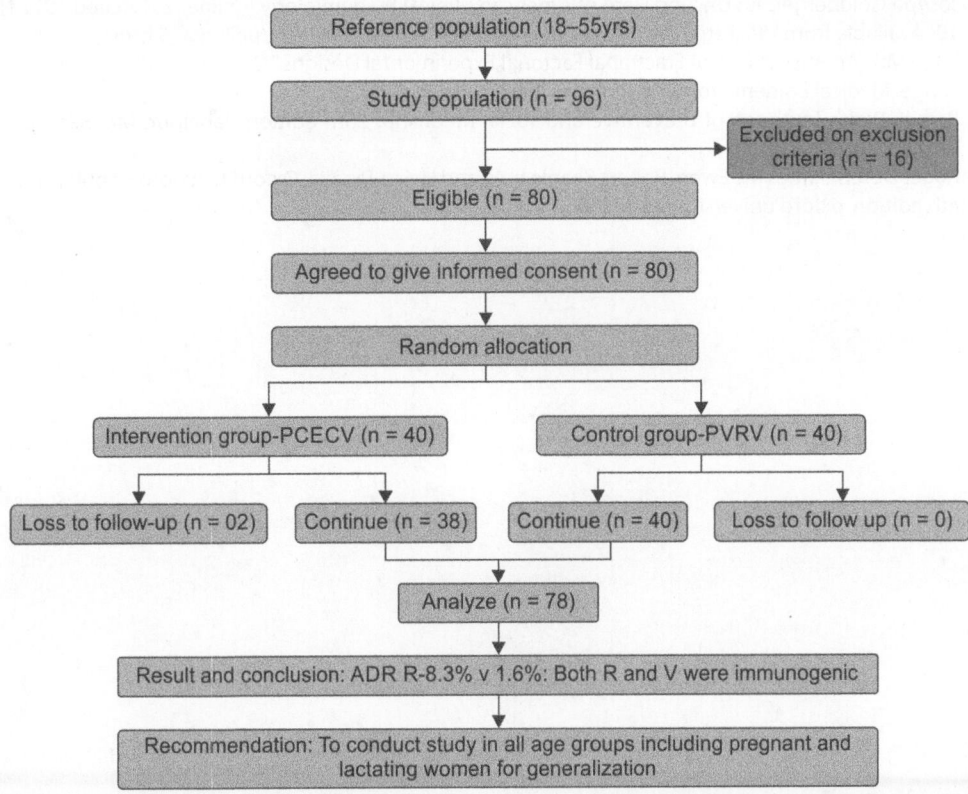

KEY POINTS

- Randomized controlled trials are prospective, comparative studies with controlled conditions and random allocation of interventions to different groups.
- Key steps include protocol preparation, selection of populations, randomization, intervention, follow-up, and assessment.
- Designs vary in a parallel group design, participants receive one intervention; in a crossover design, they receive multiple interventions sequentially.
- Techniques like allocation concealment and block randomization are used to ensure fairness and balance between groups.
- RCTs aim to minimize biases through blinding methods (single, double and triple) and mitigate selection and information biases.

BIBLIOGRAPHY

1. Ashwathnaryana DH et al. Comparative study to assess the safety and immunogenicity of PCECV and PVRV rabies vaccines administered intradermally using new one week regimen (4-4-4-0-0) in healthy volunteers. Available from: http://kimscommunitymedicine.org/sponsored-projects/.
2. Bonita R, Beagle hole R, Kjellstrom T. Basic epidemiology. 2nd edition. WHO; 2006.
3. Bowerman BL, O'Connell RT, Murphree ES. Regression Analysis: Unified Concepts, Practical Applications, and Computer Implementation. New York, NY: Business Expert Press; 2015.

4. David D.Celentano, Gordis. Epidemiology. 6th edition; 2018.
5. Hicks CR, Turner KV. Fundamental Concepts in the Design of Experiments. 5th edition. New York, NY: Oxford University Press.
6. Joseph Goldberger: An Unsung Hero of American Clinical Epidemiology [online].2012[cited 2012 Nov 10] Available from URL:http://history.nih.gov/exhibits/goldberger/docs/pellegra_5.htm
7. Kilgo MB. "An Application of Fractional Factorial Experimental Designs." Qual Eng. 1998;1:19-23.
8. Lange. Medical Epidemiology. 4th edition, 2005.
9. Park K. Park's Textbook of preventive and social medicine. 26th edition. Jabalpur: M/s Banarasidas Bhanot, Publishers; 2021.
10. Roger Detels, James Mc Ewen, Robert Beagle hole and Heizo Tanaka: Oxford text book of public health. 4th edition. oxford university press; 2006.

CHAPTER 15

Sample Size Estimation

Manjula R, Mitasha Singh, Manish Goel, Suhasini Kanyadi, Preety Tanwar, Aditi Mohta, Meely Panda

"Research means that you don't know, but are willing to find out."
—Charles F Kettering

INTRODUCTION

The sample size is the number of patients or other experimental units included in a study, and determining the sample size required to answer the research question is one of the first steps in designing a study. Choosing the correct size of sample is not a matter of preference. It is a crucial element of the research process without which you may well be spending months trying to investigate a problem with a tool which is either completely useless or unethical, or over expensive in terms of time and other resources.

An adequate sample size helps ensure that the study will yield reliable information, regardless of whether the ultimate data suggests a clinically important difference between the treatments being studied or the study is intended to measure the accuracy of a diagnostic test or the incidence of a disease. Conducting a study with an inadequate sample size is not only futile, it is also unethical. Exposing patients to the risks inherent in a research is justifiable only if there is a realistic possibility that the results will benefit those subjects, future subjects or lead to substantial scientific progress.

The formulas presented here generate estimates of the necessary sample size(s) required based on statistical criteria. However, in many studies, the sample size is determined by financial or logistical constraints. It is important to consider both statistical and clinical significance when interpreting the results of a statistical analysis; similarly, it is important to weigh both statistical and logistical issues in determining the sample size for a study.

A major purpose of doing research is to infer or generalize research objectives from a sample to a larger population. The process of inference is accomplished by using statistical methods based on probability theory. A sample is a subset of the population selected, which is an unbiased representative of the larger population. Thus, the goal of sampling is to ensure that the sample group is a true representative of the population without errors. The term 'error' includes sampling and nonsampling errors. Sampling errors that are induced by sampling design, including selection bias and random sampling error. Nonsampling errors are induced by data collection and processing problems. These include issues related to measurement, processing and data collection errors.

Why Sample Size Calculations?

The sample size calculation is to determine the number of participants needed to detect a clinically relevant treatment effect. Prestudy calculation of the required sample size is to be done in majority of quantitative studies. Usually, the number of patients in a study is restricted because of ethical, cost and time considerations. However, if the sample size is too small, one may not be able to detect an important existing effect, whereas samples that are too large may waste time, resources and money. It is therefore important to optimize the sample size. Moreover, calculating the sample size at the design stage of the study is a prerequisite when seeking ethical committee approval for a research project.

Approaches to Sample Size Calculation

There are two major classical approaches to sample size calculations in the design of quantitative studies:
1. Precision of estimation of an unknown characteristic/parameter of a population
2. Hypothesis testing of treatment effects/population parameters

Precision of Estimation: Precision Analysis

In studies concerned with estimating some parameter of a population (e.g., the prevalence of a health problem in the population), sample size calculations are important to ensure that estimates are obtained with required precision/accuracy or level of confidence. Here smaller the margin of error in the estimation, the more informative or precise the estimate. For example, a prevalence of 10% from a sample of size 20 would have a 95% confidence interval (CI) of (1%, 31%), which may not be considered very precise or informative. However, a prevalence of 10% from a sample of size 400 would have a 95% CI of (7%,13%), which may be considered more accurate or informative.

Hypothesis Testing of Treatment Effects/Population Parameters

In studies concerned with detecting an effect (e.g., a difference between two treatments, or relative risk of a diagnosis if a certain risk factor is present versus absent), sample size calculations are important to ensure that if an effect deemed to be clinically meaningful exists, then there is a high chance of it being detected, i.e., that the analysis will be statistically significant. If the sample is too small, then even if large differences are observed, it will be impossible to show that these are due to anything more than sampling variation. There are different types of hypothesis testing problems depending on the goal of the research.

The smallest difference or clinically important difference worth detecting is to be considered for calculation. Does this reflect the degree of benefit from the intervention against the control in a specified time frame? It is stated as the smallest clinically important difference? The difference that investigators think is worth detecting? The difference that investigators think is likely to be detected.

This needs to be supported by statistical methods.
1. **Test for equality:** Here the goal is to detect a clinically meaningful difference/effects when such a difference/effects exists.
2. **Test for noninferiority:** To demonstrate that the new drug is as less effective as the standard treatment (i.e., the difference between the new treatment and the standard is less than the smallest clinically meaningful difference).
3. **Test for superiority:** To demonstrate that the new treatment is more superior that standard treatment (i.e., the difference between the new treatment and the standard is greater than the smallest clinically meaningful difference).
4. **Test for equivalence:** To demonstrate the difference between the new treatment and standard treatment has no clinical importance.

Statistical Considerations for Sample Size Estimation

Null and Alternative Hypothesis

Many statistical analyses involve the comparison of two treatments, procedures or subgroups of subjects. The numerical value summarizing the difference of interest is called the *effect*. The null hypothesis $H0$ states that there is no effect and the alternative hypothesis states that there is an effect.

P-value of a Test

The p-value is the probability of obtaining the effect as extreme or more extreme than what is observed in the study if the null hypothesis of no effect is actually true. It is usually expressed as a p (e.g., p=0.05).

Type I error and Type II Error (Fig. 1)

In the process of hypothesis-testing, two fundamental errors can occur. These errors are called type I and type II errors. Each cell in the figure represents a possible relationship between the findings of the study and the 'real-life' situation in the population under investigation. Cells 1–4 represent desirable outcomes, while cells 2–3 represent potential outcomes of a study which are undesirable and need to be minimized. Type I error (α): Probability of rejecting null hypothesis when it is true, it should be no more than 5%. Type II error (β): Probability of failing to reject null hypothesis, when it is false. It is always kept below 20%. 1-Type II error is considered as Power of study.

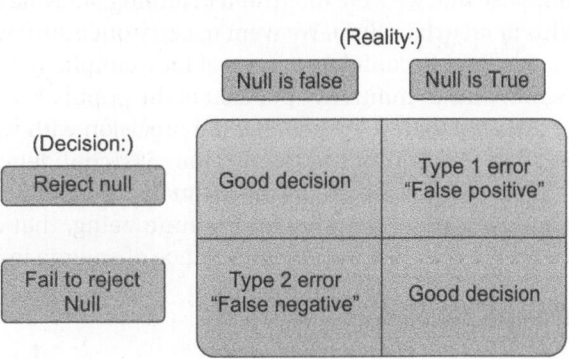

Fig. 1: Type 1 and Type 2 Errors.

Significance Level of a Test

Also called the Type 1 error probability, the significance level is a cut-off point for the p-value, below which the null hypothesis will be rejected and it will be concluded that there is evidence of an effect. The conventional significance level is $p = 0.05$ or 5%.

An important factor affecting the power of a study is the ***Effect Size (ES)*** which is under investigation in the study. This is a measure of "how wrong the null hypothesis is". For example, we might compare the efficacy of two bronchodilators for treating an asthma attack. The ES is the difference in efficacy between the two drugs. An effect size may be a difference between groups or the strength of an association between variables such as ill-health and deprivation. If an ES is small, then many studies with small sample sizes are likely to be underpowered. But if an ES is large, then a relatively small-scale study could have sufficient power to identify the effect under investigation. It is sometimes possible to increase the effect size (for example, by making more extreme comparisons or undertaking a longer or more powerful intervention). Usually this is the intractable element in the equation and accurate estimation of the effect size is essential for calculating power before a study begins to calculate the necessary sample size.

In designing studies, most people consider power of 80% or 90% (similar to our default use of 95% as the confidence level for confidence interval estimates). The inputs for the sample size formulas include the desired power, the level of significance and the effect size. The effect size is selected to represent a clinically meaningful or practically important difference in the parameter of interest.

Power of a Test

Power is the probability that the null hypothesis will be correctly rejected, i.e., when there is indeed a real difference or association, the test will detect a difference or association of a particular magnitude when it exists. The higher the power, the lower the chance of missing a real effect. Power is typically set to be at least 80%.

Examples

Example 1: Sample size to estimate a proportion/percentage

Suppose that we were interested in finding out what is the prevalence of anemia in adolescents girls in an urban slum. We want to carry out a survey, but of how many adolescent girls?

Acceptable confidence interval for example that our survey finding would reveal would lie within plus or minus five per cent of the population figure.

Assume that we decide that the precision with which we decide the prevalence of Anemia in adolescents must be plus or minus 5% (confidence interval).

In order to estimate P (the estimated percentage) we should consult previous studies or conduct a pilot. Assume, for the time being, that a similar study carried out 1.5 years ago indicated that 50% was the prevalence of anemia in adolescents.

Using the formula $N = \dfrac{4pq}{l^2}$

So, in order to be 95% confident that the true prevalence of anemia in adolescent girls within ± 5% of the answer, we will require a sample size of 400. This assumes that the prevalence would be around 50% with a range between 45% and 55%.

Example 2: Estimation of population mean

Consider an example of estimation of mean systolic blood pressure (SBP) in adults.

The sample size required to estimate the Mean SBP levels in them with the margin of error of 2 gm%. Standard deviation (σ) is known from the previous studies, which is 20.

Using formula $N = \dfrac{4\sigma^2}{l^2}$

So, in order to be 95% confident, we require sample size of 400. With allowable margin of error of 2%.

Example 3: Comparing two proportions

A placebo-controlled randomized trial proposes to assess the effectiveness of colony stimulating factors (CESS) in reducing sepsis in premature babies. A previous study has shown the underlying rate of sepsis to be about 50% in such infants around 2 weeks after birth and a reduction of this rate to 34% would be of clinical importance.

Required information:
- Primary outcome variable = presence/absence of sepsis at 14 days after treatment
- Treatment is for a maximum of 72 hours after birth.
- Hence, a categorical variable summarized by proportions.
- Size of difference of clinical importance = 16%, or 0.16 (i.e., 50%–34%)

- Significance level = 5%
- Power = 80%
- Where Zα= standard table value for 95% CI =1.96
- Z1-β = Standard table value for 80% power = 0.84
- Type of test = two-sided

The formula for the sample size for comparison of 2 proportions (two-sided) is as follows:

$$\text{Using formula } N = \frac{2(Z_\alpha + Z_\beta)^2 \, \overline{p}(1 - \overline{p})}{\Delta^2}$$

The sample size estimated is 154. This gives the number required in each of the trial's two groups. Therefore, the total sample size is double this, i.e., 308.

Example 4: Comparing two means

A randomized controlled trial has been planned to evaluate a brief psychological intervention in comparison to usual treatment in the reduction of suicidal ideation amongst patients presenting at hospital with deliberate self-poisoning. Suicidal ideation will be measured on the Beck scale; the standard deviation of this scale in a previous study was 7.7 and a difference of 5 points is considered to be of clinical importance. It is anticipated that around one third of patients may drop out of treatment

Required information:
- Primary outcome variable = The beck scale for suicidal ideation.
- A continuous variable summarized by means.
- Standard deviation = 7.7 points
- Size of difference of clinical importance = 5 points
- Significance level = 5%
- Power = 80%
- Where Zα = standard table value for 95% CI =1.96
- Z1-β = standard table value for 80% Power = 0.84
- Type of test = two-sided

The formula for the sample size for comparison of 2 means (2-sided) is as follows:

$$\text{Using formula: } N = \frac{2(Z_\alpha + Z_\beta)^2 \, \sigma^2}{\Delta^2}$$

Sample size estimated is 38. This gives the number required in each of the trial's two groups. Therefore, the total sample size is double this, i.e., 76.

Once the research question and study design are known, the following **Table 1** can be used for choosing relevant variables for calculation of sample size.

Reporting Sample Size Calculations

Sample size reporting should have the following information.
- Clear statement of the primary objective.
- The desired level of significance.
- The desired power
- The statistics that will be used for analysis.
- Whether the test would be one or two-tailed
- The smallest difference
  - Smallest clinically important difference
  - The difference that investigators think is worth detecting
  - The difference that the investigators think is likely to be detected

Table 1: Choosing relevant variables for calculation of sample size.

Type of study design		Type outcome variable	Outcome measure (assumed)	Level of significance	Precision	Specific to study design
Descriptive	Cross-sectional	Continuous	Mean and SD	Alpha	-	Relative error
		Discrete	Proportions			
Inferential	Cross-sectional	Continuous	Difference in mean and pooled SD		Beta	Relative error
		Discrete	Difference in proportions			
	Case-control	Discrete	Odds ratio			Case: Control and exposure in either
	Cohort	Discrete	Risk ratio			Gr1: Gr 2 exposure in either
	Experimental	Continuous	Difference in mean and pooled SD			Gr1: Gr 2 exposure in either
		Discrete	Difference in proportions			

❖ Justification for prior estimates used in calculations.
❖ Clear statements about the assumptions made about the distribution (Normal) or variability of the outcomes.
❖ Statement about how the sample size was adjusted.
❖ The software or formulae that were used for calculation.

Software for Sample Size Calculation

For ready reference, many sample size calculators are available on the internet. They need input of some variables and can calculate minimum sample size for different scenarios or study designs. CDC Atlanta freely provides open Epi calculator or Epi info version 7 (StatCalc section for calculation of sample size). Statulator.com also provides a sample size calculator.

Key points to remember while using software:
❖ Check whether it is the total sample size or the sample size in each group.
❖ Try software or formula against an answer you know.
❖ Use two different programs.
❖ Allow for nonresponse/loss to follow up.
❖ Play around with your calculations.

Key Points to Remember When Deciding on Sample Size

❖ We strongly recommend that researchers obtain independent advice on sample size when designing their study—and this will usually be from either a trained statistician or from a

researcher in your field who has longstanding experience of study design. This is because sample size estimation is such a crucial aspect of the design of a quantitative study, with important ethical as well as cost implications—and often very little can be done to 'salvage' the results from an insufficiently large sample.
* There is a tradeoff between committing a Type I error (false positive) and a Type II error (false negative), but historically, science has placed the emphasis on avoiding Type I errors.
* Other things being equal, increasing the sample size increases the sensitivity of the study to detect a difference between the groups being compared—and enables both alpha and beta to be set at lower levels thus reducing both Type I and Type II errors Remember that it is costly and unethical to have too large a sample size.
* To calculate statistical power, you need to estimate the effect size.
* To estimate the sample size for a descriptive study in order to estimate a mean or a proportion, it is necessary to specify the maximum acceptable margin for random error.

Real Life Examples

1. Ministry of Health and Family Welfare decided to provide vitamin supplements to school children (7-14 years) to reduce malnutrition. The malnutrition among school children was estimated to be 45%. This campaign is expected to lower the prevalence of malnutrition to 30%. Calculate the sample size needed to evaluate efficacy of campaign.

   Given: $P_0 = 0.45, P_1 = 0.30$

   Assuming: Power = 80%, $\alpha = 5\%$, $Z_{1-\beta} = 0.84$, $Z_{1-\alpha} = 1.64$

   Keeping ratio of children without malnutrition to number of children with malnutrition (r)=2 using Kelsey equation:

   $$P = \frac{(P_0 + rP_1)}{(r+1)} = \frac{[0.45 + (2*0.30)]}{(2+1)} = \frac{0.105}{3} = 0.35$$

   $$N = \frac{(r+1)}{r} \cdot \frac{(Z_{1-\alpha} + Z_{1-\beta})^2 P(1-P)}{r(P_0 - P_1)^2}$$

   $$= \frac{3*(1.64+0.84)^2(0.35*0.65)}{2*(0.45-0.30)^2} = \frac{4.198}{0.045} = 93.3 \text{ (round off to 94)}$$

   children with malnutrition = 94, children without malnutrition = 188

2. What sample size would be needed in each of the two groups for a case-control study to be 95% confident of estimating the population odds ratio to within 25% of the true value which is believed to be in the vicinity of 2.0 and the exposure rate among control is estimated to be 0.30.

   Given: $\alpha = 5\%$, relative precision (ϵ) = 0.25, OR = 2.0, $P_2 = 0.3$

   $$P_1 = \frac{OR * P_2}{[P_2(OR-1)+1]} = \frac{2*0.3}{[0.3(2-1)+1]} = 0.46$$

   $$N = \frac{Z_{1-\alpha/2}^2 [\{(1-P_1)/P_1\} + \{(1-P_2)/P_2\}]}{[\ln(1-\epsilon)]^2}$$

   $$N = \frac{(1.96)^2 [\{(1-0.46)/0.46\} + \{(1-0.3)/0.3\}]}{[\ln(1-0.25)]^2}$$

   = 423 in cases and 423 controls

3. A case-control study is planned to investigate whether bottle fed infants are at increased risk of death from ARI compared to breast fed infants. The mothers of a group of cases (infant deaths with an underlying respiratory cause named on death certificate) will be interviewed about the breast-feeding status of the child prior to the illness leading to death. The results will be compared with those obtained from mothers of a group of healthy controls regarding the current breast-feeding status of their infants. It is expected that about 40% of controls will be bottle fed and we would like to detect a difference if bottle feeding was associated with a two-fold increase of death (OR = 2). How many cases and controls need to be studied to give a 90% power of achieving 5% significance?

Given: $P_2 = 0.40$, OR = 2, $Z_{1-\beta} = 1.28$, $Z_{1-\alpha/2} = 1.96$ (for two-tailed test)
Assuming cases: control = 1:1, r = 1

$$P_1 = \frac{OR * P_2}{[P_2(OR-1)+1]} = \frac{2*0.4}{[0.4(2-1)+1]} = \frac{0.8}{1.4} = 0.57$$

$$P = (P_1+P_2)/2 = (0.40+0.57)/2 = 0.485$$

$$N = \frac{[Z_{1-\alpha/2}\sqrt{\{2P(1-P)\}} + Z_{1-\beta}\sqrt{\{P_1(1-P_1)+P_2(1-P_2)\}}]^2}{(P_1-P_2)^2}$$

$$= \frac{[1.96\sqrt{(2*0.485*0.515)} + 1.28\sqrt{\{(0.57*0.43)+(0.4*0.6)\}}]^2}{(0.57-0.4)^2}$$

$$= (1.385+0.891)^2/(0.17)^2 = 179.3 \sim 180 \text{ cases and 180 controls}$$

4. Suppose an outcome is present in 20% of the unexposed group of the cohort study, how large a sample would be needed in each of the exposed and unexposed groups to estimate the RR within 10% of the true value, which is believed to be approximately 1.75, with 95% confidence?

Given: $P_2 = 0.20$, RR = 1.75, $\alpha = 5\%$, $\epsilon = 0.10$
Since RR = P_1/P_2, therefore $P_1 = RR * P_2 = 0.35$

$$N = \frac{Z_{1-\alpha/2}^2[\{(1-P_1)/P_1\}+\{(1-P_2)/P_2\}]}{[\ln(1-\epsilon)]^2}$$

$$N = \frac{(1.96)^2[\{(1-0.35)/0.35\}+\{(1-0.20)/0.20\}]}{[\ln(1-0.10)]^2}$$

$$= 2026.95 \sim 2027 \text{ in each group}$$

5. An investigator is planning a clinical trial to evaluate the efficacy of a new drug designed to reduce systolic blood pressure. The plan is to enroll participants and to randomly assign them to receive either the new drug or a placebo. Systolic blood pressures will be measured in each participant after 12 weeks on the assigned treatment. Based on prior experience with similar trials, the investigator expects that 10% of all participants will be lost to follow up or will drop out of the study. If the new drug shows a 5 unit reduction in mean systolic blood pressure, this would represent a clinically meaningful reduction. How many patients should be enrolled in the trial to ensure that the power of the test is 80% to detect this difference?

A two-sided test will be used with a 5% level of significance. Analysis of data from the Framingham Heart Study showed that the standard deviation of systolic blood pressure was 19.0. This value can be used to plan the trial.

$$ES = \frac{|\mu_1-\mu_2|}{\sigma} = \frac{5}{19.0} = 0.26$$

$$N = \frac{2[Z_{1-\alpha/2} + Z_{1-\beta}]^2}{(ES)^2} = \frac{2*(1.96 + 0.84)^2}{(0.26)^2} = 231.95 \sim 232 \text{ per group}$$

To account for 10% attrition rate (in both groups), number to enroll will be
N_{enroll} = (desired sample size)/(proportion retained) = 232/0.90 = 258

6. It was observed that disease cure rate with drug A is 75% while that with drug B is 85%. How large should the sample size be in each group if the researcher desires to detect with a power of 90%, whether there is a difference in cure rates of the two drugs at 5% level of significance?

$P_1 = 0.75, P_2 = 0.85, \alpha = 0.05, Z_{(1-\alpha/2)} = 1.96$ (two-sided), $Z_{(1-\beta)} = 1.28$
$P_1 - P_2 = -0.10, P = (P_1 + P_2)/2 = 0.80$

$$N = \frac{[Z_{1-\alpha/2}\sqrt{\{2P(1-P)\}} + Z_{1-\beta}\sqrt{\{P_1(1-P_1) + P_2(1-P_2)\}}]^2}{(P_1 - P_2)^2}$$

$= (1.11 + 0.718)^2/0.01$

$N = 334.1 \sim 335$ per group

KEY POINTS

- The sample size is the number of cases or other experimental units included in a study and determining the sample size needed to answer the research question is one of the first ways in designing a study.
- The sample size computation is used to determine the number of agents needed to describe a clinically applicable treatment effect.
- Lower the periphery of error in the estimation, the further instructional or precise the estimate.
- The lowest difference or clinically significant difference worth detecting is to be considered for computation.
- Statistical considerations for sample size estimation: null and alternative hypothesis.
- P- value of a test, Type I error and Type II error, significance position of a test and power of a test.

BIBLIOGRAPHY

1. Altman DG. Practical statistics for medical Research. London, UK: Chapman and Hall; 1991.
2. Altman DG. Statistics and ethics in medical research: III How large a sample? Br. Med.J 1980;281:1336-8.
3. Baoliaong Z. Practical Bioststistics. How to Calculate sample size in Randomized controlled trial? J Thorac Dis. 2009;1(1):51-4.
4. Borenstein M, Rothstein H, Cohen J. Power and Precision, version 2: A computer program for statistical power analysis and confidence intervals. Englewood: Biostat Inc. 2001:287.
5. Day S, Graham D. Sample size estimation for comparing two or more treatment groups in clinical trials. Stat Med. 1991;10:33-43.
6. Freiman JA, Chalmers TC, Smith HJ, Kuebler RR. The importance of beta, the type II error and sample size in the design and interpretation of the randomized control trial survey of 71 "negative trials". N England J Med. 1978;299:690-4.
7. Lachin JM. Introduction to sample size determination and power analysis for clinical trials. Control Clin Trials. 1981;2:93-113.
8. Lemeshow S, Levy PS. Sampling of populations: Methods and Applications, 3rd edition. New York, US: John Wiley and Sons Inc; 1999.
9. Lui KJ. Sample size determination in case control studies. J clin Epidemiol 1991;44:609-12.
10. Lwanga SK, Lameshow S. Sample size determination in Health studies. A Practical Manual. World Health Organization. Geneva 1991.
11. Moussa MA. Exact, conditional and predictive power in planning clinical trials. Control Clin Trials, 1989;10:378-85
12. Noorszij M, Giovanni T, Friedo WD, Carmine Z, Michael W, Kitty JJ. Sample size calculations: Basic principles and common pitfalls. Nephrol Dial Transplant 2010:1-6.

Sampling Methods and Errors

CHAPTER 16

*Rivu Basu, Mitasha Singh, Raghavendra Huchchannavar, Ameenah H Siraja,
Aditi Mohta, Bhushan Kamble, Manjula R*

> *"By a small sample, we may judge of the whole piece."*
> —*Miguel de Cervantes*

INTRODUCTION

Whenever you're trying to look at the biochemical parameters of a particular case, what do you do? Do you take the whole quantum of blood and analyze it for glucose? No, it isn't possible. So, we take a sample. Whenever we take a sample, it is inferred that there will be some problems, some hypotheticals, some balances that need to be there. Like whenever we take a venous sample for blood sugar, it is inferred that the sugar levels will be lower than a arterial sample. Also, in the peripheral part the sugar levels shall be different from the central organs. But for the sake of feasibility, we have to accept these. We shall mention that for all practical purposes, this sample shall be taken as a measure of the entire universe, i.e., the whole body of the person. Therefore, we assume that the sample is representative of the whole body and this whole body we mention as a population.

Thus, a population in the context of statistics refers to the set of particulars—these can be people, events, homes, institutions, or commodity differently—that are the subject of research, about which a researcher would like to answer a given question. The sample is the set of data collected from the population of interest or target population, from sampling frame.

The main aim of sampling is to compare a larger population on characteristics applicable to the exploration question, to be representative so that researchers can make inferences about the larger population. However, when doing a quantitative study, the researchers should take care to draw a sample in such a way that it is representative of that population and any outcomes obtained from these studies, should be able to generalize in the normal population.

Basic Concepts in Sampling

Population

It is the entire group under study as defined by research objectives, also called the "universe." Researchers define populations in specific terms such as heads of households, individual person types, families, etc.

Sampling Frame

It is a master list of the population that helps in identifying each sampling unit by a number. Such a list or map is called sampling frame, e.g., a list of voters, a list of householders, a list of villages in a district, a list of farmers, etc.

Sample Unit or Sampling Unit

It is the basic level of investigation, the constituents of the population. They are individuals or households that are sampled from the population and cannot be further subdivided for the purpose of sampling. The research objective should define a sample unit.

Basis of Sampling

Reasons for Selecting a Sample

- Complete enumeration is practically *impossible* when the population is infinite
- When the results are required in a *short time*
- When the area of survey is *wide*
- When *resources* for survey are limited particularly in respect of money and trained persons

Principles of Sampling

- Principle of statistical regularity/Principle of inertia of large numbers
- Principle of validity
- Principle of optimization

The foremost purpose of sampling is to gather maximum information about the population under consideration at minimum cost, time and human power. This is best achieved when the sample contains all the properties of the population—representative sample.

Advantages of Sampling

Therefore, using a proper sampling technique, we will be able to make the research study:
- More economical,
- Enhance the data quality,
- Decrease the time of data collection,
- Improve the precision and accuracy of data,

A 'Representative sample' **(Fig. 1)** has all the important characteristics of the population from which it's drawn. A good sample should be 'representative, free from bias, complete and have applicable size'.

When using qualitative research approaches, however, the representativeness of the sample is NOT a primary concern. In exploratory studies which aim at getting a rough print of how certain variables manifest themselves in a study population or at relating and exploring therefore far unknown variables, you may try to select those study units which give you the richest possible information.

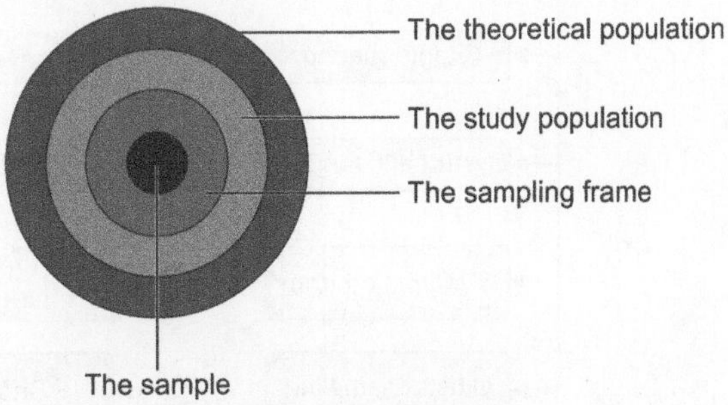

Fig. 1: Representative sample.

Sampling Methods

For better understanding the sampling can be divided into the following three types (**Flowchart 1**):
1. Nonprobability Sampling designs
2. Probability Sampling designs
3. Mixed Sampling designs

Probability Sampling

Simple Random Sampling

The probability of being selected is "equal" for all members of the population. A simple random sample from a finite population is a sample selected such that each possible sample combination has equal probability of being chosen. It is also called unrestricted random sampling. Simple random sampling (SRS) may be with or without replacement and is considered the gold standard.

It may be done using:
* Blind Draw Method (e.g., "lottery method")
* Random Numbers Method (all items in the sampling frame given numbers, numbers then drawn using table or computer program)
* Computer Aided-Simple random sample by excel.

Some example of random number series are Tippett's series comprising 41,600 numbers, Fisher and Yates' series comprising 15,000 digits, Kendall and Smith's series comprising 100,000 digits.

Example of using random number table method (**Fig. 2**):

Advantages of SRS

* Known and equal chance of selection
* Easy method when there is an electronic database

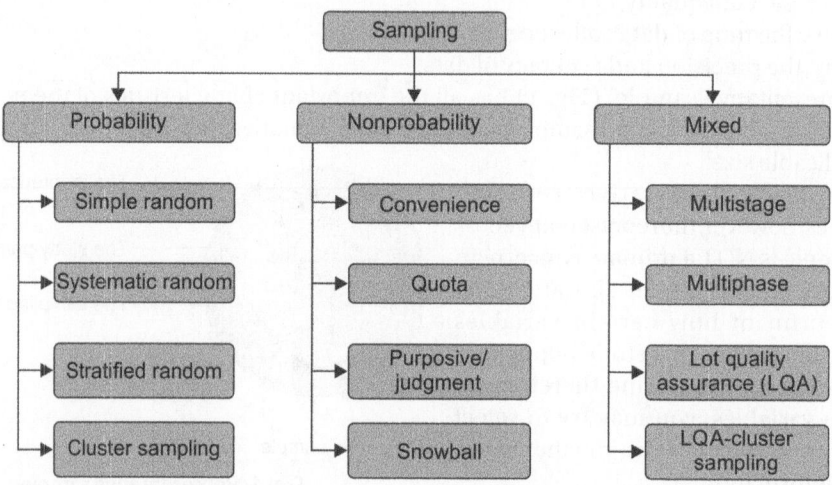

Flowchart 1: Broad classification of sampling procedures.

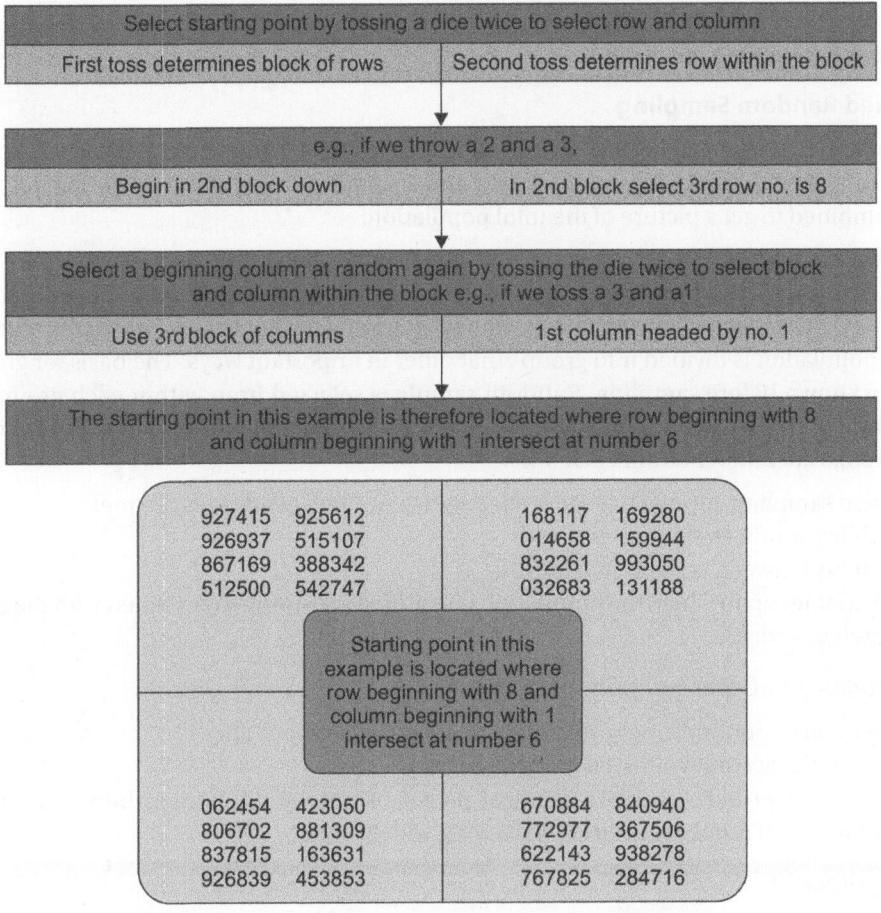

Fig. 2(Top and bottom): Using random number table.

Disadvantages of SRS

- Complete accounting of population needed
- Cumbersome to provide unique designations to every population member

Systematic Random Sampling

This method is widely employed because of its ease and convenience. A frequently used method of sampling when a complete list of the population is not available is systematic sampling. The whole sample selection is based on a random start. The first unit is selected with the help of random numbers and the rest get selected automatically according to a predesigned pattern.

Sampling interval (SI) = Population size (N)/Sample size (n)

Advantages

- Known and equal chance of any of the SI "clusters" being selected
- Efficiency does not need to designate (assign a number to) every population member, just those early on the list (unless there is a very large sampling frame).
- Less expensive and faster than SRS

Disadvantages

Small loss in sampling precision

Stratified Random Sampling

This method is used when the population is not homogenous. The given population is separated into homogeneous groups/segments/strata and a sample is taken from each. The results are then combined to get a picture of the total population.

There are two methods:
- Proportional method (stratum share of total sample is stratum share of total population)
- Disproportionate method (variances among strata affect sample size for each stratum)

The population is divided into groups that differ in important ways. The basis for grouping must be known before sampling. Random sample is selected from within each group. For a given sample size, this sampling method reduces error compared to simple random sampling if the groups are different from each other.

A stratified sampling approach is most effective when three conditions are met:
1. Variability within strata is minimized
2. Variability between strata is maximized
3. The variables upon which the population is stratified are strongly correlated with the desired dependent variable.

Advantages Over Other Sampling Methods

1. Focuses on important subpopulations and ignores irrelevant ones.
2. Improves the accuracy/efficiency of estimation.
3. Permits greater balancing of statistical power of tests of differences between strata by sampling equal numbers from strata varying widely in size.

Disadvantages

1. Requires selection of relevant stratification variables which can be difficult.
2. Is not useful when there are no homogeneous subgroups.
3. Can be expensive to implement.

Cluster Sampling

If done correctly, this is a form of random sampling. Population is divided into groups with similar characteristics (Clusters). Some of the groups are randomly chosen. In pure cluster sampling, the whole cluster is sampled. In simple multistage clusters, there is random sampling within each randomly chosen cluster. For a given sample size, a cluster sample is prone to higher error than a simple random sample. Cost savings of clustering may permit larger samples. Error is smaller if the clusters are like each other.

Nonprobability Sampling

Qualitative research methods are typically used when focusing on a limited number of informants, whom we select strategically so that their in-depth information will give optimal insight into an issue about which little is known. This is called purposeful sampling. There are several possible strategies that a researcher can choose. Most frequently different strategies are combined, depending on the content under study and the type of information required by the researcher.

Convenience Sampling

Sample is selected from units that are conveniently available or those population groups in which it is easy to conduct surveys or investigations are chosen irrespective of representativeness of population, e.g., person interviewed at random in a shopping center for a television program, students in class, people on state street, friends. Biases are maximum in this sampling method and the results obtained are unsatisfactory in terms of drawing conclusions. If there is little variation in the population, the possible bias problems are less important. It is generally used for making pilot studies to have just a basic idea about the study variables. Convenience sampling is a method of sampling wherein the study units are selected based on convenience. This may happen at the beginning of a study when researchers are merely orienting themselves, or when there are many similar informants and the researchers do not (yet) prefer specific categories. When there seems no other choice (no one else available for an interview) researchers may also sample conveniently.

Quota Sampling

Quota sampling is a nonprobability sampling method that relies on the nonrandom selection of a predetermined number or proportion of units. This is called a quota. You first divide the population into mutually exclusive subgroups (called strata) and then recruit sample units until you reach your quota. These units share specific characteristics, determined by you prior to forming your strata. The aim of quota sampling is to control what or who makes up your sample. Your design may:
❖ Replicate the true composition of the population of interest
❖ Include equal numbers of different types of respondents
❖ Over-sample a particular type of respondent, even if population proportions differ

Purposive Sampling

It is also known as judgmental sampling. In this process whereby the researcher selects a sample based on experience or knowledge of the group to be sampling. The researcher chooses units because of certain characteristics and usually used when working with very small samples. Purposive Sampling refers to a group of nonprobability slice ways in which units are named because they've characteristics that you need in your sample. In other words, units are named "on purpose" in purposive sampling. Sometimes it is also called as Judgmental sampling, as the sampling method relies mostly on the researcher's judgment when relating and opting the individualities, cases or events that can give the best possible information in order to achieve the objectives of the study. Purposive sampling is the most commonly used sampling technique for qualitative research and mixed methods research. It is particularly useful if you need to find information-rich cases or make the most out of limited resources, but is at high threat for exploration impulses like observer bias. The types of purposive sampling are as follows.

Extreme case sampling

Selection of extreme cases, like good or extreme poor compliers to treatment, is an important and best strategy to identify contributing factors to poor compliance. In the same way, selection of well-nourished children of the same age will help to identify contributing factors for malnutrition and methodical comparison of a inadequately and a very well-functioning district health team (DHT) will give insight into factors that may contribute to the satisfactory functioning of DHTs. Also "thick"(elaborate) description of single, deviant cases may be useful.

Maximum variation sampling

If the researcher wants to gain insight as complete as possible in a particular issue in all its variations, this method is useful. Purposeful sampling shouldn't be erratic. Care should be taken that for different orders of informants, selection rules are developed to help the researcher in using personal choice of study participants.

Homogeneous Sampling

Occasionally the researcher would like to have specific information about one particular group only, for illustration, a group that, for unclear reasons, is more at threat than others. In focus group discussion (FGDs), we generally elect homogeneous groups because participants relate freely when they're amongst people of analogous social status.

Critical Case Sampling

Critical cases are those who can make the difference with respect to an intervention you want to introduce or to estimate.

P.S: *Purposeful sampling is NOT the same as convenience sampling.*

Snowball Sampling

It is used when the desired sample characteristic is rare, wherein it may be extremely difficult or cost prohibitive to locate respondents in these situations. Snowball sampling relies on referrals from initial subjects to generate additional subjects. While this technique can dramatically lower search costs, it comes at the expense of introducing bias because the technique itself reduces the likelihood that the sample will represent a good cross-section from the population. One or two cases are contacted in the population. The cases are asked to identify further cases. The new cases further identify new cases. The snowballing is stopped when either no new cases are given or the sample is as large as is manageable.

Mixed Sampling Methods

Multistage Sampling (Fig. 3)

It is applied where an extensive area is required to be studied within limited resources. To bring down the cost involvement, size of the sample is reduced progressively in stages by drawing a series of sub-samples till a conveniently small yet representative sample is obtained which can be studied within limited resources. For, e.g., Multistage sampling for estimating prevalence of ascariasis in preschool children in district of northern India is given in the figure below. Their prevalence shall reflect prevalence of ascariasis in all districts of north India.

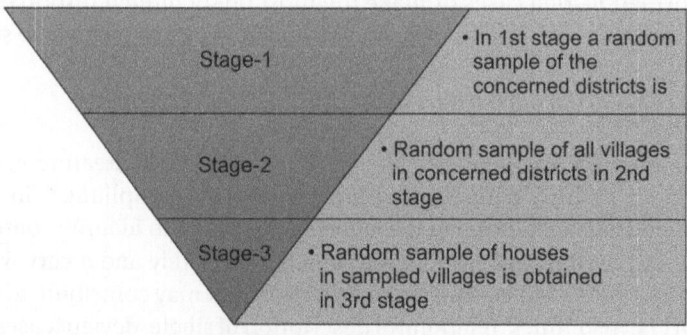

Fig. 3: Multistage sampling.

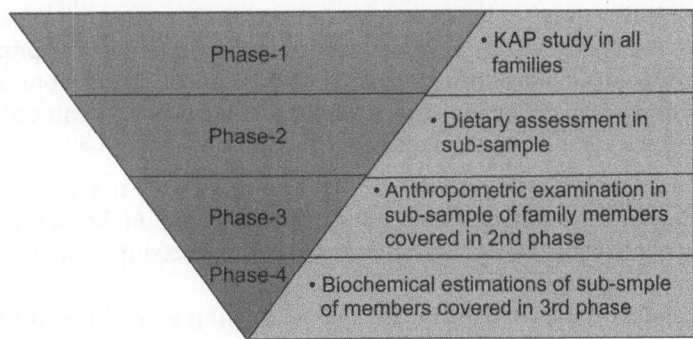

Fig. 4: Multiphase sampling.

Multiphase Sampling (Fig. 4)

Number of units get reduced in every succeeding phase, which also reduces magnitude of complicated procedures reserved for last phase. Study procedures are applied in phases of increasing complexity so that, the most complex and the most expensive procedures are reserved for the last phase or the smallest sample. Therefore, this sampling makes the studies less expensive, less time-consuming, less laborious and more purposeful. For example:

Lot Quality Assurance Sampling (LQAS)

These surveys are carried out in two or more sets or lots with same objective. Results obtained are compared. Lot giving unfavorable result is considered for interventions, e.g., maternal and neonatal tetanus elimination surveys.

Random Samples and Randomization

Random samples and randomization are two different concepts. Although both involve the use of the probability sampling method, random sampling determines who will be included in the sample. Randomization or random assignment, determines who will be in the treatment or control group. Random sampling is related to sampling and external validity (generalizability), whereas random assignment is related to design and internal validity.

In experimental research, failure to assign subjects randomly to groups is generally more serious than having a nonrandom sample. Failure to randomize (the former error) invalidates the experimental findings. A nonrandom sample (the latter error) simply restricts the generalizability of the results.

Biases in Sampling

There are several possible sources of bias that may arise when sampling. The most well-known source is nonresponse. Nonresponse can occur in any interview situation but it is mostly encountered in large-scale surveys with self-administered questionnaires. Respondents may refuse or forget to fill in the questionnaire. The problem lies in the fact that nonrespondents in a sample may exhibit characteristics that differ systematically from the characteristics of respondents.

There are several ways to deal with this problem and reduce the possibility of bias:
- Data collection tools (including written introductions for the interviewers to use with potential respondents) should be pretested. If necessary, adjustments should be made to ensure better co-operation.
- If nonresponse is due to absence of the subjects, follow-up of nonrespondents may be considered.

- If nonresponse is due to refusal to co-operate, an extra, separate study of nonrespondents may be considered in order to identify to what extent they differ from respondents.
- Another strategy is to include additional people in the sample, so that nonrespondents who were absent during data collection can be replaced. However, this can only be justified if their absence was very unlikely to be related to the topic being studied.

Studying volunteers only: The fact that volunteers are motivated to participate in the study may mean that they are also different from the study population on the factors being studied. Therefore, it is better to avoid using nonrandom selection procedures that introduce such an element of choice.

Sampling of registered patients only: Patients reporting to a clinic are likely to differ systematically from people seeking alternative treatments.

Missing cases of short duration. In studies of the prevalence of disease, cases of short duration are more likely to be missed. This may mean missing fatal cases, cases with short illness episodes and mild cases.

Seasonal bias: It may be that the problem under study, for example, malnutrition, exhibits different characteristics in different seasons of the year. For this reason, data should be collected on the prevalence and distribution of malnutrition in a community during all seasons rather than just at one point in time. When investigating health services performance, to take another example, one has to consider the fact that towards the end of the financial year shortages may occur in certain budget items which may affect the quality of services delivered.

Tarmac bias: Study areas are often selected because they are easily accessible by car. However, these areas are likely to be systematically different from more inaccessible areas.

KEY POINTS

- A good sample should be 'representative, free from bias, complete and have applicable size'.
- Sampling is a technique of selecting individual members or a subset of the population to make statistical inferences from them and estimate the characteristics of the whole population.
- Sampling methods are divided into nonprobability Sampling designs and probability sampling designs.
- Probability sampling is a more reliable way of selecting people for a study as it gives everyone in the group an equal and fair chance of getting selected.

BIBLIOGRAPHY

1. Altman DG, Machi D, Bryant TN, Gardner MJ. Statistics with Confidence, 2nd edition. BMJ Publishing.
2. Brett Jackson. Business Research Methods. Ed-Tech Press; 2019
3. Corlien MV, Pathmanathan I, Brownlee A. Designing and conducting health systems research projects. KIT Publishers International Development Research Centre and World Health Organization; 2003;1.
4. Fleetwood D. Sample: Definition, types, Formula and Examples [Internet]. 2023 [cited 2023 Jun 22]. Available from: https://www.questionpro.com/blog/sample/
5. Goyal RC. Research Methodology for health Professionals. Sampling Methods. Jaypee publishers; 2013.
6. Hauschke D, Steinijans V, Pigeo, I. Bioequivalence Studies in Drug Development. John Wiley and Sons. New York; 2007.
7. Nikolopoulou K. What Is Quota Sampling?|Definition and Examples, 2002. Scribbr. https://www.scribbr.com/methodology/quota-sampling/
8. Sampling [Internet]. National Institutes of Health; [cited 2023 Jun 22]. Available from: https://www.nlm.nih.gov/nichsr/stats_tutorial/section2/mod1_sampling.html
9. Sundaram KR, Dwivedi SN, Sreenivas V. Medical statistics: Principles and practice, 2nd edition. Wolters Kluwer (India) Pvt. Ltd. New Delhi; 2015.

Basic Statistics

CHAPTER 17

Rashmi Kundapur, Sumit Chawla, Archisman Mohapatra, Aditi Mohta,
Suhasini Kanyadi, Preety Tanwar, Manjula R, Bhushan Kamble

> *"If we knew what we were doing, it would not be called research, would it?"*
> —Albert Einstein

"The problem of statistical errors in the medical literature is long standing, wide-spread, potentially serious, relatively unknown, and not well addressed, despite the fact that most errors occur in the more common application of statistics."–Lang T

INTRODUCTION

Important terms in statistics
- **Datum/Data:** Collection of variables
- **Statistics**: Science of numbers
- **Descriptive statistics:** Collection, compilation, presentation, and summarization of data
- **Inferential statistics:** Drawing inferences from set of data
- **Biostatistics:** Use of statistical methods in health-related fields
- **Variable:** Logical grouping of characteristics derived from data, e.g., gender, temperature, religion, blood group, socioeconomic status, etc.
- **Characteristics:** Attribute of a variable, e.g., male/female are characteristics while gender is variable

Statistics is a mathematical science of collecting, organizing, presenting, analyzing, and interpreting numerical data to assist in making more effective decisions. Statistics implies both data and statistical methods. The word statistics is derived from the Latin word statista; a person dealing with the affairs of the state. Statistics would be one of the most used subjects, having its application in practically every field for instance, in functional fields such as physical and social sciences, humanities, business, industries and also in various academic fields.

Why Statistics?

Numerical information is everywhere. The data collected is of no use if some information regarding their characteristics cannot be derived or any actionable intelligence cannot be gained from them. Statistical techniques are thus used to help take action or to make decisions that affect our daily lives.

Statistics provides methods for
1. **Design:** Planning and carrying out research studies.
2. **Description:** Summarizing and exploring data.
3. **Inference:** Making projections and generalizing about events represented by the data.

Science is a measurement. Therefore, the "who, what, when, where, and why" of the measurements must be clearly stated and appropriate for the study. The most common error is assuming that we know how something was measured.

Population in the field of statistics is described as the summation of the individual values about which understandings are to be made. Note that a population can be a collection of any effects, like books, creatures or insensible thus it doesn't inescapably deal with people.

A sample is a subset of the population recruited for study. Sample drawn should be representative of the entire population so that consequences drawn from a sample relate to the defined population from which sample is drawn **(Fig. 1)**.

Description of population is in parameter and from this population we take the sample, the figures we get from sample is called data, statistics is applied to the data either descriptive or deducible and its results are inferred as parameter to the population **(Fig. 2)**.

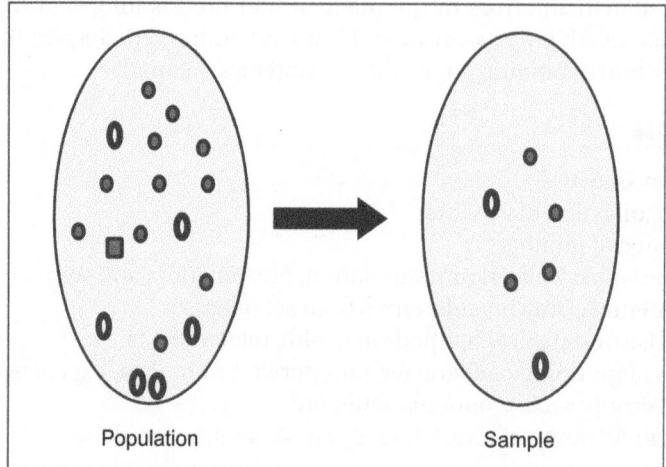

Fig. 1: Population and sample.

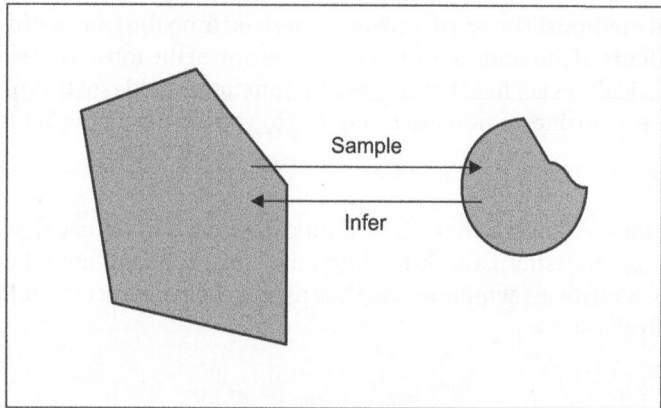

Fig. 2: Population vs. sample.

Example: Consider the exploration problem of finding out what is the chance of scholars going to library at least once a week.
Parameter: The proportion p of time 1 MBBS scholars going to library at least once a week.
Statistic: The proportion p̂ of scholars going to library at least once a week calculated from the sample time 1 MBBS scholars.

Statistical Analysis

It can generally be classified in two divisions as given below.

Descriptive Statistics

Summarization of a collection of data in a clear and accessible way. The measures used to describe the data set are measures of central tendency and measures of variability or dispersion.

Inferential Statistics

Draws conclusion from data taking into account arbitrary variation and probability. It generally requires the slice to be arbitrary.

Two main styles used in deducible statistics
1. **Estimation:** The sample statistic is used to estimate a population parameter and a confidence interval about the estimate is constructed.
2. **Hypothesis testing:** A null hypothesis is put forward. Analysis of the data is also used to determine whether to reject or accept the null hypothesis.

Variables and Its Different Types

There are two objectives when presenting data: convey your story and establish credibility.
- Edward Tufte
1. Data is obtained by observing the values of the variables for one or further people. Each individual piece of data is known as an observation and the collection of all compliances for particular variables is called a data set or data matrix.
2. Before starting any data analysis, it is important to know what type of variables you are working with. The types of variables tell **(Fig. 3)** you which estimates you can calculate and latterly, which types of statistical tests you should use.

Qualitative or Categorical Variables

They cannot be measured but can only be described. They can be counted as number of individuals having same characteristics/attributes. For example, gender is qualitative variable,

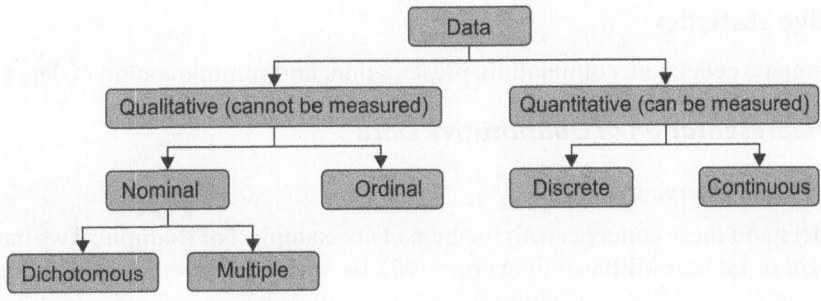

Fig. 3: Types of data or variables.

but its characteristics like male/female can be counted. Here, we would like to stress that qualitative data depends on the variable to be studied, not its characteristics.

Types of Qualitative Variables

Nominal

It is simple categorization in characteristics of a qualitative variable. It can be of two types:
- Dichotomous (binary), i.e., two categories, e.g., Gender (male/female) and test positive/negative
- Multiple, i.e., more than two categories, e.g., blood group (A/B/AB/O)

Ordinal

There is an implied order/rank in characteristics of a qualitative variable. For example, pain scale: attributes are ranked from 1 to 10; socioeconomic status: its attributes are in order like lower, middle, upper middle and upper.

Quantitative Variables

These variables can be measured, and are represented by a number or quantity.

Types of Quantitative Variables

Discrete

Variable with perfect values and no fractions, e.g., platelet count, heart rate, etc.

Continuous

Variable with all values in range or with fractions, e.g., height (1.1 m), weight (95.5 kg), etc.

Quantitative data can be converted to qualitative data (categorical variables) for simplicity of analysis and interpretation, but not vice versa. For example, individuals may be classified into various age groups depending on their age, adolescents (10–19); adults (>18); geriatric (>60).

Quantitative data can also be measured in terms of interval and ratio scales.
- **Interval scale:** An interval scale has an order, data is measurable (unlike ordinal qualitative variable) and the difference between two values is meaningful. There is no clear definition of zero, e.g., temperature (fahrenheit), temperature (celsius), pH. The difference between pH 1 and 2 is equal to difference between pH 2 and 3.
- **Ratio scale:** A ratio variable has all the properties of an interval variable and also has a clear definition of zero. Here, both the ratio and interval between two measurements are meaningful, e.g., weight of 4 grams is twice as heavy as a weight of 2 grams. However, a temperature of 10° C should not be considered twice as hot as 5°C.

Descriptive Statistics

They encompass collection, compilation, presentation, and summarization of data **(Table 1)**.

Tabular Representation of Quantitative Data

Range and Class Intervals

Let us understand these concepts with the help of an example. For example, if we have details of the weight of 1st year MBBS students (n = 100), we divide the data into suitable groups by

Table 1: Methods of presentation of data.	
Qualitative data	**Quantitative data**
Tabular	*Tabular*
One way table Two way table K way table/high order table	Frequency distribution Cumulative frequency distribution
Graphical	*Graphical discrete*
Bar diagram Pie chart Pictogram	Bar diagram Histogram Polygon Box and whisker Stem and leaf plot
	Graphical continuous
	Histogram Frequency polygon Cumulative frequency polygon (ogive) Stem and leaf plot
Others: Line diagram, funnel plot, forest plot	

weight (hypothetical), of 60–70, 70–80, 80–90, 90–100, 100–110 and 110–120. These groups are called class intervals (CI), and the width/interval of each CI is 10.

Range = highest value–lowest value = 120–60 = 60
K = number of class intervals= 1+ (3.322 x log n) = 7.6
Width = range/K = 60/7.6 = approximately 8
But the researcher may assume another K, such as K = 6 in this example.
Here we have 6 CI, i.e., 60–70, 70–80, 80–90, 90–100, 100–110, 110–120.
Width = 60/6 = 10.

Class intervals can be of two types:
- **Inclusive type:** Can be used only for discrete variables. Lower and upper limit of CI are included in data, e.g., (60–69, 70–79, 80–89, 90–99, 100–109, 110–119).
- **Exclusive type:** Can be used for both discrete and continuous variables. Either lower limit or upper limit is excluded from each of the class interval, e.g., (60–70, 70–80, 80–90, 90–100, 100–110, 110–120).

Frequency Distribution Table (Discrete Data)
Example: Table 2.

Table 2: Frequency distribution table.		
Socioeconomic status	*Total (n)*	*Frequency*
Lower	5	⌊⌊⌊⌊⌊
Lower middle	10	⌊⌊⌊⌊⌊ ⌊⌊⌊⌊⌊
Upper middle	20	⌊⌊⌊⌊⌊ ⌊⌊⌊⌊⌊ ⌊⌊⌊⌊⌊ ⌊⌊⌊⌊⌊
Upper	15	⌊⌊⌊⌊⌊ ⌊⌊⌊⌊⌊ ⌊⌊⌊⌊⌊
Total	50	

Table 3: K way table.

Status of hypertension	Hypertensive		Nonhypertensive		Total(N)
Gender	Males (n)	Females (n)	Males (n)	Females (n)	
Socioeconomic status					
Lower	4	6	4	6	20
Lower middle	6	14	6	14	40
Upper middle	29	11	29	11	80
Upper	20	10	20	10	60
Total	59	41	59	41	200

Tabular Representation of Qualitative Data

One way table: One characteristic to be studied
Two way table: Two characteristics to be studied
K way table/high order tables (Table 3): More than two characteristics to be studied, e.g., K way table depicting socioeconomic status, gender, and status of hypertension.

Graphical Representation of Data

Bar Diagram (Figs. 4 and 5)

Types: Simple, Multiple, Component bar diagram

Pie Diagram (Fig. 6)

A circle is used for the presentation of qualitative data, and area enclosed by it is 100%. Area of each sector varies with the corresponding frequency or percentage. Since full angle at the

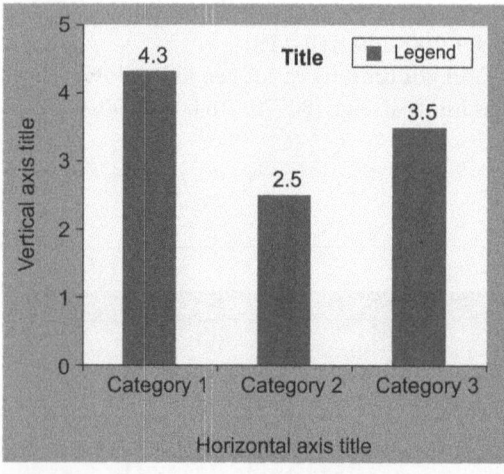
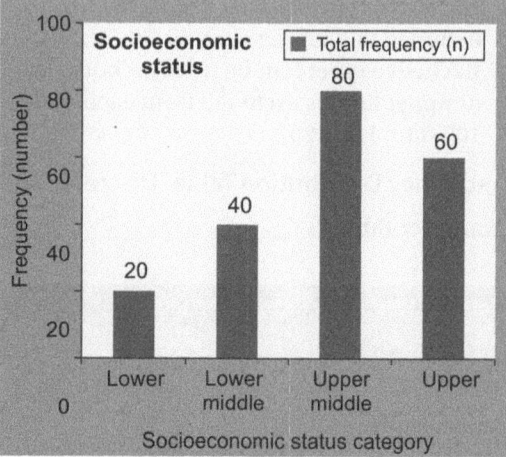

Fig. 4: Elements of a *simple bar diagram* (vertical or horizontal orientation) are title, legend, horizontal axis title (X axis), vertical axis title (Y axis), data labels, defining categories. The width of the bars is kept constant for all the categories and the space between the bars also remains constant throughout.

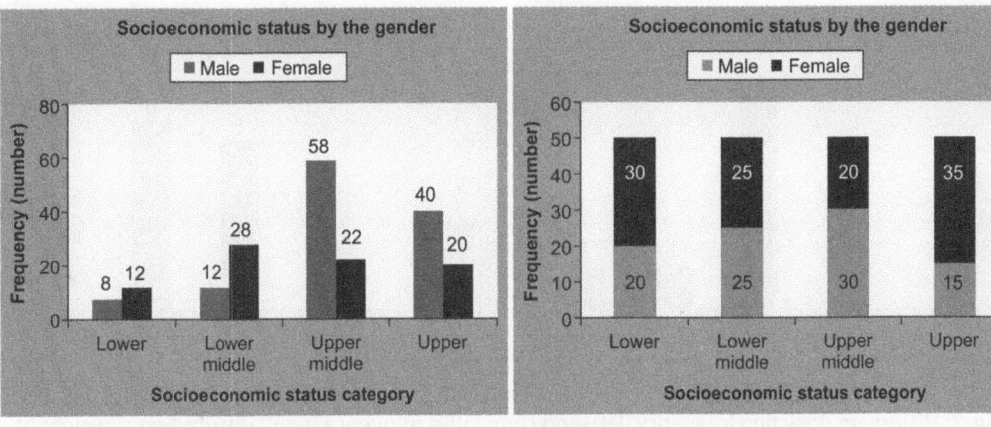

Fig. 5: *Multiple bar diagram* (left) and *Component bar diagram* (right). The latter is chosen when the total of all bars is the same (50 in this example).

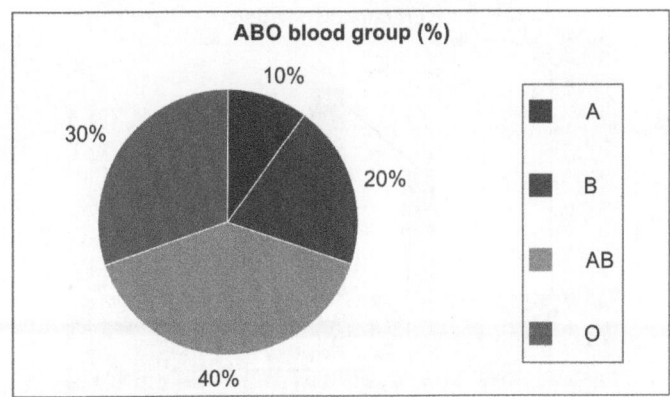

Fig. 6: Pie diagram representing distribution of blood group in a population sample

center is 360 degrees, it is clear that for any particular category the angle should be 3.6 times corresponding frequency or percentage.
- Angle of a sector = (frequency/total) × 360 degree
- It is better represented when categories are less than six.

Histogram (Table 4 and Fig. 7)
Example:

Table 4: Frequency distribution of weight of students.	
Class interval (excluding lower limit)	*Frequency*
60–70	3
70–80	5
80–90	1
90–100	1

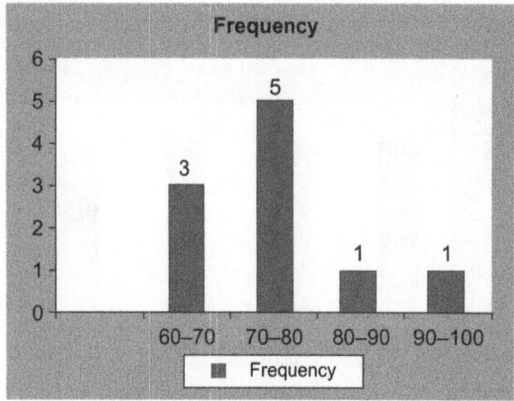 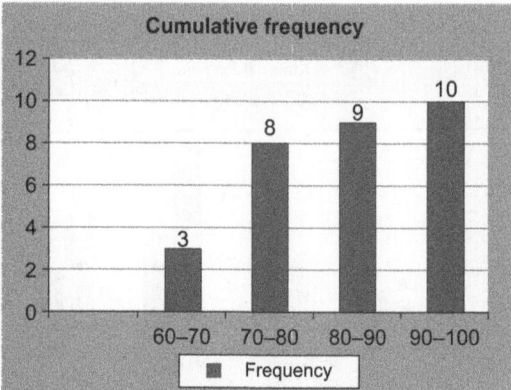

Fig. 7: Histogram depicting frequency (left) and cumulative frequency (right) distribution of weight of students.

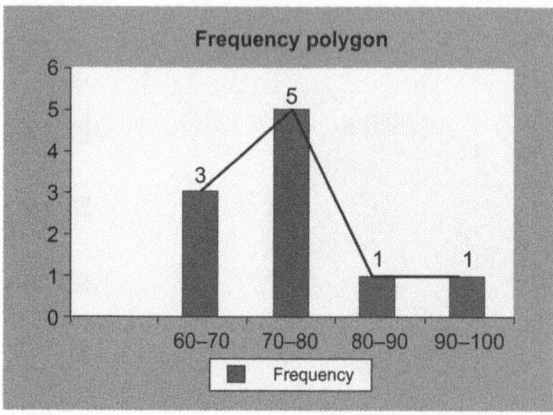

Fig. 8: Frequency polygon.

Polygon (Fig. 8)

It can be superimposed on the histogram by connecting the midpoints of the tops of each of the rectangles by straight lines.

Pictogram (Fig. 9 and Table 5)

Suitable symbol is chosen to represent certain number of units of variable. Then, each value in the given series of data is represented either by taking similar symbol, its size being proportional to the value or by taking number of symbols of same size. For example, for data given in the table below, a pictogram is made on the right.

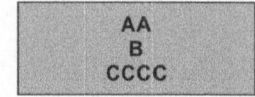

Fig. 9: Pictogram depicting frequency of different symbols.

Table 5: Frequency of different symbols.

Frequency	Symbol	Units of
20	A	2
10	B	1
40	C	4

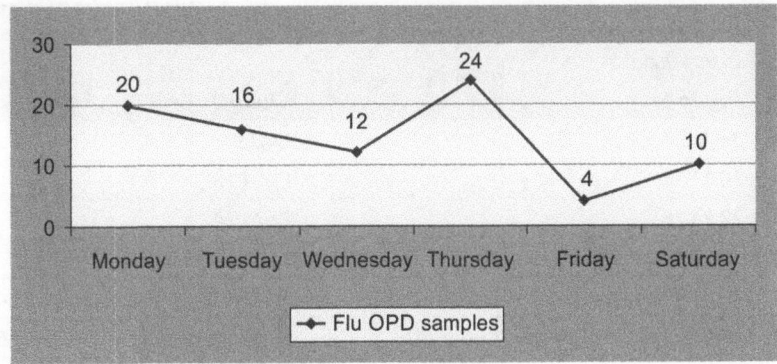

Fig. 10: Line diagram.

Line Diagram (Fig. 10)

It is used to depict time trends.

Box and Whisker Plot

It is used to represent discrete type of quantitative data. To understand the plot, let us understand the concept of quantiles, first.

Quantiles divide the total data into equal parts after arranging the data in ascending order of magnitude. Quartile divides the total data into 4 equal parts. Let Q_1, Q_2 and Q_3 denote first, second and third quartiles respectively. If $X_1, X_2, \ldots X_n$ are n observations arranged in ascending order of magnitude then quartiles are:

- ❖ $Q_1 = X_{(n+1)/4}$ indicates that 25% of observations are less than or equal to Q_1.
- ❖ $Q_2 = X_{2(n+1)/4}$ indicates that 50% of observations are less than or equal to Q_2 or median.
- ❖ $Q_3 = X_{3(n+1)/4}$ indicates that 75% of observations are less than or equal to Q_3.

In a box and whisker plot (given below **Fig. 11**), the box represents the interquartile range (Q_3-Q_1). In case of skewed data, the median will not lie in the center of the box, but towards one end of the box. The whiskers are made from Q_1 and Q_3 to the minimum and maximum values of the dataset, which are the most distant points lying within or at the fences, *but not beyond them*. The upper fence lies 1.5 times IQR towards the upper quartile. The lower fence lies 1.5 times IQR towards the lower quartile. Beyond the fences (not visible in the plot), the data points are considered *outliers*.

Stem and Leaf Plot

It is used to represent discrete and continuous type of quantitative data. It can be used to compare the distribution of two or more distributions by studying their shapes. For example, **Table 6 and Figure 12.**

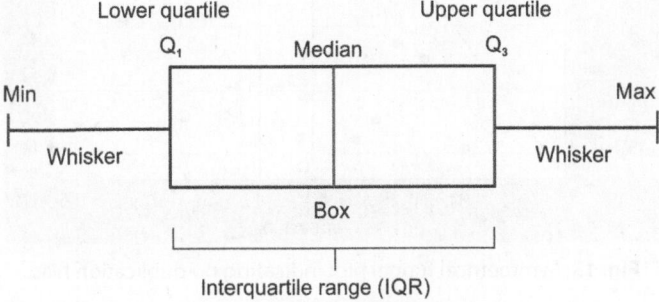

Fig. 11: Box and whisker plot.

Section 2: Quantitative Research Methodology

Table 6: Distribution of age of individuals in two groups (discrete data).

	Discrete data	
CI	Group 1	Group 2
0–10	3,4,5,6,7	2,4,7,9
10–20	10,11,12	13,14,15
20–30	22,24,26	22,23,24
30–40	30,32,32,33,34,35,36,36,37,38,39	30,31,31,32,38,39
40–50	40,41,44,44,45,45,45,46,47,48,49	40,42,43,44,44,44,45,46,46,48,48,49,49
50–60	50,50,51,53,55,55,59	50,50,51,53,54,54,56,56,57,57,59

Leaf (group 2)	Stem	Leaf (group 1)
9742	0	34567
543	1	012
432	2	246
982110	3	02234566789
9988665444320	4	01445556789
97766443100	5	0013559

Fig. 12: Stem and leaf plot for age distribution of individuals in two groups.

Funnel Plot (Fig. 13)

Funnel plot is used to check for publication bias, which arises when larger studies with statistically significant results are more likely to be published and cited and are preferentially published in English language journals and those indexed in Medline. In funnel plot, the effect estimates of intervention from different studies are plotted on X axis, against a measure of study size or precision on Y axis. Thus, smaller trials will be plotted more widely at the bottom of the

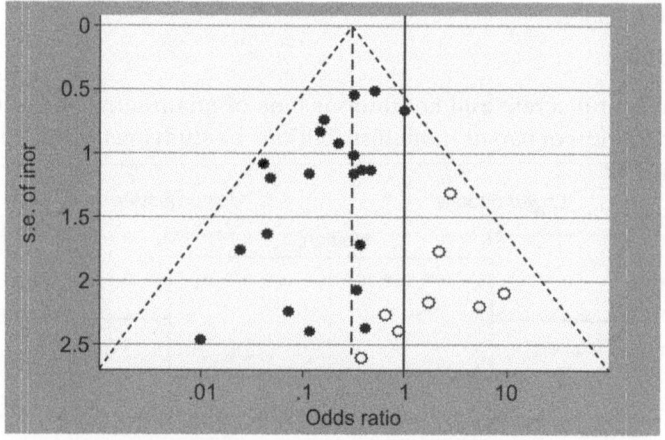

Fig. 13: Symmetrical funnel plot indicating no publication bias.
(*Source*: Higgins et al., 2011).

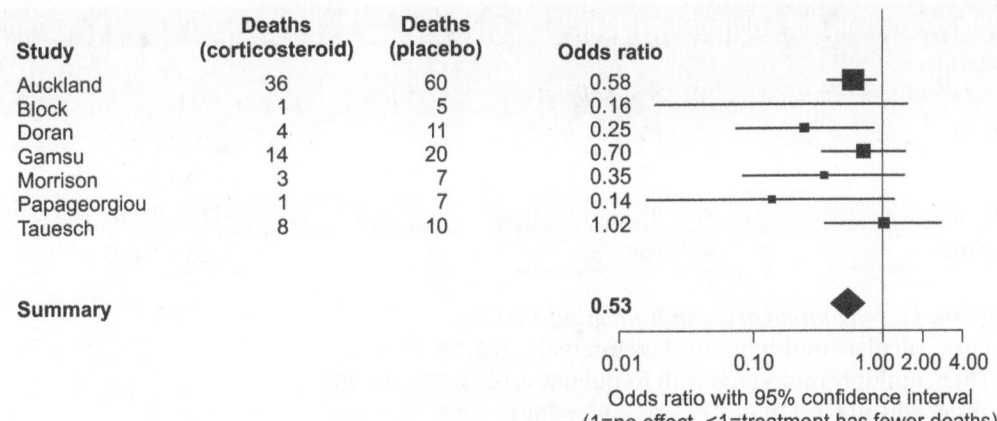

Fig. 14: Forest plot.
(*Source:* Roberts et al., 2017)

graph. If there is no publication bias, the shape of the plot resembles a symmetrical inverted funnel. If smaller studies with statistically insignificant results are not published, there will be a gap in one of the bottom corners of the funnel plot and it will be asymmetrical. The summary effect is, thus, overestimated in such meta-analysis.

Forest Plot (Blobbogram) (Fig. 14)

It is a graphical display of estimated results from a number of scientific studies addressing the same question, along with the overall results.

Measures of Statistical Averages and Variation

Summary measures provide description of data in terms of concentration of data and variability existing in data. They help in drawing certain conclusions about the reference population from which the sample data has been drawn. We will discuss two kinds of summary measures: measures of central tendency and measures of variability.

Measures of Statistical Averages or Central Tendency or Location

These are used to give idea about the center point of quantitative data and distributions. There are three measures of central tendency: mean, median and mode.

Mean/Arithmetic Mean

It is most appropriate measure for normally distributed data. It is calculated by summation of values of all observations and then dividing it by total number of observations.

$$\bar{x} = \frac{\sum x}{n}$$

It is less suitable for skewed distributions. It is influenced by extreme values/outliers and hence gives a poor 'typical' value in such samples. It depends on all values of the data set, but is affected by the fluctuations of sampling.

Example: If the age (in years) of 2nd year MBBS students practical batch are as follows: 21,19,20,21,23, 21,20,19,22, 20,

Mean =21+19+20+21+23+21+20+19+22+20= 206/10 = 20.6 years

This value describes the entire data in one value **(Table 7)**.

Table 7: Distribution of weight of individuals.

Class interval (excluding lower limit)	Mid-point of CI (x)	Frequency (y)	x*y
60–70	65	3	65 × 3 = 195
70–80	75	5	75 × 5 = 375
80–90	85	1	85 × 1 = 85
90–100	95	1	95 × 1 = 95

Example for calculation of mean from grouped data:
- First, calculate mid-point of class interval x. (65, 75, 85, 95)
- Then, multiply midpoints with frequency y. (195, 375, 85, 95)
- Then, add all x*y. (195 + 375 + 85 + 95 = 750)
- Then, divide the above sum by the totally (750/10 = 75)
- Hence, mean of the above grouped data is 75.

Geometric Mean (GM)

If $x_1, x_2, \ldots, x_n$ are n observations, then GM $(x) = (x_1 x_2 \ldots x_n)^{1/n}$. It is less affected by extreme values, but cannot be used when observation is either negative or zero. For example,
Geometric mean of $(12, 14, 18) = (12 \times 14 \times 18)^{1/3} = 14.46$

Harmonic Mean

If $x_1, x_2, \ldots, x_n$ are n observations, then harmonic mean (HM) is defined as reciprocal of mean of reciprocals. It cannot be used when observation is either negative or zero. It gives less weightage to largest observation and more to lowest observation. It is less affected by fluctuation in sampling.

$$H(x_1, x_2, \ldots x_n) = \frac{n}{\frac{1}{x_1} + \frac{1}{x_2} + \ldots \frac{1}{x_n}} = \frac{n}{\sum_{i=1}^{n} \frac{1}{x_i}}$$

Example: If the age (in years) of 2nd year MBBS students practical batch are: 21,19,20,21,23, 21,20,19,22, 20, the harmonic mean = 10/0.488= 20.5.

Median

When the data is skewed, median is used. Median is a locative measure which is the middle observation after all the values are arranged in ascending or descending order. In other words, median is that value which divides the entire data set into two equal parts, when the data set is ordered in an ascending (or descending) fashion. When there are odd n number of observations, we have a single middle value [(n+1)/2] which is the median value. When there are even n number of observations, there are two middle values and the median is calculated by taking the mean of these two middle observations $1/2[(n/2$ observation + $(n/2 +1)$ observation]. For example, the following are the pulse rate per minute of 10 healthy individuals:
82,79,60,76, 63,81,68,74,60,75.
  To calculate the median, first arrange the given data in ascending order of magnitude:
60,60,63,68,**74,75**,76,79,81,82
Here n =10
Hence median = (74+75)/2= 74.5

  Median can be calculated even if values of extremes are not known, if n is known. It can be used for qualitative data, which cannot be measured quantitatively but can be arranged in ascending or descending order of magnitude. If lowest and highest observations are wide apart, then median is a better measure of central tendency than mean. It is likely to be affected by the fluctuation of the sampling than mean.

Mode

Mode is the most common value that repeats itself in the data set. Though mode is easy to calculate, at times it may be impossible to calculate mode if we do not have any value repeating itself in the data set. It may also happen that we come across two or more values repeating themselves same number of times, indicating bimodal or multimodal distribution. For example, the following are blood pressure readings of 11 hypertensive patients aged 50 y. 184,170,16 8,188,162,164,174,172,178,166,188. The observation 188 has occurred twice while all other observations have occurred only once. Hence, mode = 188.

Mode is not based on all the observations. It is likely to be affected by the fluctuation of the sampling than mean and median. Mode is generally not used, since it is not amenable to statistical analysis.

Measures of Variability or Dispersion or Scatteredness or Spread

We measure variability in order to gather information concerning the relative position of other data points in the sample, e.g., **Table 8**.

Various measures of dispersion are as follows:
- Range (already discussed under 'Descriptive statistics')
- Interquartile range (already discussed under 'box and whisker plot')
- Mean deviation
- Variance
- Standard deviation
- Coefficient of variation.

Range

One of the simplest measures of variability is range. Range is the difference between the two extremes, i.e., the difference between the maximum and minimum observation (already discussed under 'Descriptive statistics'). One of the drawbacks of range is that it uses only extreme observations and ignores the rest. This variability measure is easy to calculate but it is affected by the fluctuations of sampling. It gives rough idea of the dispersion of the data.
For example, sample of weight (in kg) of 10 MBBS students: 72, 80, 70, 65, 55, 63, 80, 50, 55, 74
Range = 80–50 = 30 kg

Table 8: Comparison of marks obtained by three students in three subjects.

Students	Marks obtained		
	Subject 1	Subject 2	Subject 3
Student 1	100	101	150
Student 2	100	100	100
Student 3	100	99	50
Mean	100	100	100
Variation	Nil	+	+++
Range	0	2	100

Mean Deviation

It is the average of absolute deviations from the mean.

Mean deviation = $[\Sigma |x - \mu|]/n$

It is based on all the observations. It is a better measure of dispersion than range. However, it ignores the plus/minus signs of the deviations.

Variance

It is the sum of squared deviations divided by the sample size. It may be remembered as MSD: mean square deviation.

Steps to calculate variance:
1. Calculate mean of the observations (mean)
2. Find out the difference between each observation and the mean (absolute deviation)
3. Square the differences (square of absolute deviations)
4. Sum of the squared deviations
5. Divide by sample size n or (n -1) (adjustment for the fact that the mean is just an estimate of the true population mean).

Standard Deviation (SD or σ)

It is the square root of variance or root mean square deviation (RMSD).

$$SD = \sqrt{\frac{\Sigma |x - \bar{x}|^2}{n}}$$

The denominator of SD is n for population and (n-1) for a sample.

Standard deviation of zero, indicates that all the observations are identical. *Example:* Number of lab tests performed under different departments of a medical college in a day have been given in the table below. Calculate mean, mean deviation, variance and standard deviation **(Table 9)**.

Coefficient of Variation

It is used to compare the variability in two or more series of data, which differ in their averages or have different units of measurement. It measures the variation/spread of the data relative to the size of the mean. It is independent of unit of measurement. If the coefficient of variation is greater for one data set it suggests that the data set is more variable than the other data set.
- CV = (SD/Mean) * 100
- Let us take an example **(Tables 10 and 11)**.

Table 9: Number of lab tests performed under different departments of a medical college in a day.

Department	Lab tests performed (LT)	Deviation from mean	Absolute deviation	Square deviation
Physiology	10	10−9 = 1	1	$1^2 = 1$
Micro	8	8−9 = −1	1	$−1^2 = 1$
Biochem	6	6−9 = −3	3	$−3^2 = 9$
Pathology	12	12−9 = 3	3	$3^2 = 9$
Community medicine	9	9−9 = 0	0	$0^2 = 0$
Total	45	0	8	20
Mean = 45/5 = 9 (LT) Variance = (20/(5-1)) = 20/4 = 5 (LT)			Mean deviation = 8/5=1.6 (LT) Standard deviation = $\sqrt{5}$ = 2.2	

Table 10: Distribution of blood sugar values of 10 prediabetic patients estimated using three different techniques.

S. No.	Technique 1	Technique 2	Technique 3
1	132	138	132
2	131	128	131
3	133	133	133
4	134	134	132
5	132	137	132
6	133	136	134
7	132	122	132
8	133	126	131
9	132	129	132
10	128	137	131

Table 11: Summary measures of blood sugar estimates of 10 prediabetic patients done using three different techniques.

	Technique 1	Technique 2	Technique 3
Mean	132 mg/dL	132 mg/dL	132 mg/dL
SD	1.63 mg/dL	5.46 mg/dL	0.94 mg/dL
CV	1.24	4.13	0.71

In above example, mean is the measure of central tendency, standard deviation indicates precision and coefficient of variance allows us to compare the variability of entire dataset.

Normal Distribution or Gaussian Distribution

If we draw a smooth curve passing through the mid points of the bars of histogram or frequency polygon (when a large number of observations of any characteristic are considered at a time), and if the curve is bell-shaped, then the data is said to be roughly following normal distribution.

Characteristics of a Normal Distribution Curve (Fig. 15)

- It is a bell-shaped symmetrical curve.
- Mean, mode, and median coincide (= 0).
- The curve on either side of the mean is mirror image of the other side.
- Area under the curve is 1.
- Area enclosed between mean and multiple of SD is constant.
  - Mean ± 1 SD ------- Encloses 68.3% of the total area.
  - Mean ± 2 SD ------- Encloses 95.4% of the total area.
  - Mean ± 3 SD ------- Encloses 99.7% of the total area.

A normal curve is determined entirely by the mean and the standard deviation. It is possible to have various normal curves with different standard deviations but same mean and various normal curves with different means but same standard deviation.

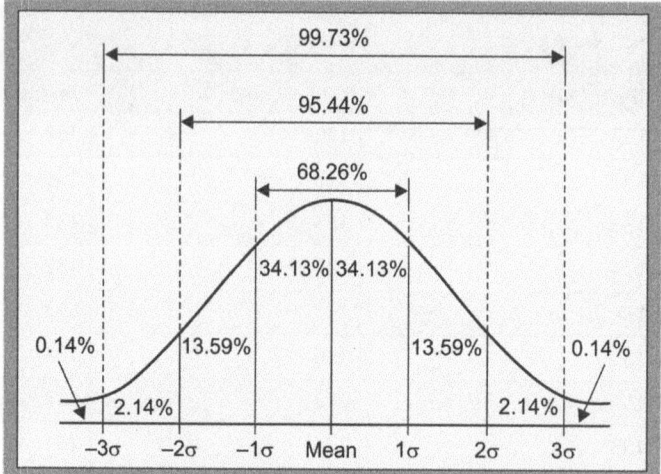

Fig. 15: Area under a normal distribution curve.

Central Limit Theorem

Different samples would give different estimates of a population mean, due to sampling variation. According to the central limit theorem, this sampling distribution of the sample means approximates a normal distribution as the sample sizes get larger, even if the population's actual distribution is non normal.

Standardizing a Normal Distribution: Standard Normal Variate (Z)

On standardization of a normal distribution, the mean becomes zero and the standard deviation becomes one. This allows for easy calculation of the probability of certain values occurring in the distribution or to compare data sets with different means and standard deviations. While data points are referred to as in a normal distribution, they are called z or z-scores in the z-distribution.

$$z = \frac{x - \mu}{\sigma}$$

A z-score is a standard score that tells us how many standard deviations away from the mean an individual value (x) lies.
- A positive z-score means that x-value is greater than the mean.
- A negative z-score means that x-value is less than the mean.
- A z-score of zero means that x-value is equal to the mean.

Converting a normal distribution into the standard normal distribution allows us to:
- Compare scores on different distributions with different means and standard deviations.
- Normalize scores for statistical decision-making (e.g., grading on a curve).
- Find the probability of observations in a distribution falling above or below a given value.
- Find the probability that a sample mean significantly differs from a known population mean.

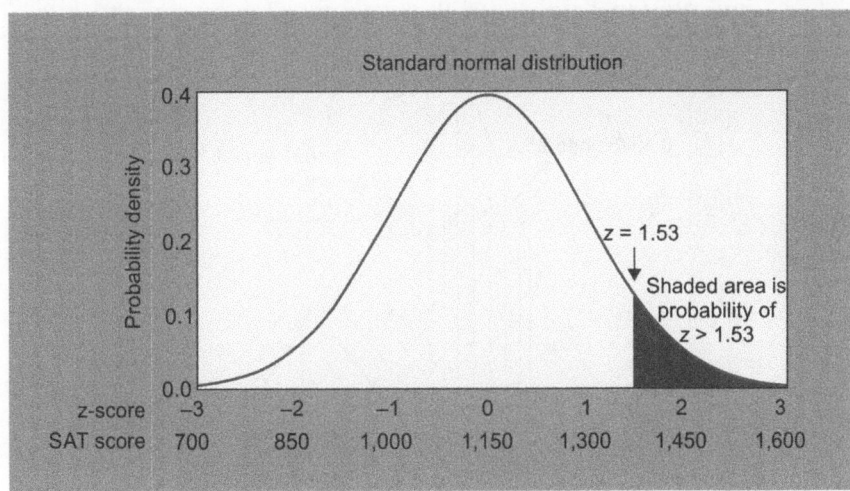

Fig. 16: Standard normal distribution of SAT scores.

Example 1: You collect scores from students in a new test preparation course. The data follows a normal distribution with a mean score (M) of 1,150 and a standard deviation (SD) of 150. You want to find the probability that scores in your sample exceed 1,380.
Solution: To standardize your data, you first find the z-score for 1,380. The z-score tells you how many standard deviations away 1,380 is from the mean.
- Step 1: Subtract the mean from the x value. x – M = 1,380–1,150 = 230
- Step 2: Divide the difference by the standard deviation. z = 230 ÷ 150 = 1.53
  That means 1380 is 1.53 standard deviations from the mean of your distribution.
- Step 3: Find the probability of this score using a z-table. For a z-score of 1.53, the p-value is 0.937. This is the probability of scores being 1380 or less (93.7%), and it is the area under the curve left of the shaded area.
  To find the shaded area, you subtract 0.937 (p value) from 1 (total area under the curve).
  Probability of x >1,380 = 1 – 0.937 = 0.063 **(Fig. 16)**
  That means it is likely that only 6.3% of scores in your sample exceed 1,380.

Example 2: Assume that among diabetics the fasting blood level of glucose is approximately normally distributed with a mean of 105 mg/100 mL and SD of 9 mg/100 mL. What proportion of diabetics has levels between 90 and 125 mg/100 mL?
Solution: Transform values 90 and 125 mg/100 mL into standardized z score.
- $z_1 = [(90-105)/9] = -1.67$
- $z_2 = [(125-105)/9] = 2.2$

Proportion of diabetics who have levels between 90 and 125 mg/100 mL is equal to area enclosed between z_1 and z_2 in the standard normal curve, which is 0.9386 or 93.86% **(Fig. 17)**.

Standard Error of Mean

The standard deviation of sample means from the population mean is called standard error of mean. Total 95% of the sample means in the distribution obtained by repeated sampling, lie within 1.96 standard errors above or below the population mean.

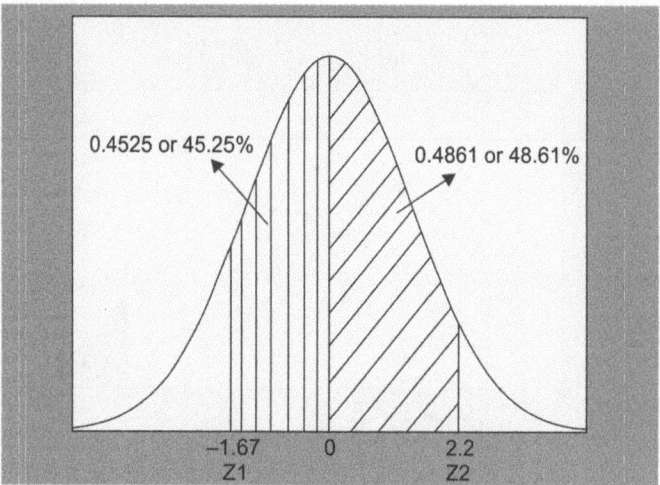

Fig. 17: Standard normal curve.

KEY POINTS

- A sample is a selected subset of a larger population used in studies to analyze broader trends or characteristics.
- The normal distribution is foundational for significance testing in statistical analysis.
- Identifying variable types is a crucial first step in data analysis, guiding the choice of statistical methods.
- Central tendency, measured by arithmetic mean, median and mode, indicates where data values tend to center.
- Variation in data is assessed using five measures: range, quartile deviation, mean deviation, standard deviation and standard error, facilitating hypothesis testing about population characteristics based on sample data.

BIBLIOGRAPHY

1. Agresti A, Finlay B., Statistical Methods for the Social Sciences, 3th Edition. Prentice Hall, 1997
2. Bali J, Anil K. Describing the Data. Basics of Biostatistics: A Manual for the Medical Practitioners. The Health Sciences Publisher; 2017;87-114.
3. Bali J, Bali RT, Gupta YK. Essentials of Biostatistics. Delhi J Ophthalmol, 2018;28;58-63.
4. Daly L, Bourke GJ. Interpretation and uses of medical statistics. 5th edition. UK: Wiley-Blackwell & Sons; 2000. p. 588.
5. Emerson JD, Colditz GA. Use of statistical analysis. N Engl J Med. 1983;309:709-13.
6. Higgins JP, Green S. Cochrane handbook for systematic reviews of interventions Version 5.1.0 [updated March 2011]. London: The Cochrane Collaboration; 2011.
7. Lane, D. 2003, Levels of Measurement. OpenStax CNX. Retrieved May 1, 2013, from http://cnx.org/content/m10809/latest/)
8. Lang T, Secic M. How to Report Statistics in Medicine: Annotated Guidelines for Authors, Editors, and Reviewers. Philadelphia, PA: American College of Physicians; 1997.
9. L Satyanarayana. "Introduction to Biostatistics". Biostatistics—A Manual of Statistical Methods for Use in Health, Nutrition and Anthropology. Ed. K. Visweswara Rao (Ed), New Delhi, Jaypee Brothers Medical Publishers Ltd., 1996;1-11.
10. Probability and Statistics [PROBABILITY & STATISTICS 3 - OS] by Morris H. (Author); Schervish, Mark J. (Author) DeGroot, (Jan. 31, 2002).
11. Roberts D, Brown J, Medley N, Dalziel SR. Antenatal corticosteroids for accelerating fetal lung maturation for women at risk of preterm birth. Cochrane Database Syst. Rev. 2017:(3).
12. Watkins JC. "Organizing and Producing Data". An Introduction to the Science of Statistics: From Theory to Implementation Preliminary Edition; 3-4.

18

CHAPTER

Test of Significance

*Malatesh Undi, Rachana AR, Raghavendra Huchchannavar,
Ameenah H Siraja, Manjula R*

"There are two possible outcomes: if the result confirms the hypothesis, then you have made a measurement. If the result is contrary to the hypothesis, then you have made a discovery."
—*Enrico Fermi*

INTRODUCTION

Hypothesis testing is a fundamental concept in research methodology that involves using statistical methods to determine whether there is sufficient evidence to reject or accept a proposed hypothesis. A hypothesis is an informed and testable statement or proposition that attempts to explain a phenomenon or a relationship between variables. Hypothesis testing allows researchers to draw conclusions about populations based on samples and involves formulating a null hypothesis and an alternative hypothesis, collecting data, and then using statistical tests to determine whether the data provides sufficient evidence to reject the null hypothesis in favor of the alternative hypothesis.

In hypothesis testing, a null hypothesis (H_0) and an alternative hypothesis (H_1 or H_A) are formulated. The null hypothesis is the statement that there is no significant difference between two groups being compared or that the observed effect is due to chance. The alternative hypothesis is the statement that there is a significant difference between the two groups or that the observed effect is not due to chance.

To test a hypothesis, researchers collect data and use statistical tests to analyze it. The statistical tests provide a measure of the likelihood that the observed effect could be due to chance alone. If the results of the statistical tests provide sufficient evidence to reject the null hypothesis, then the alternative hypothesis is accepted. On the other hand, if the statistical tests do not provide sufficient evidence to reject the null hypothesis, then the null hypothesis is accepted.

Why Should one Test the Hypothesis?

Researcher helps the administrators/clinicians/policy makers in making evidence-based decisions by testing the hypothesis and answering the following questions:
- Is the difference real?
- Is the difference due to chance?
- Is the difference due to study design and nonsampling error?

Hypothesis testing is a crucial step in the research process, as it allows researchers to draw conclusions based on empirical evidence. By testing hypotheses, researchers can evaluate the effectiveness of interventions, explore relationships between variables, and make informed decisions based on the data. It is an important tool for advancing knowledge and understanding in a variety of fields.

Let us see some of the examples.

Example 1: Suppose if a researcher wants to assess if there is an association between smoking and the risk of developing lung cancer.
Null hypothesis (H_0): There is no significant association between smoking and the risk of developing lung cancer.
Alternative hypothesis(H_1): There is a significant association between smoking and the risk of developing lung cancer.
Statistical test: A case-control study can be conducted, and the results can be analyzed using statistical tests such as the *chi-square test* to determine whether there is a significant association between smoking and the risk of developing lung cancer.

Example 2: Suppose if a researcher wants to find out if there is a difference in the prevalence of hypertension between urban and rural populations.
Null hypothesis (H_0): There is no significant difference in the prevalence of hypertension between urban and rural populations.
Alternative hypothesis(H_1): There is a significant difference in the prevalence of hypertension between urban and rural populations.
Statistical test: A cross-sectional study can be conducted, and the results can be analyzed using statistical tests such as (a) *t-test* to determine whether there is a significant difference in the blood pressure measurement between rural and urban population and (b) *chi-square test* to know the difference in prevalence of hypertension between urban and rural populations.

Steps in Testing a Hypothesis

The following steps are involved in testing of a hypothesis:

Identify the Research Question

The first step is to clearly define the research question and identify the variables involved in the study. The research question should be specific and worth answering.

Formulate the Null and Alternative Hypothesis

Based on the research question, the null hypothesis and alternative hypothesis should be formulated. The null hypothesis represents the default assumption (no significant difference), while the alternative hypothesis represents the researcher's hypothesis (significant difference). The alternate hypothesis can be one-sided or two-sided hypothesis.

Determine the Level of Significance

The level of significance is the probability threshold used to determine whether to reject the null hypothesis. Typically, a significance level of 0.05 (5%) is used in hypothesis testing.

Select an Appropriate Statistical Test

The appropriate statistical test should be selected based on the type of data being analyzed and the research question. Commonly used statistical tests include t-tests, ANOVA, chi-square tests, and regression analysis.

Collect and Analyze the Data

Data should be collected and analyzed using the selected statistical test. The results of the test will provide a p-value, which represents the probability of observing the results if the null hypothesis were true.

Interpret the Results

The results of the statistical test should be interpreted in the context of the research question. If the p-value is less than the level of significance assumed before the start of the study, the null hypothesis is rejected, and the alternative hypothesis is accepted. If the p-value is greater than the level of significance, then the null hypothesis is accepted (failed to reject) and the alternate hypothesis rejected.

Conclusions

Based on the results of the statistical test, conclusions should be drawn about the research question. The conclusions should be based on the evidence provided by the data analysis and should be stated in a clear and concise manner.

Communicate the Findings

The findings of the study should be communicated to the relevant audience, such as peers, policymakers, or the general public. The communication should be clear and understandable, and the limitations of the study should be acknowledged.

Hypothesis

A hypothesis is an informed and testable statement or proposition that attempts to explain a phenomenon or a relationship between variables. In simpler terms, a hypothesis is a statement yet to be proved, and this statement is to be based on scientific evidence obtained from earlier studies or the scientific observations from currently available information.

It is an *assertion* or *statement* regarding a parameter of the population
Note *that it is the null hypothesis(H_0) that is always being tested.*

Null Hypothesis (H_0)

It is based on the assumption that the **external factor has no role to play or there is no difference in the effect or outcome** due to the factor of interest.

Thus, it is an assumption stating that **there is no significant difference between two values** obtained from two sample groups or between a sample and the population

$$H_0 : \mu_1 = \mu_2$$

Hypothesis (H_1)

It is based on the assumption that **there is a difference between the two groups and this difference is not due to chance** but because of some external factor or intervention.

Thus, it is an assumption stating that **there is a significant difference between two values** obtained from two sample groups or between a sample and the population.

$$H1 : \mu1 \neq \mu2$$

The null hypothesis (H0) is a statement that suggests there is no significant relationship between two variables, or no significant difference between two groups being compared. It is a statement of no effect or no change. The null hypothesis is typically the default assumption in a study unless there is evidence to support an alternative hypothesis.

For example, in a study comparing the effectiveness of two treatments for a particular medical condition, the null hypothesis would be that there is no significant difference in the effectiveness of the two treatments. This means that any observed difference in the effectiveness of the two treatments would be due to chance alone.

The alternative hypothesis (H1 or Ha) is a statement that suggests there is a significant relationship between two variables or a significant difference between two groups being compared. It is the opposite of the null hypothesis and represents the researcher's hypothesis that there is an effect or change.

Continuing with the above example, the alternative hypothesis would be that there is a significant difference in the effectiveness of the two treatments. This means that any observed difference in the effectiveness of the two treatments is not due to chance alone and could be attributed to a difference between the two treatments.

In hypothesis testing, researchers collect data and use statistical tests to determine the probability of observing the results if the null hypothesis were true. If the probability is very low (usually less than 5% or 0.05), the null hypothesis is rejected, and the alternative hypothesis is accepted. However, if the probability is high (greater than 5%), the null hypothesis is not rejected, and the alternative hypothesis is not supported.

Errors

Type I and type II errors are two types of errors that can occur in statistical hypothesis testing (Table 1).

Type I Error

Observing a difference when in truth there is none. Type I error occurs when we reject the null hypothesis even though it is true. This is also known as a false positive. The probability of making a type I error is denoted by alpha (α) and is typically set at 0.05 or 0.01, depending on the level of stringency required by the research question.

Type II Error

Failing to observe a difference when there is one. Type II error occurs when we fail to reject the null hypothesis even though it is false. This is also known as a false negative. The probability of making a type II error is denoted by beta (β) and is typically set at 0.2 or 0.1, depending on the level of acceptable risk for the research question.

Table 1: Summary of the two types of errors.

Your decision	REALITY	
	H_0 True (no association)	H_1 True (association)
Accept H_0/fail to reject H_0 (no statistically significant difference)	Correct decision	Type II error (beta)
Reject H_0 (Statistically significant difference)	Type I error (alpha)	Correct decision

Note: H_0 denotes null hypothesis

Examples

Suppose a researcher is interested in testing whether a new drug is more effective than a placebo in reducing blood pressure. The null hypothesis (H0) is that there is no difference between the two groups (one group receiving new drug and the other group receiving placebo), and the alternative hypothesis (Ha) is that there is a difference between the two groups **(Fig. 1)**.

If the researcher conducts a study with a significance level (α) of 0.05, and the statistical test results in rejecting the null hypothesis (p value <0.05), but in reality, the drug is not more effective than the placebo, this is a type I error. The researcher has concluded that there is a difference between the two groups when there is none.

If the researcher conducts a study with a significance level (α) of 0.05, and the statistical test results in failing to reject the null hypothesis (p value $\geq$ 0.05), but in reality, the drug is more effective than the placebo, this is a type II error. The researcher has failed to detect a difference between the two groups that actually exists.

It is important for researchers to be aware of the possibility of type I and type II errors in their research, and to choose an appropriate significance level and statistical power to minimize the risk of making these errors.

Setting a Criterion

Tailed Test

A one-tailed test is used when an alternative hypothesis specifies a direction. This is when the alternative hypothesis states that the parameter is either bigger or smaller than the value specified in the null hypothesis.

❖ If H_1 state μ is < μ_0, the critical region occupies the left tail *(left-tailed test)*
  $H_0 : \mu = \mu_0$
  $H_1 : \mu < \mu_0$
❖ If H_1 state μ is > μ_0, the critical region occupies the right tail *(right-tailed test)*
  $H_0 : \mu = \mu_0$
  $H_1 : \mu > \mu_0$

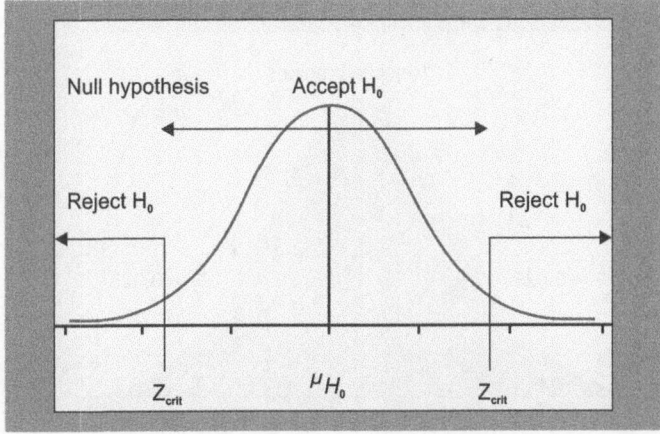

Fig. 1: Normal distribution illustrating rejection and nonrejection regions for null hypothesis testing.

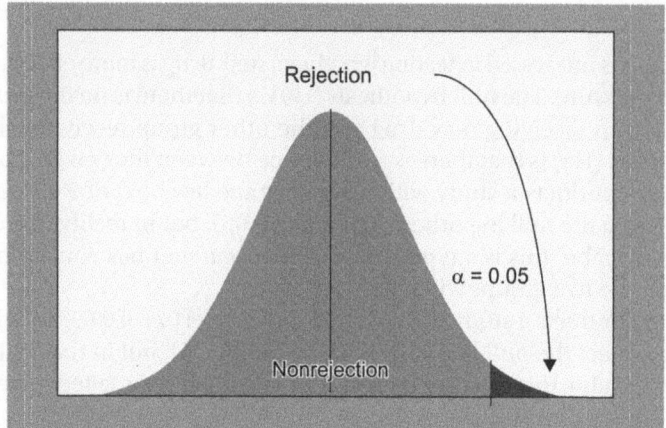

Fig. 2: One-tailed hypothesis test with a 5% significance level rejection region.

For example, a drug manufacturer claims that Drug A reduced blood pressure on an average by 20mm Hg. If a researcher is interested in knowing whether drug A reduces blood pressure lesser than 20 mm Hg, he/she can use one tailed test.

A diagram of the level of significance can be illustrated using a normal distribution curve **(Fig. 2)**. The area under the curve represents the probability of obtaining a particular test statistic, assuming the null hypothesis is true.

The shaded area represents the level of significance (α). If the test statistic falls within this shaded area, the null hypothesis is rejected. If the test statistic falls outside this shaded area, the null hypothesis is not rejected. In this example, the shaded area represents the level of significance (α) set at 0.05. If the test statistic falls within this shaded area (i.e., to the left of −1.96 or to the right of 1.96), the null hypothesis is rejected. If the test statistic falls outside this shaded area (i.e., between −1.96 and 1.96), the null hypothesis is not rejected.

Two-tailed Test

A two-tailed test is used when an alternative hypothesis does not specify a direction, i.e., when the alternative hypothesis states that the null hypothesis is wrong **(Fig. 3)**.

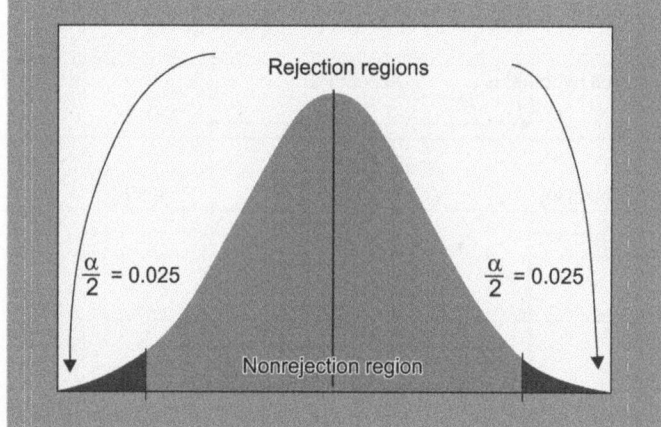

Fig. 3: Two-tailed hypothesis test with rejection regions at a 5% significance.

- If H_1 state that μ is either greater or less than μ_0
  $H_0 : \mu = \mu_0$
  $H_1 : \mu \neq \mu_0$
  α is divided equally between the two tails of the critical region.

For example, a drug manufacturer claims that drug A reduced blood pressure on an average by 20mm Hg. If a researcher is interested in knowing whether Drug A reduces blood pressure greater or lesser than 20 mm Hg, he/she can use two tailed test.

The main difference between one-tailed and two-tailed tests is that one-tailed tests will only have one critical region whereas two-tailed tests will have two critical regions.

Acceptance and Rejection of H_0

Type I error: Rejecting H_0 when H_0 is true

α: Type I error rate –level of significance (l.o.f)

The level of significance, also known as alpha (α), is the probability threshold used in hypothesis testing to determine whether to reject the null hypothesis. It represents the maximum probability of making a type I error, which occurs when the null hypothesis is rejected when it is actually true. The level of significance is typically set at 0.05 (5%), meaning that the probability of making a type I error is 5% or less. However, depending on the study, the level of significance may be set at a different value, such as 0.01 (1%) or 0.10 (10%).

Type II error: Accepting/failing to reject H_0 when H_0 is false (H_1 true)

β: Type II Error Rate

1-β: Power of the test—The power of a hypothesis test is the probability of making the correct decision if the alternative hypothesis is true, i.e., the probability of rejecting the null hypothesis when the alternative hypothesis is the hypothesis that is true.

To minimize the type I and type II error, they are fixed at some levels by the researcher and most common choice is:

Type I error, $\alpha = 5\%$ Type II error, $\beta = 20\%$

Type I and Type II Errors

- Common choices for most of studies
  - Alpha error = 5%
  - Beta error = 20%
- Exploratory study
  - Alpha error = 10%
  - Beta error = 10%
- Confirmatory study
  - Alpha error = 1%
  - Beta error = 10%

p-value

While hypothesis testing, a result is said to be statistically significant if it is unlikely to have occurred by chance.

The probability of a result due to chance is called its p-value
- Smaller the p-value, more significant is the result
- If a test of significance gives a p-value < α, the null hypothesis is rejected (difference is significant)

How to decide when to reject the null hypothesis?
(H_0 rejected using reported *p-value*)
- If $Z \leq Z\alpha$ **or** p-value > 0.05 – H_0 accepted (nonsignificant) at 5% l.o.f
- If $Z > Z\alpha$ **or** p value ≤ 0.05 – H_0 rejected/H_1 accepted (significant) at 5% l.o.f
- $Z\alpha = 1.96$ for $\alpha = 5\%$
- $Z\alpha = 2.58$ for $\alpha = 1\%$
- $Z\alpha = 3.29$ for $\alpha = 0.1\%$

Illustration:
A researcher is investigating whether a new drug X is effective in reducing blood pressure. The null hypothesis is that there is no significant difference in blood pressure between the group receiving the drug A and the placebo group. The alternative hypothesis is that there is a significant difference in blood pressure between the two groups.

The researcher conducts a statistical test and obtains a p-value of 0.03. If the level of significance is set at 0.05, the researcher can reject the null hypothesis and accept the alternative hypothesis, since the p-value is less than 0.05. This means that there is evidence that the drug X is reducing blood pressure as compared to placebo.

Tests of Statistical Significance

Parametric Test of Significance

Parametric tests are statistical tests that assume that the data being analyzed follows a certain distribution, usually the normal distribution and are continuous variables. The test is applied to estimate at least one population parameter from sample statistics, e.g., t-test, ANOVA, and Pearson correlation. These tests can be applied on data sets that fulfil certain assumptions otherwise the nonparametric counterpart of these tests have to be utilized to know statistical significance.

Assumptions: The below mentioned assumptions must be fulfilled for application of parametric tests
1. Data must be in interval and ratio scale.
2. The sample must be normally distributed. Normality can be checked by looking at the distribution curve for skewness and kurtosis, inspection of the histogram or by application of tests such as Kolmogorov-Smirnov tests or Shapiro-Wilk test.
3. The selected population should be representative of the target population to which you are planning to generalize your results. This can be achieved by enrolling adequate number of study subjects (based on calculated sample size) and adopting appropriate sampling method.

Nonparametric Test of Significance

Nonparametric tests are *distribution free*, make no assumption about the distribution of the variable in the population. These tests are used when the data being analyzed is not normally distributed or when the sample size is too small to rely on the central limit theorem. **For example, Wilcoxon signed-rank test, the Mann-Whitney U test, and the Kruskal-Wallis test.** It's important to note that the choice of whether to use a parametric or nonparametric test depends on the specific characteristics of the data being analyzed and the research question being asked. If the data meets the assumptions of parametric tests, these tests tend to be more powerful. If the data does not meet these assumptions, nonparametric tests may be more appropriate.

Tests of Significance (for Quantitative Data) are Basically Discussed Under Two Heads

1. Z-test for large samples
2. t-test for small samples
   - Unpaired t-test (for two independent samples) and
   - Paired t-test (for single sample with correlated observations)

For application of Z or t test, initially standard error (chance variation) has to be studied:

Statistic	Mean	Standard error
Sample Mean	μ	$\sigma/\sqrt{n}$
Difference of means	$\mu_1 - \mu_2$	$\sqrt{(\sigma_1^2/n_1) + (\sigma_2^2/n_2)}$
Sample proportion (p)	P	$\sqrt{PQ/n}$ where, Q=1-P
Difference of proportions (P1–P2)	P1–P2	

For large samples (with sample size, n>30) which are usually assumed as normally distributed, Z-tests are applied:

- One sample Z-test/normal test (to test the statistical significance of the difference in sample and population means)
- Two sample Z-test (to test the statistical significance of the difference in two population means)
- To test the statistical significance of difference in sample and population proportions (Z-test for proportions)
- To test the statistical significance of the difference in proportions between two independent populations

Z-tests	Hypotheses	Test statistic
For single mean ($\bar{X}$)	H_0: There is no significant difference between sample mean and population mean H_1: There is significant difference between sample mean and population mean	$Z = \|\bar{X} - \mu SDn\|$
For difference of means ($\bar{X}_1 - \bar{X}_2$)	H_0: There is no significant difference between mean value of 2 groups H_1: There is significant difference between mean value of 2 groups	$Z = \|\bar{X}_1 - \bar{X}_2 SE\|$ $SE = \sqrt{(SD_1^2/n_1) + (SD_2^2/n_2)}$
For Sample Proportion(p)	H_0: There is no significant difference between sample and population proportions H_1: There is significant difference between sample and population proportions	$Z = \|p - Ppqn\|$
For difference of proportions (p1-p2)	H_0: There is no significant difference between the 2 proportions H_1: There is significant difference between the 2 proportions	$Z = \|p_1 - p_2 p_1 q_1 n_1 + p_2 q_2 n_2\|$

For small samples with sample size n≤30, small sample tests (t-tests) are used:

- One sample 't' test
- Two independent samples 't' test or unpaired 't' test
- Paired-samples t-test

t-tests	Hypotheses	Test statistic
One sample t-test	H_0: There is no significant difference between sample mean and population mean H_1: There is significant difference between sample mean and population mean	$t = \|\overline{X} - \mu SDn\|$ with d.f = n-1
Independent samples t-test	H_0: There is no significant difference between the means of 2 groups H_1: There is significant difference between the means of 2 groups	$t = \|\overline{X}_1 - \overline{X}_2 SD\sqrt{1n1 + 1n2}\|$ with d.f $= n_1 + n_2 - 2$ where, SD $= n1-1SD12+n2-1SD2\wedge2n1+n2-2$
Paired-sample t-test	H_0: There is no significant difference before and after the treatment (intervention). H_1: There is significant difference before and after the treatment (intervention).	$t = \|d\sqrt{n}S\|$ with d.f = n-1 where, d-mean of the differences S- SD of the differences * d.f – degrees of freedom (no. of independent values)

PARAMETRIC TESTS

Type of data	Number of groups compared	Type of test	Examples
Continuous	1	Pearson's correlation	Comparison of changes in blood pressure with age
Continuous	2 (matched) or 1 group before-after study	Paired t-test	Comparison of blood pressure among two group of patients (matched for baseline parameters) receiving two different treatment or in one-group before after study
Continuous	2 (unmatched)	Two-sample t-test (unpaired t-test)	Comparison of blood pressure in patients receiving a new medication versus a control group
Continuous	>2	Analysis of variance (ANOVA)	Comparison of cholesterol levels in patients receiving different doses of a medication

NONPARAMETRIC TESTS

Type of data	Number of groups compared	Type of test	Examples
Continuous	1	Spearman's correlation	Comparison of changes in pain perceived with dosage of analgesia
Continuous	2	Mann-Whitney U test	Comparison of pain scores in patients receiving a new medication versus a control group
Continuous	>2	Kruskal-Wallis test	Comparison of anxiety levels in patients receiving different doses of a medication
Categorical	2	McNemar's test	Comparison of the prevalence of a disease before and after a treatment

Categorical	>2	Friedman test	Comparison of the effectiveness of three different treatments on symptoms of a disease
Categorical	2	Chi-square test or Fisher's exact test	Comparison of the prevalence of smoking in patients with lung cancer versus those without lung cancer
Categorical	>2	Chi-square test or Fisher's exact test	Comparison of the prevalence of hypertension in patients with diabetes, obesity, or both

KEY POINTS

- Note the eight steps of testing a hypothesis.
- If the probability is less than 0.05, the null hypothesis is rejected, and the alternative hypothesis is accepted. However, if the probability is high (greater than 5%), the null hypothesis is not rejected, and the alternative hypothesis is not supported.
- A type I error (false-positive) occurs if an investigator rejects a null hypothesis that is actually true in the population; a type II error (false-negative) occurs if the investigator fails to reject a null hypothesis that is actually false in the population.

BIBLIOGRAPHY

1. Altman DG, Bland JM. Statistics Notes: The significance level. BMJ. 1994;309(6948):996. doi:10.1136/bmj.309.6948.996
2. Armitage P, Berry G, Matthews JNS. Statistical Methods in Medical Research. 4th edition. Wiley; 2008.
3. Hulley SB, Cummings SR, Browner WS, Grady DG, Newman TB. Designing Clinical Research. 4th edition. Lippincott Williams & Wilkins; 2013.
4. Kline RB. Principles and Practice of Structural Equation Modeling. 4th edition. Guilford Press; 2016.
5. Sullivan GM, Feinn R. Using Effect Size-or Why the P Value Is Not Enough. J Grad Med Educ. 2012;4(3):279-82. doi:10.4300/JGME-D-12-00156.1

CHAPTER 19

Advanced Statistics

Soumya Swaroop Sahoo, Kamal Kishore, Aditi Mohta, Bhushan Kamble

"Research is formalized curiosity. It is poking and prying with a purpose."
—*Zora Neale Hurston*

INTRODUCTION

One-way analysis of variance (ANOVA) is one of the most common statistical techniques to test the equality of three or more means in medical research. ANOVA is also called the Fisher analysis of variance, and it is the extension of the t- and z-tests. The term became well-known in 1925, after appearing in Fisher's book, "Statistical Methods for Research Workers."(Fisher R). It was employed in experimental psychology and later expanded to subjects that were more complex.

In ANOVA, the test gets a common P value. A significant P value of ANOVA test indicates the presence of at least one pair, between which the mean difference was statistically significant. To identify that significant pair(s), posthoc test (multiple comparisons) is used. In ANOVA test, when at least one covariate (continuous variable) is adjusted to remove the confounding effect from the result, it is called analysis of covariance (ANCOVA). ANOVA test (F test) is called "analysis of variance" rather than "analysis of means" because inferences about means are made by analyzing variance.

Hypothesis building: Like other tests, there are two kinds of hypotheses; null hypothesis and alternative hypothesis. The alternative hypothesis assumes that a statistically significant difference exists between the means, whereas the null hypothesis assumes that there is no statistically significant difference between the means.

The first step is to calculate the test statistic, i.e., *F value* in ANOVA test, **(Fig. 1)** also called *calculated value*. It is calculated after inserting inputs (from the samples) in statistical test formula. Calculated F value is ratio of the variability between groups with the variability of the observations within the groups.

- F = Explained variance/unexplained variance, or
- F= Between group variability/within group variability

At degree of freedom of the given observations and desired level of the confidence (usually two-sided test, which is more powerful than one-sided test), corresponding tabulated value of the F test is selected.

Comparison of calculated value with tabulated value and null hypothesis: If the calculated value is greater than the tabulated value, then reject the null hypothesis. As the sample size increases, corresponding degree of freedom also increases. For a given level of confidence,

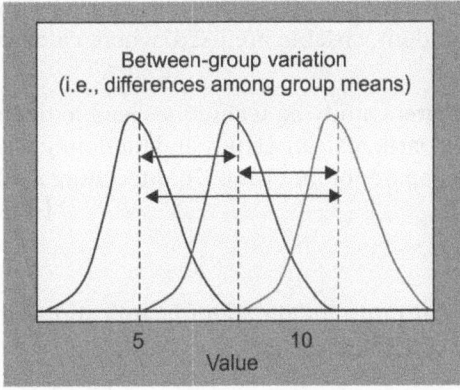 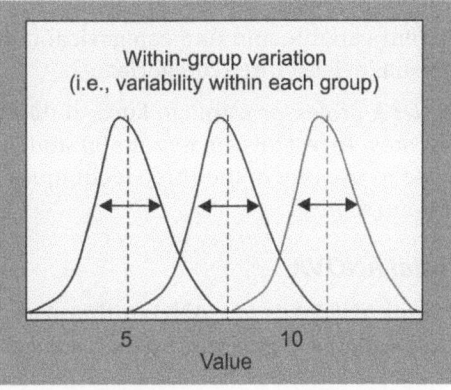

Fig. 1: Understanding F statistic in ANOVA.

higher degree of freedom has lower tabulated value. That is why, when the sample size increases, its significance level also improves (i.e., P value is decreasing).

Assumptions for ANOVA

1. The data from group has common mean. This means that there are no sub-populations with different means.
2. **Homoskedasticity:** The data from all groups have common variance. That is, the variability in the data does not depend on group membership.
3. **Independence:** The subjects are independently sampled.
4. **Normality:** The data are normally distributed.

Classification of ANOVA test (Flowchart 1)

There are different types of ANOVA test, with varying objectives. The two main types are *one-way ANOVA* and *one-way repeated measures ANOVA*. The former is used for independent observations, and the latter for dependent observations. When used for one categorical independent variable. it is called *one-way ANOVA*, whereas for two categorical independent variables, it is called *two-way ANOVA*.

One-way ANOVA

The One-way ANOVA is extension of independent samples t test (in independent samples t test, means between two independent groups are compared, whereas in one-way ANOVA, means are compared among three or more independent groups). A significant P value of this test refers

Flowchart 1: Broad classification of ANOVA test.

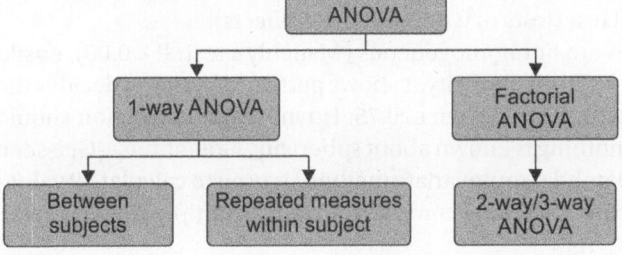

to multiple comparisons test to identify the significant pair(s). In this test, one continuous dependent variable and one categorical independent variable are used, where categorical variable has at least three categories.

Example: A professor wants to know if three different studying techniques lead to different exam scores. To test this, he recruits 30 students to participate in a study and randomly assigns each one to use one of the three techniques to prepare for an exam. Does teaching method affect exam scores?

Factorial ANOVA

A factorial ANOVA is any ANOVA that uses two or more independent factors and a single response variable. A two-way ANOVA is a type of factorial ANOVA.

Two-way ANOVA

The two-way ANOVA is extension of one-way ANOVA. In one-way ANOVA, only one independent variable is used, whereas in two-way ANOVA, two independent variables are used. The primary purpose of a two-way ANOVA is to understand whether there is any interrelationship between two independent variables on a dependent variable. In this test, a continuous dependent variable (approximately normally distributed) and two categorical independent variables are used.

Example: A professor wants to understand how class time and teaching method affect exam scores. He uses two different teaching methods and two different teaching times (early morning and early afternoon) and records the average exam scores of each student at the end of the semester.

Response variable: exam score, factors: teaching method and teaching time
- Does teaching method affect exam scores?
- Does teaching time affect exam scores?
- Is there an interaction effect between teaching method and teach time?

We could use a factorial ANOVA for this analysis because he wants to understand how two factors affect a single response variable.

One-way Repeated Measures ANOVA

Repeated Measures ANOVA (RMA) is the extension of the paired t test. RMA is also referred to as within-subjects ANOVA or ANOVA for paired samples. Repeated measures design is a research design that involves multiple measures of the same variable taken on the same or matched subjects either under different conditions or more than two time periods.

In RMA, the means between three or more dependent groups are compared. Before calculating the significance level, Mauchly's test is used to assess the homogeneity of the variance (also called sphericity) within all possible pairs. When P value of Mauchly's test is insignificant (P ≥ 0.05), equal variances are assumed and P value for RMA would be taken from sphericity assumed test (tests of within-subjects effects).

In case variances are not homogeneous (Mauchly's test: P < 0.05), epsilon (ε) value (which shows the departure of the sphericity, 1 shows perfect sphericity) decides the statistical method to calculate P value for RMA. When ε≥0.75, Huynh-Feldt correction should be applied; while for ε<0.75 or when nothing is known about sphericity, Greenhouse-Geisser method (univariate method), or Wilks' lambda (multivariate method) is used to calculate P value for the RMA. When the RMA is significant, pair-wise comparison using multiple paired t tests with a Bonferroni correction is used.

Two-way Repeated Measures ANOVA

Two-way Repeated Measures ANOVA is combination of between-subject and within-subject factors. A two-way RMA (also known as a two-factor RMA or a two-way "Mixed ANOVA") is extension of one-way RMA.

In one-way RMA, use one dependent variable under repeated observations (normally distributed continuous variable) and one categorical independent variable (i.e., time points), whereas in two-way RMA, one additional categorical independent variable is used.

The primary purpose of two-way RMA is to understand if there is an interaction between these two categorical independent variables on the dependent variable (continuous variable). The distribution of the dependent variable in each combination of the related groups should be approximately normally distributed, where second independent variable will be included as between subjects' factor.

Example: You want to measure the resting heart rate of subjects one month before they start a training program, during the middle of the training program and one month after the training program to see if there is a significant difference in mean resting heart rate across these three time points. We repeatedly measured the same subjects, hence the reason why we used a repeated measures ANOVA.

One-way Analysis of Covariance (One-way ANCOVA)

One-way ANCOVA is extension of one-way ANOVA. In one-way ANOVA, we do not adjust the covariate, whereas in one-way ANCOVA, we adjust at least one covariate. Thus, one-way ANCOVA tests find out whether the independent variable still influences the dependent variable after the influence of the covariate(s) has been removed (i.e., adjusted). In this test, one continuous dependent variable, one categorical independent variable and at least one continuous covariate for removing its effect/adjustment are used.

One-way Repeated Measures ANCOVA

One-way repeated measures ANCOVA is the extension of the One-way RMA. In one-way RMA, we do not adjust the covariate; whereas, in the one-way repeated measures ANCOVA, we adjust at least one covariate. Thus, the one-way repeated measures ANCOVA is used to test whether means are still statistically equal or different after adjusting the effect of the covariate(s).

Although ANCOVA is usually used when there are differences between your baseline groups (Senn, 1994; Overall, 1993), it can also be used in pre-test/post-test analysis when regression to the mean affects your post-test measurement (Bonate, 2000). The technique is also common in nonexperimental research (e.g., surveys) and for quasi-experiments (when study participants cannot be assigned randomly). However, this particular application of ANCOVA is not always recommended (Vogt, 1999).

ANCOVA can explain within-group variance. It takes the unexplained variances from the ANOVA test and tries to explain them with confounding variables (or other covariates).

Example: A professor wants to know if three different studying techniques lead to different exam scores. To test this, he recruits 30 students to participate in a study and randomly assigns each one to use one of the three techniques to prepare for an exam. But he wants to account for the grade that the student already has in the class. He can use their current grade as a covariate and conduct an ANCOVA to determine if there is a statistically significant difference between the mean exam scores of the three groups. This allows him to test whether or not studying technique has an impact on exam scores after the influence of the covariate has been removed.

Multivariate Analysis of Variance

Multivariate analysis of variance (MANOVA) is an extension of the univariate analysis of variance. In ANOVA, we examine for statistical differences on one continuous dependent variable by an independent grouping variable. The MANOVA extends this analysis by considering multiple continuous dependent variables and bundles them together into a weighted linear combination or composite variable.

MANOVA will compare whether or not the newly created combination differs by the different groups or levels, of the independent variable. In this way, the MANOVA essentially tests whether or not the independent grouping variable simultaneously explains a statistically significant amount of variance in the dependent variable.

Example: A clinical psychologist recruits 100 people who suffer from panic disorder into her study. Each subject receives one of four types of treatment for eight weeks. At the end of treatment, each subject participates in a structured interview, during which the clinical psychologist makes three ratings: physiological, emotional, and cognitive. She wants to know which type of treatment reduces the symptoms of the panic disorder the most, as measured on the physiological, emotional, and cognitive scales.

Illustrated Examples

Illustrated Example No. 1

Three popular weight loss programs are considered. The first is a low-calorie diet. The second is a low-fat diet and the third is a low carbohydrate diet. For comparison purposes, a fourth group is considered as a control group. Participants in the fourth group are told that they are participating in a study of healthy behaviors with weight loss as only one component of interest. The control group is included here to assess the placebo effect. A total of 20 patients agree to participate in the study and are randomly assigned to one of the four diet groups. Weights are measured at baseline and patients are counseled on the proper implementation of the assigned diet (with the exception of the control group). After 8 weeks, each patient's weight is again measured and the difference in weights is computed by subtracting the 8-week weight from the baseline weight. Positive differences indicate weight losses and negative differences indicate weight gains. For interpretation purposes, we refer to the differences in weights as weight losses and the observed weight losses are shown below.

Low calorie	Low fat	Low carbohydrate	Control
8	2	3	2
9	4	5	2
6	3	4	-1
7	5	2	0
3	1	3	3

Step 1. Set up hypotheses and determine level of significance
H0: $\mu1 = \mu2 = \mu3 = \mu4$;   H1: Means are not all equal $\alpha = 0.05$

Step 2. Select the appropriate test statistic
The test statistic is the F statistic for ANOVA, F=MSB/MSE.

Step 3. Set up decision rule
In this example, df 1 = k-1 = 4-1=3 and df2=N-k=20-4=16. The critical value is 3.24 and the decision rule is as follows: Reject H0 if F > 3.24.

Step 4. Compute the test statistic.

	Low calorie	Low fat	Low carbohydrate	Control
N	5	5	5	5
Group mean	6.6	3.0	3.4	1.2

If we pool all N = 20 observations, the overall mean $\bar{X} = 3.6$

Sum of squares between $SSB = \sum n_j (\bar{X}_j - \bar{X}_j)^2$

So, in this case: $SSB = 5(6.6 - 3.6)^2 + 5(3.0-3.6)^2 + 5(3.4-3.6)^2 + 5(1.2-3.6)^2$

$SSB = 45.0 + 1.8 + 0.2 + 28.8 = 75.8$

$$SSE = \sum\sum(X - \bar{X}_j)^2$$

Sum of squares of error (SSE) requires computing the squared differences between each observation and its group mean. We will compute SSE in parts. For the participants in the low-calorie diet:

Low calorie	(X - 6.6)	(X - 6.6)²
8	1.4	2.0
9	2.4	5.8
6	–0.6	0.4
7	0.4	0.2
3	–3.6	13.0
Total	0	21.4

Thus, $\sum(X - \bar{X}_1)^2$ 21.4

For the participants in the low-fat diet:

Low fat	(X - 3.0)	(X - 3.0)²
2	–1.0	1.0
4	1.0	1.0
3	0.0	0.0
5	2.0	4.0
1	–2.0	4.0
Totals	0	10.0

Thus, $\sum(X - \bar{X}_2)^2 = 10.0$

For the participants in the low carbohydrate diet:

Low carbohydrate	(X - 3.4)	(X - 3.4)²
3	–0.4	0.2
5	1.6	2.6
4	0.6	0.4
2	–1.4	2.0
3	–0.4	0.2
Totals	0	5.4

Thus, $\sum(X - \bar{X}_3)^2 = 5.4$

For the participants in the control group:

Control	(X - 1.2)	(X - 1.2)²
2	0.8	0.6
2	0.8	0.6
−1	−2.2	4.8
0	−1.2	1.4
3	1.8	3.2
Totals	0	10.6

Thus, $\sum(X - \bar{X}_4)^2 = 10.6$

Therefore,

$$SSE = \sum\sum(X - \bar{X}_j)^2 = 21.4 + 10.0 + 5.4 + 10.6 = 47.4$$

We can now construct the ANOVA table.

Source of variation	Sums of squares (SS)	Degrees of freedom (df)	Means squares (MS)	F
Between Treatment	SSB=75.8	4-1=3	75.8/3=25.3	25.3/3.0=8.43
Error (or Residual)	SSE=47.4	20-4=16	47.4/16=3.0	
Total	SST=123.2	20-1=19		

Step 5. Interpretation

We reject H_0 because 8.43 ≥3.24. We have statistically significant evidence at $\alpha = 0.05$ to show that there is a difference in mean weight loss among the four diets.

In this example, participants in the low-calorie diet lost an average of 6.6 pounds over 8 weeks, as compared to 3.0 and 3.4 pounds in the low fat and low carbohydrate groups, respectively. Participants in the control group lost an average of 1.2 pounds which could be called the placebo effect because these participants were not participating in an active arm of the trial specifically targeted for weight loss.

Illustrated Example No. 2

Consider the clinical trial in which three competing treatments for joint pain are compared in terms of their mean time to pain relief in patients with osteoarthritis. Because investigators hypothesize that there may be a difference in time to pain relief in men versus women, they randomly assign 15 participating men to one of the three competing treatments and randomly assign 15 participating women to one of the three competing treatments (i.e., stratified randomization). Participating men and women do not know to which treatment they are assigned. They are instructed to take the assigned medication when they experience joint pain and to record the time, in minutes, until the pain subsides.

Table of Time to Pain Relief by Treatment and Sex

Treatment	Male	Female
A	12	21
	15	19
	16	18
	17	24
	14	25
B	14	21
	17	20
	19	23
	20	27
	17	25
C	25	37
	27	34
	29	36
	24	26
	22	29

The analysis in two-factor ANOVA is similar to that illustrated above for one-factor ANOVA. The computations are again organized in an ANOVA table but the total variation is partitioned into that due to the main effect of treatment, the main effect of sex and the interaction effect. The results of the analysis are shown below (and were generated with a statistical computing package; here, we focus on interpretation).

ANOVA Table for Two-factor ANOVA

Source of variation	Sums of squares (SS)	Degrees of of freedom (DF)	Mean squares (MS)	F	P value
Model	967.0	5	193.4	20.7	0.0001
Treatment	651.5	2	325.7	34.8	0.0001
Sex	313.6	1	313.6	33.5	0.0001
Treatment * Sex	1.9	2	0.9	0.1	0.9054
Error or residual	224.4	24	9.4		
Total	1191.4	29			

There are 4 statistical tests in the ANOVA table above. The first test is an overall test to assess whether there is a difference among the 6 cell means (cells are defined by treatment and sex).

The F statistic is 20.7 and is highly statistically significant with p=0.0001. When the overall test is significant, focus then turns to the factors that may be driving the significance (in this example, treatment, sex or the interaction between the two). The next three statistical tests assess the significance of the main effect of treatment, the main effect of sex and the interaction effect. In this example, there is a highly significant main effect of treatment (p = 0.0001) and a highly significant main effect of sex (p = 0.0001). The interaction between the two does not reach statistical significance (p = 0.91). The table below contains the mean times to pain relief in each of the treatments for men and women (note that each sample mean is computed on the 5 observations measured under that experimental condition).

Mean Time to Pain Relief by Treatment and Gender

Treatment	Male	Female
A	14.8	21.4
B	17.4	23.2
C	25.4	32.4

Treatment A appears to be the most efficacious treatment for both men and women. The mean times to relief are lower in Treatment A for both men and women and highest in Treatment C for both men and women. Across all treatments, women report longer times to pain relief (see below).

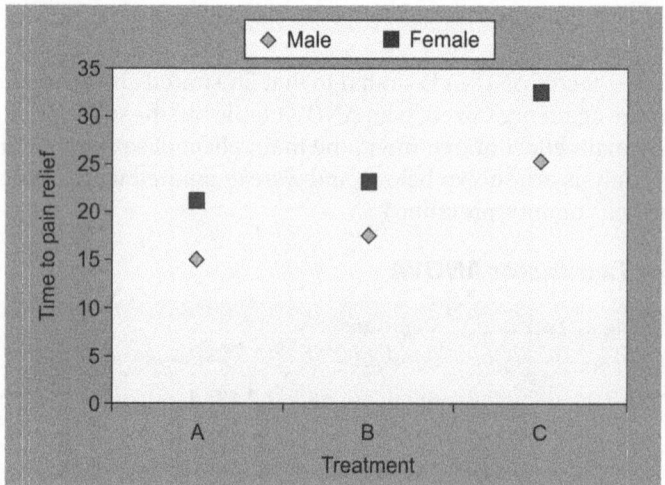

Notice that there is the same pattern of time to pain relief across treatments in both men and women (treatment effect). There is also a sex effect-specifically, time to pain relief is longer in women in every treatment.

Suppose that the same clinical trial is replicated in a second clinical site and the following data are observed.

Time to pain relief by treatment and sex–clinical site 2		
Treatment	Male	Female
A	22	21
	25	19
	26	18
	27	24
	24	25
B	14	21
	17	20
	19	23
	20	27
	17	25
C	15	37
	17	34
	19	36
	14	26
	12	29

The ANOVA table for the data measured in clinical site 2 is shown below.

Summary of two-factor ANOVA–clinical site 2.					
Source of variation	Sums of Squares (SS)	Degrees of freedom (DF)	Mean squares (MS)	F	P value
Model	907.0	5	181.4	19.4	0.0001
Treatment	71.5	2	35.7	3.8	0.0362
Sex	313.6	1	313.6	33.5	0.0001
Treatment * sex	521.9	2	260.9	27.9	0.0001
Error or residual	224.4	24	9.4		
Total	1131.4	29			

Notice that the overall test is significant (F=19.4, p=0.0001), there is a significant treatment effect, sex effect and a highly significant interaction effect. The table below contains the mean times to relief in each of the treatments for men and women.

Mean time to pain relief by treatment and gender—clinical site 2.		
Treatment	Male	Female
A	24.8	21.4
B	17.4	23.2
C	15.4	32.4

Notice that now the differences in mean time to pain relief among the treatments depend on sex. Among men, the mean time to pain relief is highest in Treatment A and lowest in Treatment C. Among women, the reverse is true. This is an interaction effect (see below).

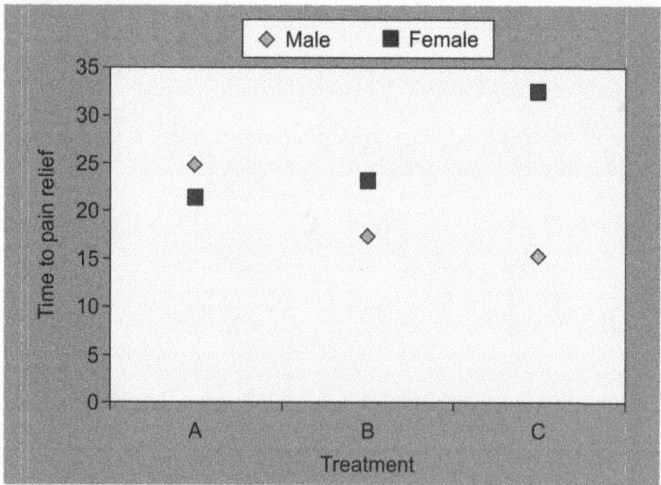

Notice above that the treatment effect varies depending on sex. Thus, we cannot summarize an overall treatment effect (In men, treatment C is best, in women, treatment A is best).

Limitations of ANOVA

1. It often happens that the parent populations do not follow the normal distribution. In such cases, ANOVA cannot be used.
2. It rarely happens that all the population variances are equal. If the assumption of homoscedasticity is violated, then the use of ANOVA cannot be justified.
3. If the null hypothesis is rejected, we can only conclude that some population means are unequal. The ANOVA test does not tell us anything about which of them are unequal. Then, a few post hoc tests must be carried out.

Chi-square Test

The chi-square test, developed by Karl Pearson, is the simplest and most widely used non parametric test. It tests whether there is an association between categorical variables. However, it does not provide any inference about causation.

Logic of Chi-square Test

- The total number of observations in each column and the total number of observations in each row are given or fixed.
- If we assume that columns and rows are independent, we can calculate expected frequencies.
- We compare the observed frequency in each cell with the expected frequency.

Data Requirement for Chi-square Test

- Two categorical variables.
- Two or more categories (groups) for each variable.
- Independence of observations.
  - There is no relationship between the subjects in each group.
  - The categorical variables are not "paired" in any way (e.g., pre-test/ post-test observations).

- Relatively large sample size.
  - Expected frequencies for each cell are at least 1.
  - Expected frequencies should be at least 5 for the majority (80%) of the cell

Chi-square tests are carried out only on the number of occurrences, not on percentages, proportions, means of observations or other derived statistics.

Steps of Chi-square Test

- Define null and alternate hypothesis
- State alpha value (α)
- Calculate degree of freedom
- State decision rule
- Calculate test statistic
- State and interpret results

The test statistic for the chi-square test of independence is denoted as χ^2, and is calculated as:

$$\chi^2 = \sum_i \frac{(O_i - E_i)^2}{E_i}$$

Where:
O = Observed value (the actual count of cases in each cell of the table)
E = Expected value (calculated below)
χ^2 = The cell chi-square value
$\sum \chi^2$ = Formula instruction to sum all the cell chi-square values

The calculated χ^2 value is then compared with the critical value from the χ^2 distribution table with degrees of freedom df = (R - 1) (C - 1) and chosen confidence level. If the calculated χ^2 value is greater than the critical χ^2 value, then we reject the null hypothesis.

Types of Chi-square Test

There are two commonly used types of chi-square tests:
1. **Chi-square goodness of fit:** It is an inferential procedure used to determine whether a frequency distribution of a single variable follows a claimed distribution. For example, sudden infant death syndrome (SIDS) is seasonal or not? Null hypothesis: The proportion of cases of SIDS is identical in winter, summer, autumn, and spring.
2. **Chi-square test of independence:** It is the most commonly used type which gives an association between two variables. For example, is there a difference between various degrees of anemia (mild, moderate, severe) and gender (male, female)?

Illustrated Example of Chi-square Test

Let us take an example related to vector borne disease cases in three districts of a state and conduct a chi-square test to find the P value.

Observed frequencies:

Region	Malaria	Chikungunya	Dengue	Total
District A	21	32	40	93
District B	10	12	31	53
District C	15	10	12	37
Total	46	54	83	183

Expected frequencies (variables perfectly independent):

	Malaria	Chikungunya	Dengue	Total
District A	19	21	30	70
District B	12	10	26	48
District C	11	8	20	39
Total	42	39	76	157

Chi-square points = $[(\text{Observed } (O_i) - \text{Expected } (E_i)]^2 / \text{Expected } (E_i)$

Parameters	Malaria	Chikungunya	Dengue	Total
	Observed	Expected	$(O_i - E_i)^2$	$(O_i - E_i)^2/E_i$
District A	93	70	529	7.557142857
District B	53	48	25	0.520833333
District C	37	39	4	0.102564103
Chi-square				8.180540293

Critical value of Chi-square = 7.814727903
P value is 0.002817847, which is <0.05, so null hypothesis is rejected.

KEY POINTS

- Planning a research well and choosing the right research question precedes statistical analysis.
- Use appropriate measures of association in conjunction with statistical tests of significance, to quantify the strength of association.
- Analysis of variance, or ANOVA, is a statistical method that separates observed variance data into different components to use for additional tests.
- ANOVA is used for three or more groups of data, to gain information about the relationship between the dependent and independent variables.
- If no true variance exists between the groups, the ANOVA's F-ratio should be close to 1.

BIBLIOGRAPHY

1. Bonate, P. Analysis of Pretest-Posttest Designs. CRC Press. Horn, R. (n.d.). Understanding Analysis of Covariance. 2000. (Last accessed on 29th July, 2022) Available from: http://oak.ucc.nau.edu/rh232/courses/eps625/
2. Leech, N. et. al. SPSS for Intermediate Statistics: Use and Interpretation. Psychology Press. 2005.
3. Overall, J. Letter to the editor: The use of inadequate correlations for baseline imbalance remains a serious problem. J.Biopharm. 1993. Stat. 3, 271.
4. Ronald Fisher. "Statistical Methods for Research Workers." Springer-Verlag New York, 1992.
5. Senn, S. Testing for baseline balance in clinical trials. Statistics in Medicine. 1994; 13:17.
6. Vogt, W. P. Dictionary of Statistics and Methodology: A Nontechnical Guide for the Social Sciences (2nd ed.). Thousand Oaks, CA: Sage Publications.1999.

Referencing and Discussion

CHAPTER 20

Rock D Britto, Raghavendra Huchchannavar, Sridevi Kulkarni, Manjula R

Always be willing to look at both sides of the argument. Understanding the other side is the best way to strengthen your own.
—*Jim Rohn*

INTRODUCTION
Scientific research has a standard order of representing information. IMRaD style is a commonly used format, under the anatomy of scientific research. IMRaD style is followed widely for both journal articles and thesis/dissertations, the most common products of healthcare research in India. The following **Figure 1** represents the anatomy of scientific research,

Discussion
Having a good discussion is like having riches. —*African Proverb*
Discussion is the crucial section in the research, involving a profound understanding of the research problem, critical thinking about the issue, and providing deeper and creative solutions to the problem based on the findings. Paradoxically, it is given the least importance in research. Discussion not only involves the consolidation and interpretation of results. But also effectively filling the void/gap in the literature and indicating the future direction of the research.

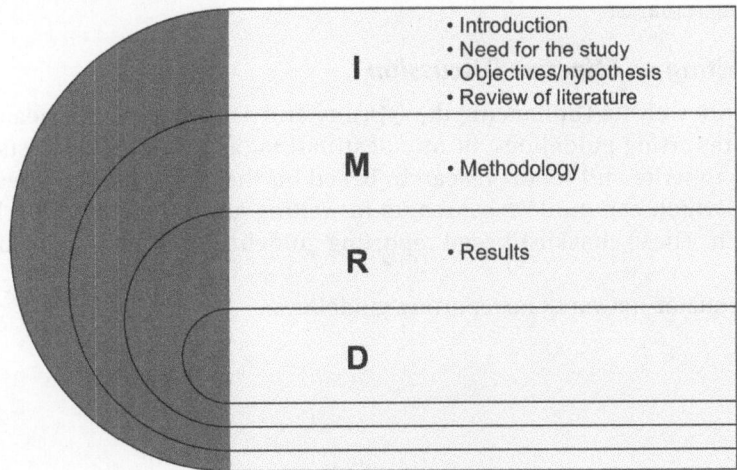

Fig. 1: Anatomy of scientific research.

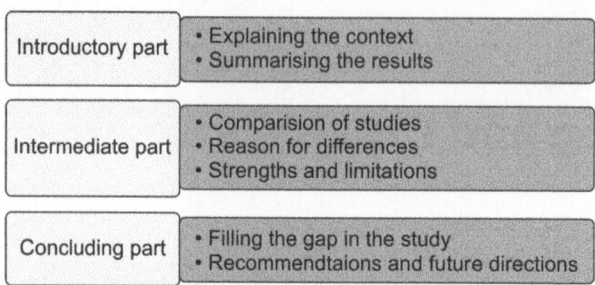

Fig. 2: Components of a discussion.

Components of a Discussion (Fig. 2)

"To solve a big problem, divide it." —*Unknown*

Discussion comprises of three important components. The first part is introductory part that summarizes the overall results. The second part compares the findings of the present research with previous work. It addresses the reason for the differences in the study results. It also explains the strengths and limitations of the study. The third is the concluding part and it focuses on the significance of the study to fill the gap in the field of the study. It also provides recommendations and future directions to the research.

Checklist for Discussion

1. Summary of the most important findings (not the repeat of results section).
2. Discuss and interpret the results in relation to the research questions.
3. Comparison of the relevant literatures with respect to the results.
4. Identify the possible reasons for difference in the study results.
5. Clearly explain the significance of the results in the study.
6. Identify the strengths of the study.
7. Evaluate and acknowledge the limitations of the research (usually bias).
8. State the relevant recommendations for individuals, healthcare providers and policy makers.
9. Future directions of the research.
10. Concluding remarks.

Protip for Writing an Effective Discussion

Equator network website (Enhancing the QUAlity and Transparency Of health Research) provides the reporting guidelines, at one destination, as a set of checklists for various study designs to write and report research. Based on the study designs, these checklists are available, which can guide researchers in writing and publishing in a high impact health research. These checklist-based reporting guidelines will help in making a perfect discussion.

https://www.equator-network.org/reporting-guidelines/

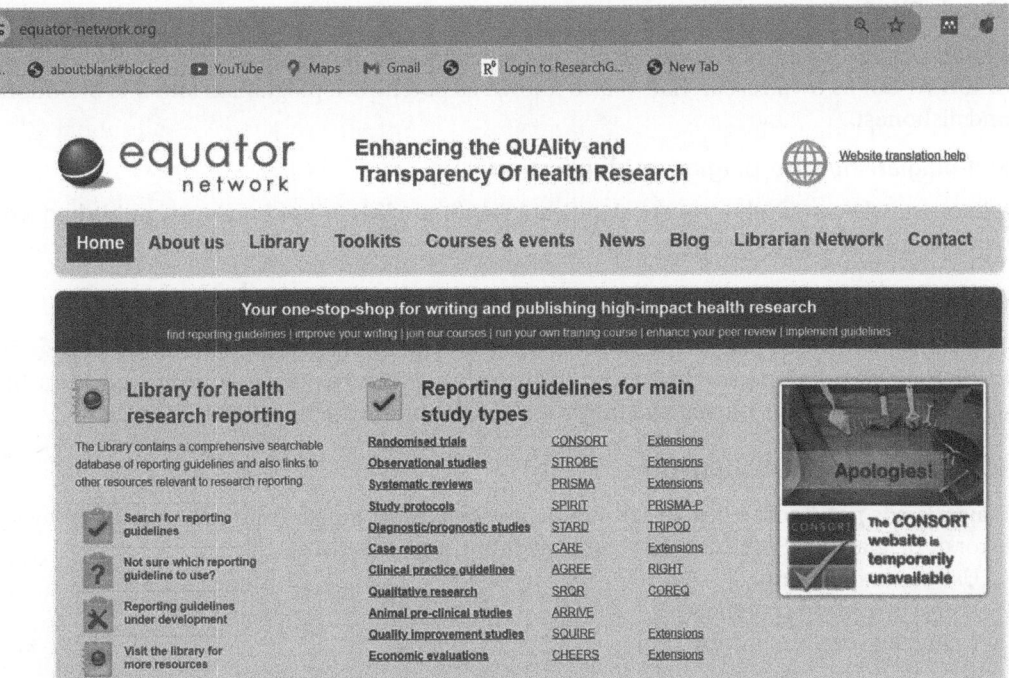

Plagiarism

To steal ideas from one person is plagiarism; to steal from many is research." — Steven Wright

Plagiarisms is an act of fraud. It involves both stealing someone else's work and lying about it afterward. It is the close paraphrasing of another person's ideas (whether intentionally or not) by simply changing a few words or altering the order of presentation and without any acknowledgement of the source.

Types of Plagiarism in Research

There are many types of plagiarism in research. Some of the common types are:

Complete Plagiarism

It is the most severe form of plagiarism. In this, a person steals the entire work or manuscript of another author and publishes if under his name.

Verbatim/Direct Plagiarism

It is a form of complete plagiarism. It occurs when an author copies the text of another author, word for word, without the use of quotation marks or attribution, thus passing it on as his or her own.

Paraphrasing Plagiarism

This is the most common type of plagiarism. It involves the use of someone else's writing with some minor changes to the sentences and using it as one's own.

Mosaic Plagiarism

Mosaic plagiarism may be more difficult to detect because it interlays someone else's phrases or text within its own research. It is also known as patchwork plagiarism and it is intentional and dishonest.

Self-plagiarism/Auto-plagiarism/duplication

It happens when an author reuses significant portions of his or her previously published work without attribution.

Consequences of Plagiarism

The consequences of plagiarism depends on the type of plagiarism, amount of plagiarism, institutional regulations, and legislation of the country. When a plagiarism is proved, the article will be retracted in the journal and the name of the author will be defamed forever.

Methods to Avoid Plagiarism

Plagiarism is not a crime but an error to be avoided. Most journal allows a minimum level of error or plagiarism. Some crucial ways of avoiding plagiarism are,
1. Use of paraphrasing,
2. Use of own word sentences,
3. Citing the source of information.

Referencing

Referencing is a method to demonstrate to your readers that you have conducted a thorough and appropriate literature research. It's the way of giving credit to one's work in the form of citation. Citation is the form of number/ text that correlates with your source to reference list. Reference list contains details only of those works (sources) cited in the text. The entries in the reference list are made in the same order that they have been cited. While the bibliography lists sources that are not cited in the text, but which are relevant to the subject and were used for background reading. The bibliography is arranged alphabetically by author or title.

Need and Importance of Referencing

- To credit a person's work.
- To make work more informative and provide supporting evidence for the hypothesis.
- To get recognition and authentication of the work.
- To avoid plagiarism by differentiating one's own idea from someone else.
- To identify the source of information in an article.

Sources of Information

There are a variety of sources of information that can be used as a citation in research. The most common sources are:
- Books, Journals and Newspaper magazines.
- Conference paper and annual reports.

- Institutional and Governmental publications.
- Electronic sources—websites, databases.

Elements in the Reference List

Most reference lists require the elements in the following order i.e., author's name; date (year of publication); title of document/ publication; edition; periodicity (volume/ issue/part number); series; page numbers.

Referencing Style

There are several different styles of referencing:
- The Vancouver style (most important numeric style)
- The Harvard style (most important author date style)
- Chicago manual of style
- American Medical Association (AMA) style
- American Psychological Association (APA) style
- Modern Language Association (MLA) style
- Chicago/Turabian style

Most journals prefer NLM's International Committee of Medical Journal Editors (ICMJE) Recommendations for the conduct reporting, editing and publication of scholarly work in medical journals.

Reference Management Software

Reference management software helps to download and store references including abstracts, keywords and notes with the references and also with full text. It automatically inserts citation of references/bibliography while typing (cite while you write). It helps to change the reference order hassle free and it produces a list of references based on different styles asked for.

Some of the different management software are: Mendeley referencing software, Zotero referencing software, End Note Basics, RefWorks, Citeulike. Among them, the best reference management software is Mendeley due to its many free services.

Mendeley Referencing Software

Mendeley is a free reference manager and academic social network that can help you collect references and organize your citations.

Importance of Mendeley

- Mendeley helps to minimize the mistakes and improve the chance of acceptance.
- It helps to highlight and take notes of the articles we have collected.
- It showcases our research profile to various researchers worldwide and get connected to persons with similar expertise.
- It helps to track the performance in research through metrics.
- Use Datasets to find figures, images, tables, graphs, videos among million datasets from different open research data repositories.
- It helps to find career and funding opportunities worldwide with the career future option.

Steps for Using Mendeley Software

Step 1: Install free Mendeley reference managing software from Mendeley website. (Mendeley.com)

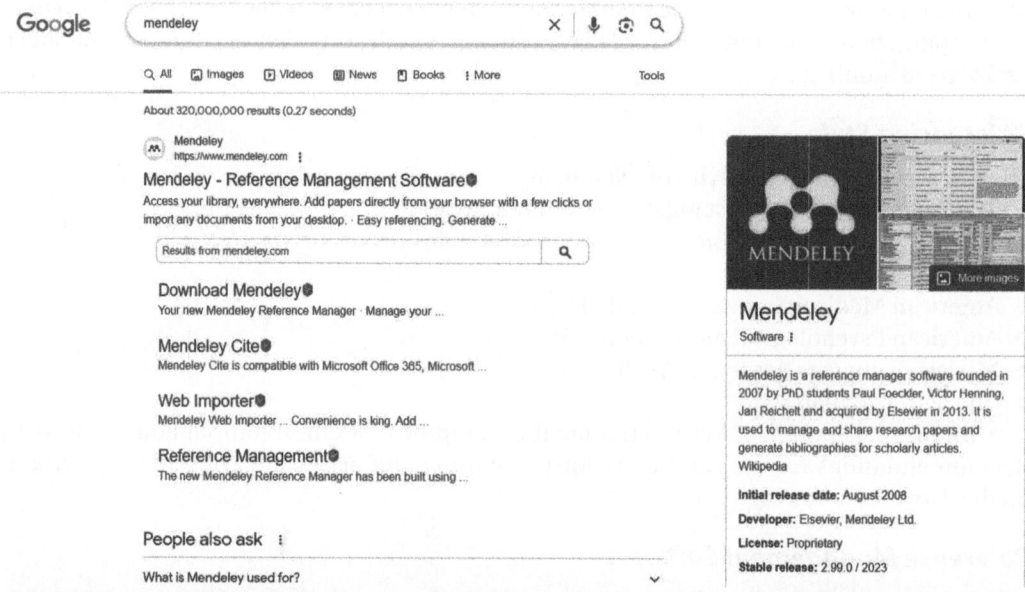

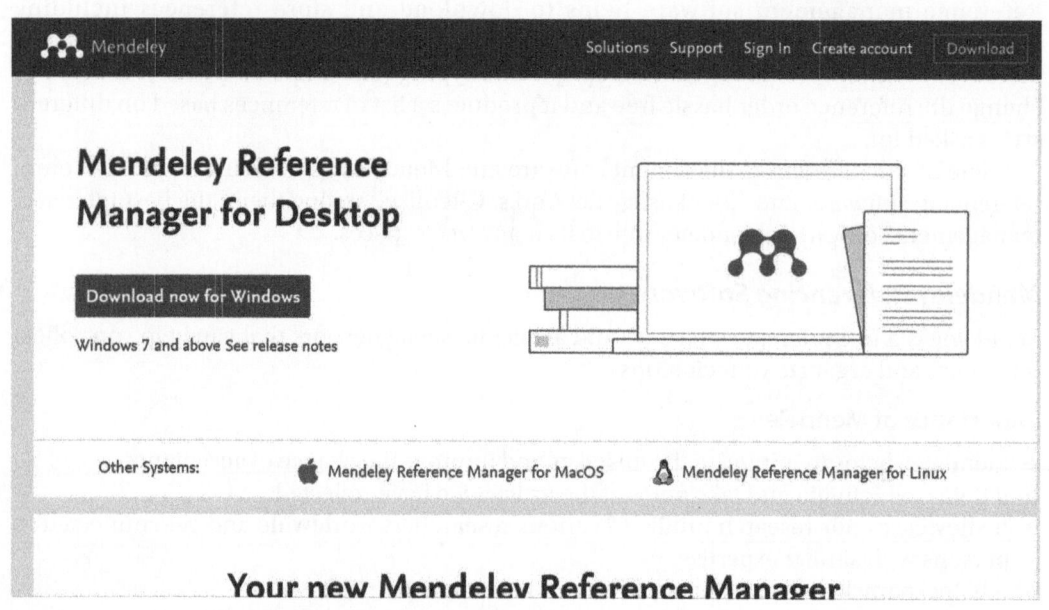

Chapter 20: Referencing and Discussion

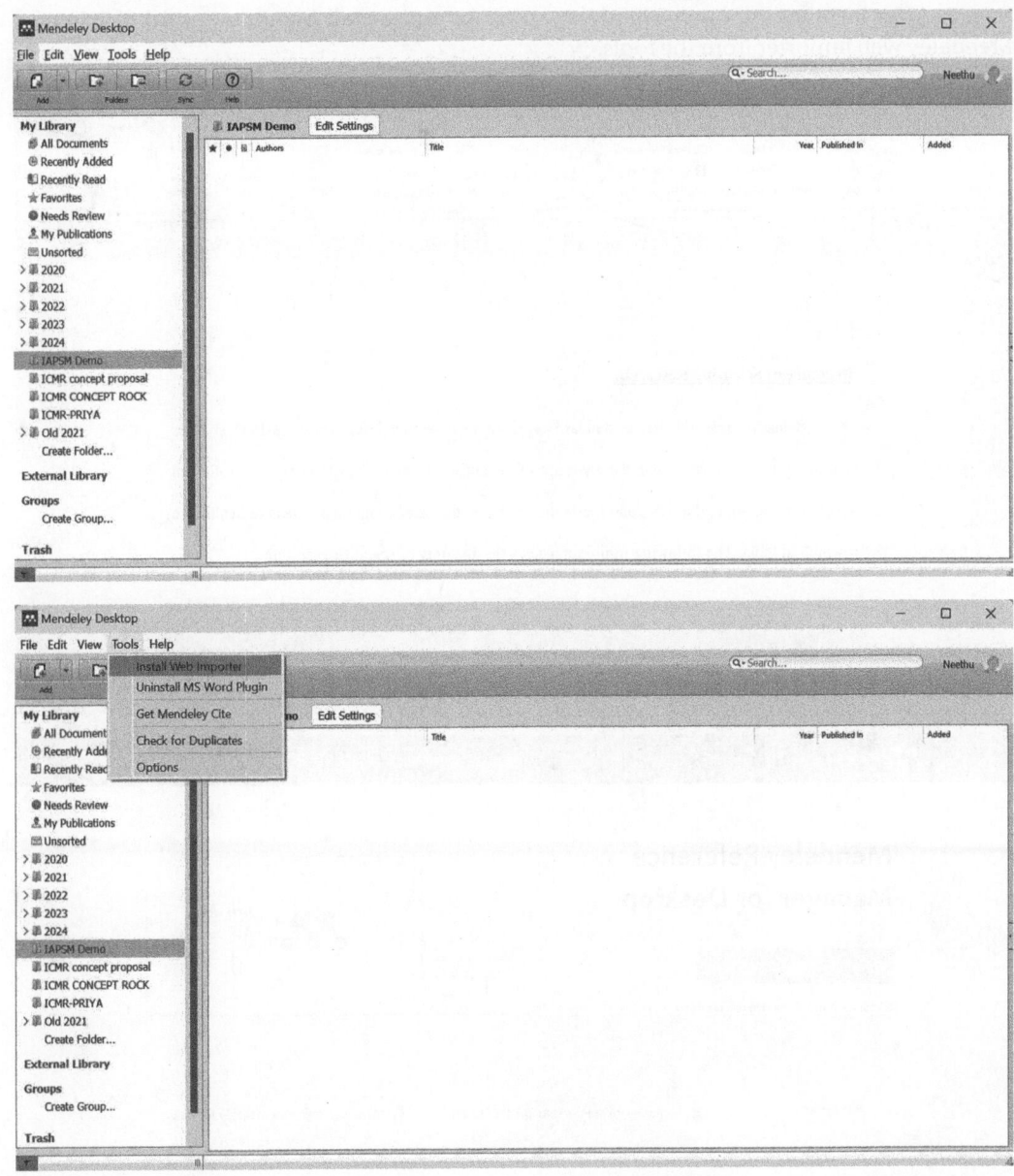

Section 2: Quantitative Research Methodology

Step 2: After installation, open Mendeley software and install Mendeley word plugin and Mendeley web importer from the tools.

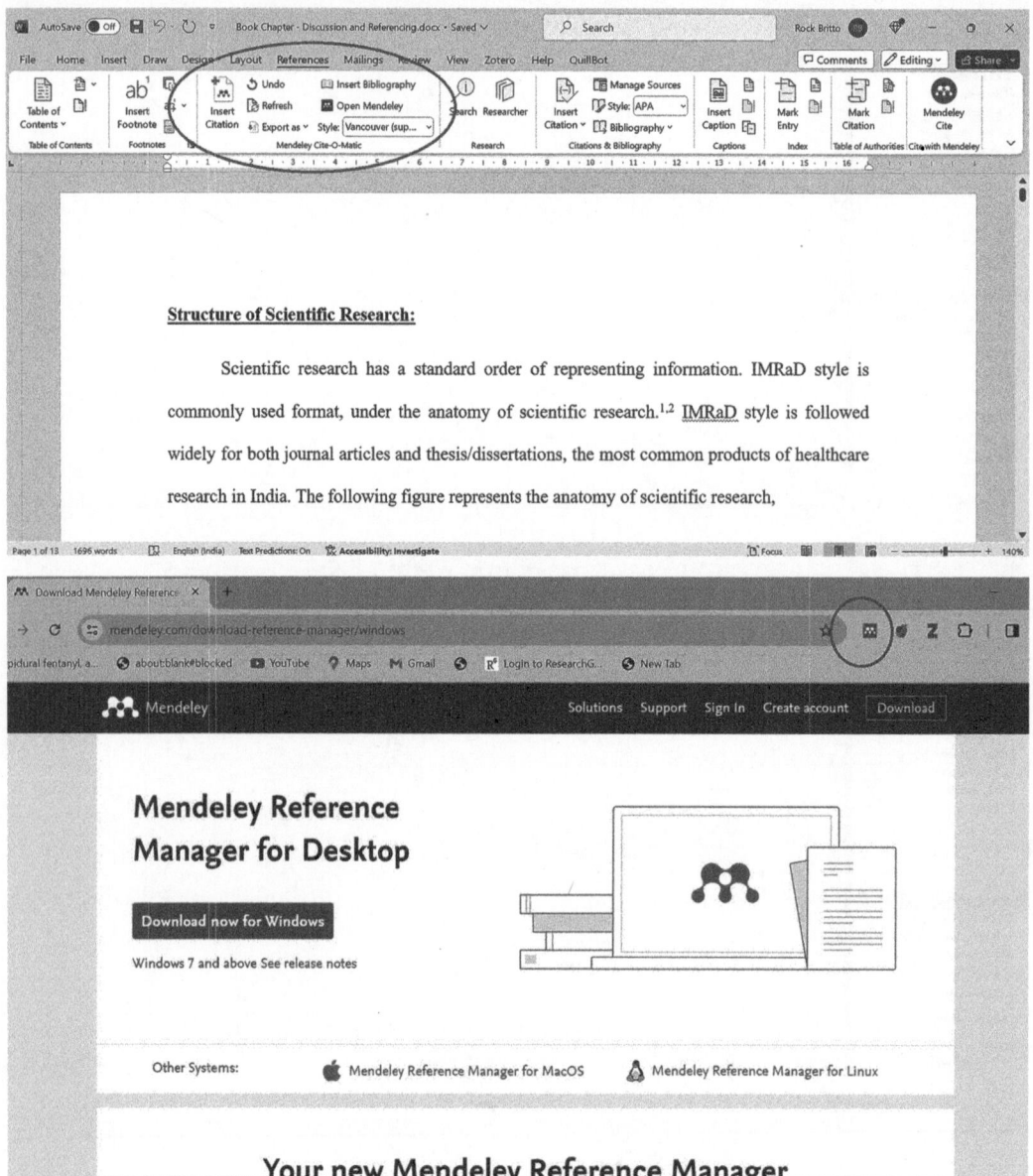

Chapter 20: Referencing and Discussion

Step 3: After installation of Mendeley word plugin and web importer, ensure that the icons are present as it appears as below.

Step 4: Importing references into Mendeley. This can be performed by 4 methods.

Step 4a: Importing references manually

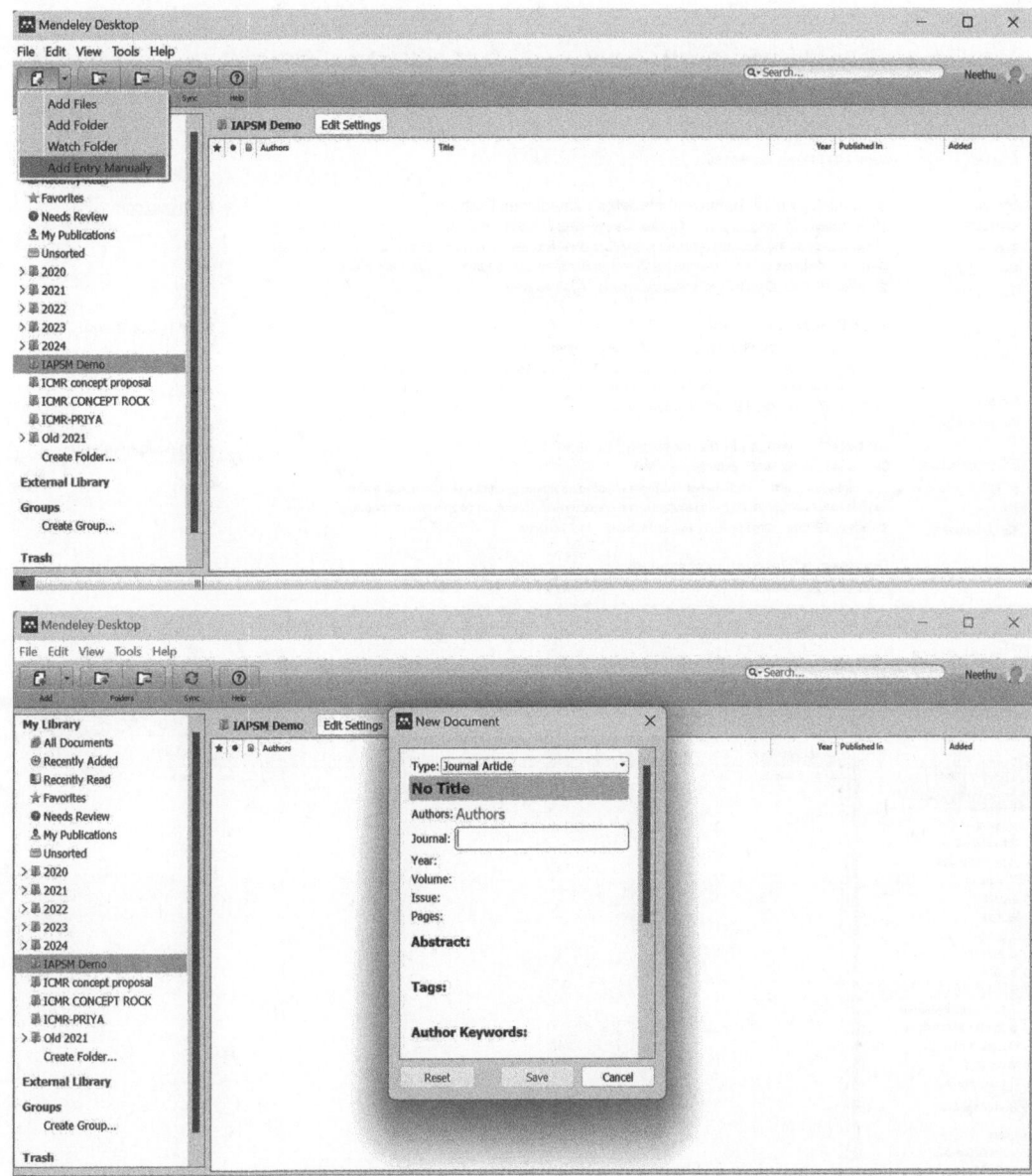

Section 2: Quantitative Research Methodology

Step 4b: Importing references with the help of any databases (e.g., Google scholar). In this method, the required article is downloaded from database and the downloaded article is dragged and inserted into Mendeley.

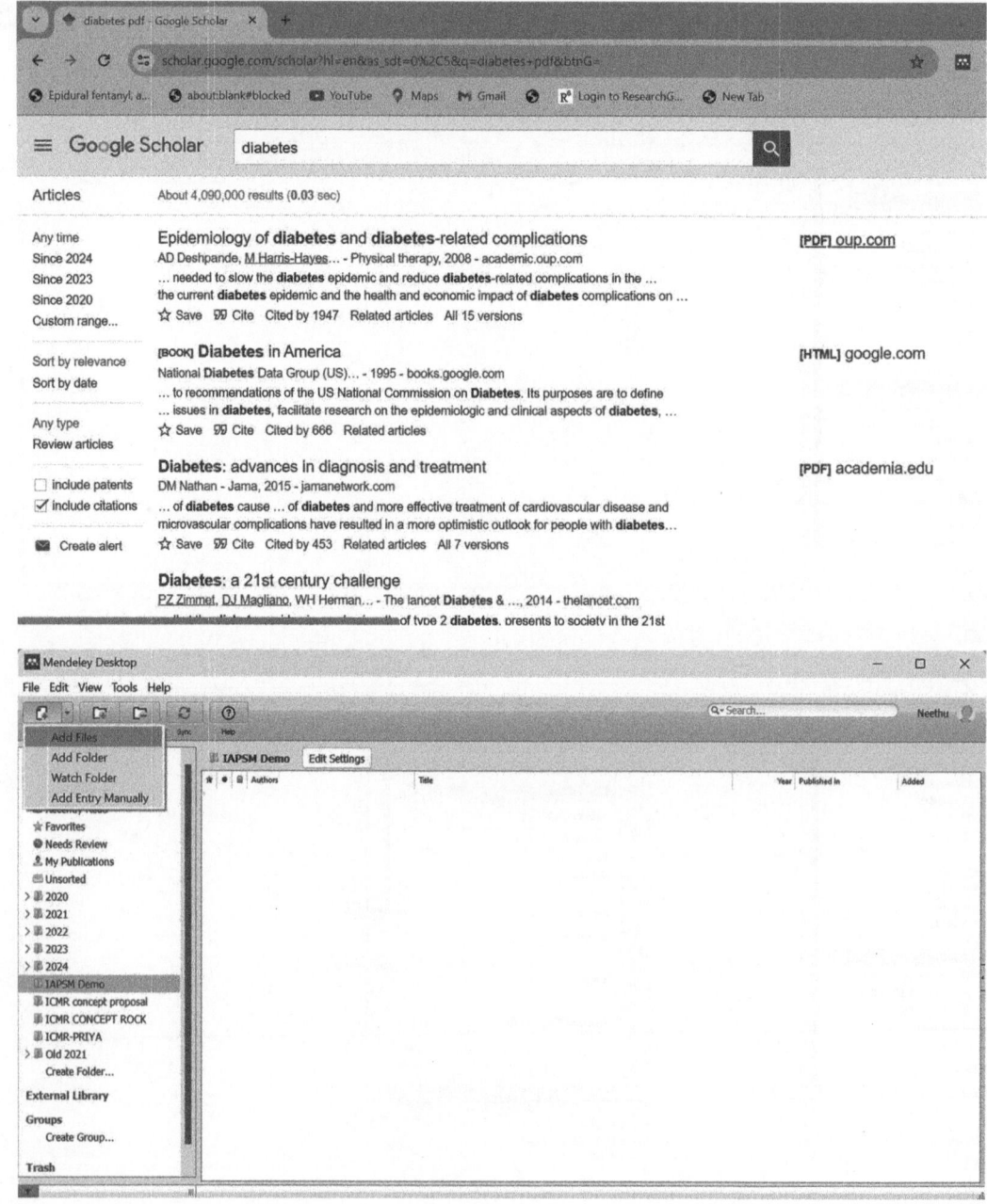

Step 4c: The third method is directly downloading the citation (in RIS or BibTex format) from the journal and insertion into Mendeley.

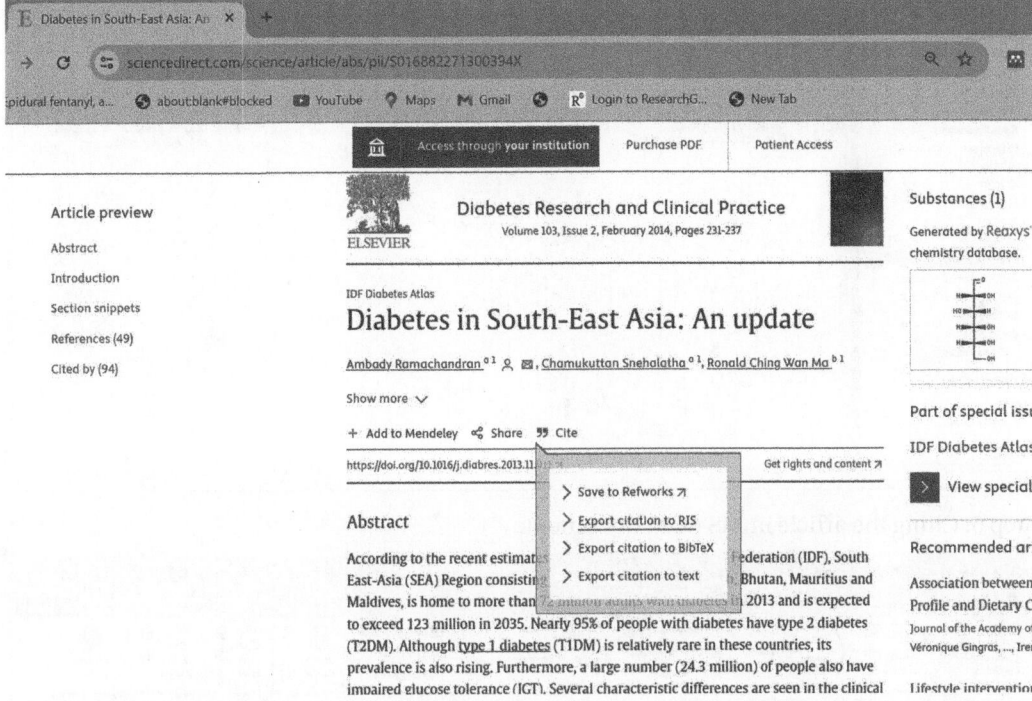

Step 4d: Direct addition of the reference with the help of Mendeley web importer and synchronization in Mendeley referencing manager.

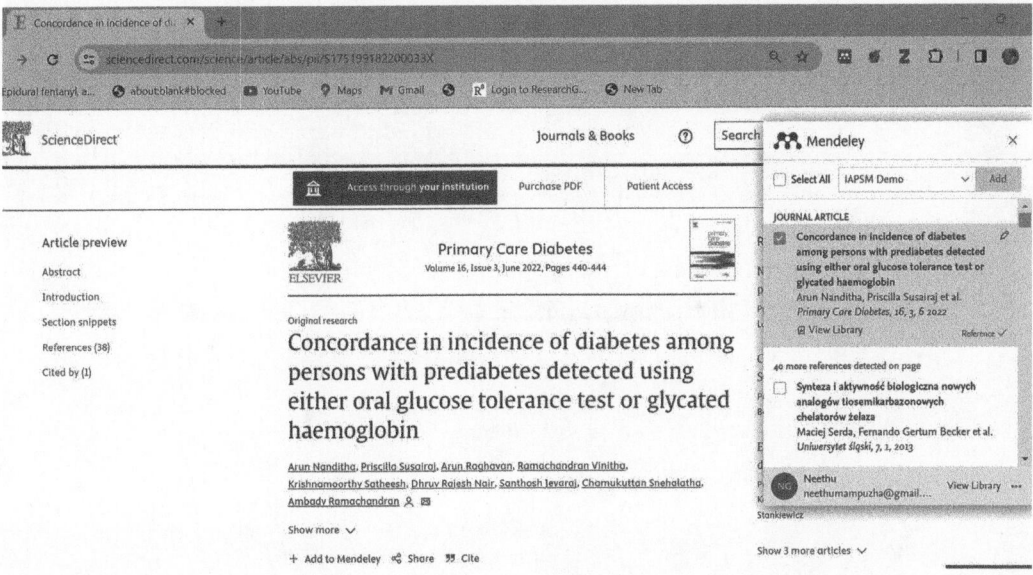

Section 2: Quantitative Research Methodology

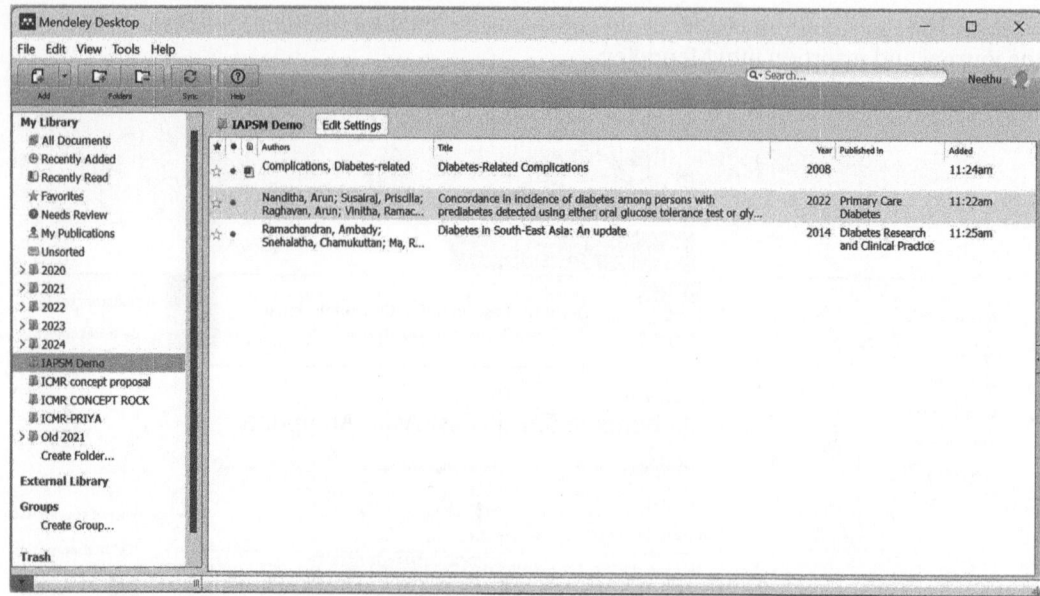

Step 5: Citing the article in MS word document.

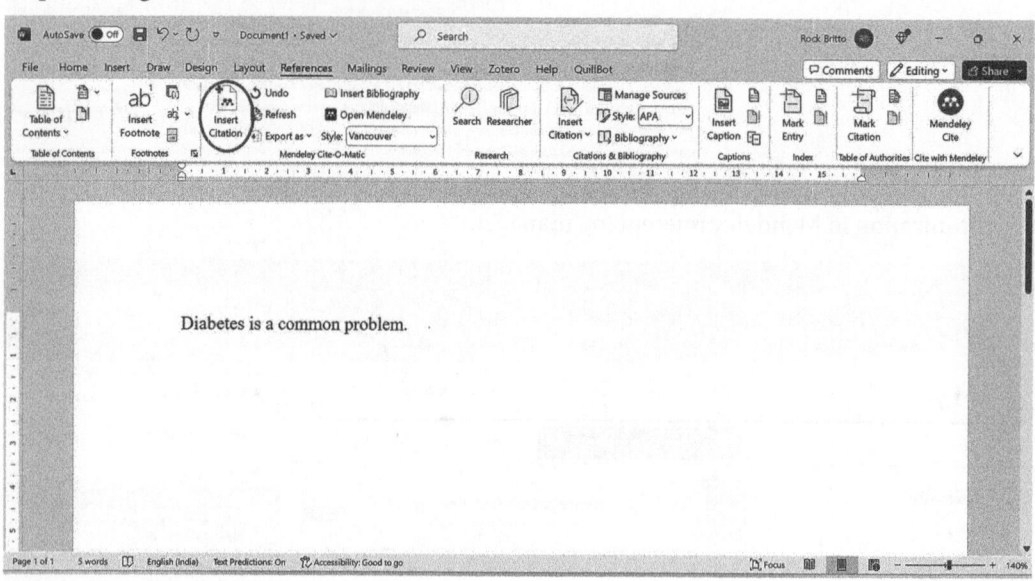

Chapter 20: Referencing and Discussion 161

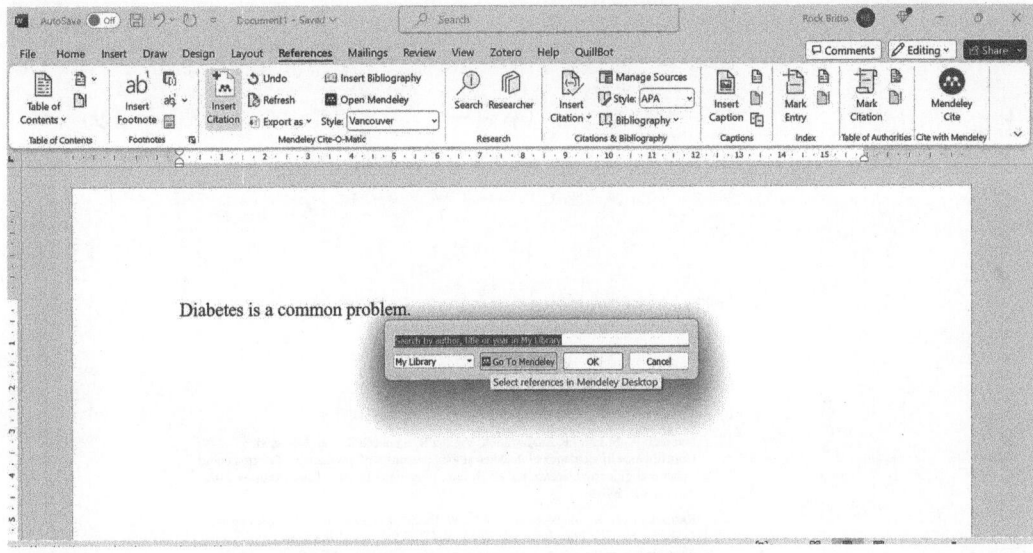

Step 6: Insert bibliography in the reference section in your manuscript.

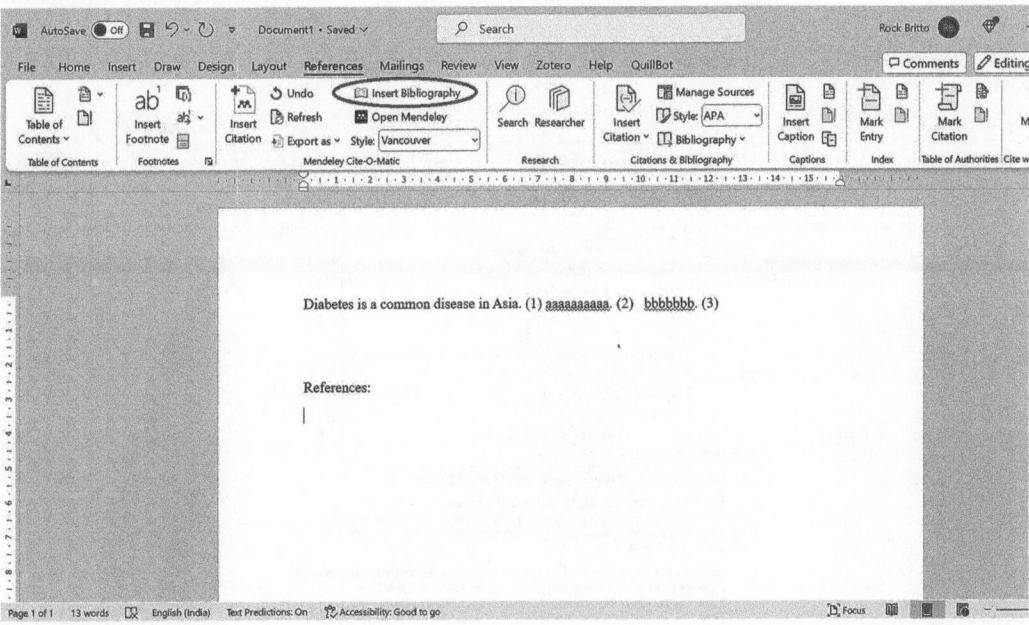

Section 2: Quantitative Research Methodology

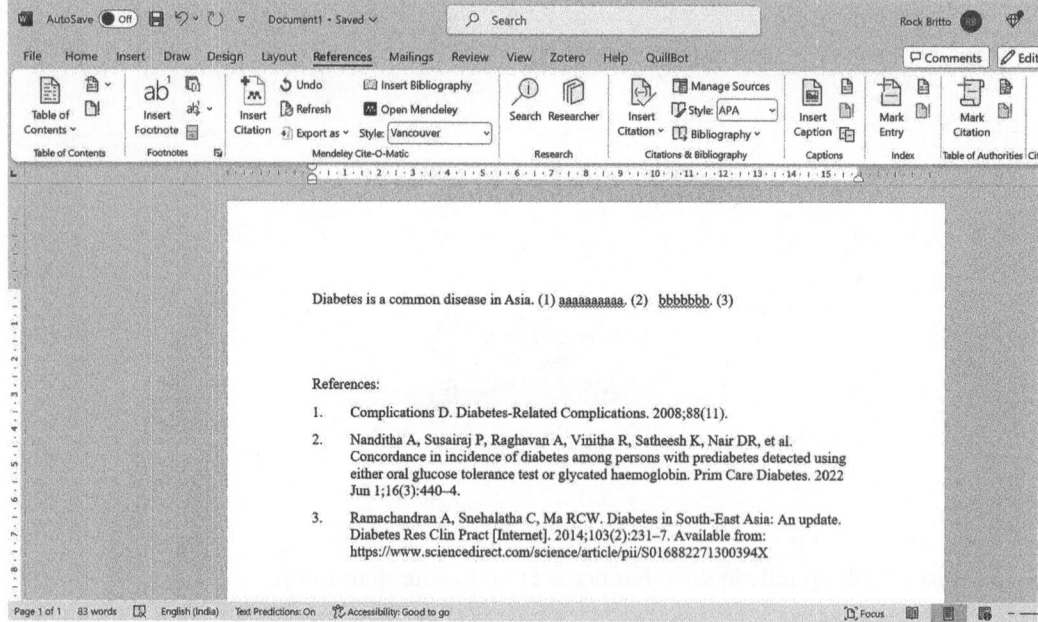

Step 7: Choosing the appropriate reference style as per the journal instructions and citing the article.

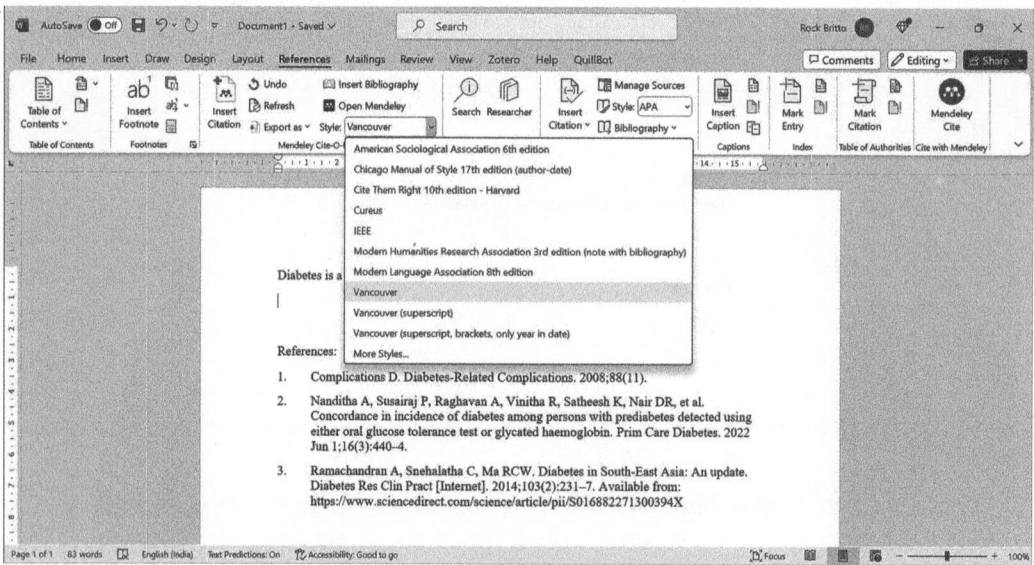

KEY POINTS

- Discussion starts with key results of your study in line with objectives stated. It is not repetition of the results.
- The findings of the current study are compared with the previous study and reasons for similarity or differences in the findings are compared.
- A good discussion helps the research to make conclusions and reach at implications of the study.
- References are the way of giving credit to one's work in the form of citation.
- Reference managers like Zotero, Mendeley, Endnote, etc., help in easy retrieval of scientific information stated in the study.

BIBLIOGRAPHY

1. Article S. Uniform requirements for manuscripts submitted to biomedical journals: Writing and editing for biomedical publication. J Pharmacol Pharmacother. 2010;1(1):42-58.
2. Dhammi I, Ul Haq R. What is plagiarism and how to avoid it? Indian J Orthop [Internet]. 2016 Nov 1 [cited 2022 Jan 31];50(6):581. Available from: /pmc/articles/PMC5122250/
3. Docherty M, Smith R. The case for structuring the discussion of scientific papers. Br Med J. 1999;318(7193):1224-5.
4. Gilmour R, Cobus-Kuo L. Reference management software: A comparative analysis of four products. Issues Sci Technol Librariansh. 2011;66.
5. Hernandez DA, El-Masri MM, Hernandez CA. Choosing and using citation and bibliographic database software (BDS). Diabetes Educ. 2008;35(5):463-6.
6. Mendeley–Citation Management and Writing Tools–LibGuides at MIT Libraries [Internet]. [cited 2022 Jan 29]. Available from: https://libguides.mit.edu/cite-write/mendeley
7. Shubrook JH, Kase J, Norris M. HOW TO WRITE A SCIENTIFIC ARTICLE. Int J Sports Phys Ther [Internet]. 2012 Sep [cited 2022 Jan 31];7(5):512. Available from: /pmc/articles/PMC3474301/
8. Steele SE. Bibliographic citation management software as a tool for building knowledge. J Wound Ostomy Cont Nurs. 2008 Sep;35(5):463–6.
9. The EQUATOR Network | Enhancing the QUAlity and Transparency Of Health Research [Internet]. [cited 2022 Jan 28]. Available from: https://www.equator-network.org/
10. Vieira RF, De Lima RC, Mizubuti ESG. How to write the discussion section of a scientific article. Acta Sci - Agron. 2019;41(1).
11. Wachtel RE. Personal bibliographic databases. Science (80-). 1987;235(4792):1093-6.

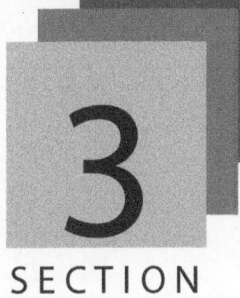

Qualitative Research Methodology

SECTION OUTLINE

Chapter 21: Introduction to Qualitative Research
Chapter 22: Types of Qualitative Research
Chapter 23: Sampling in Qualitative Research
Chapter 24: Analysis and Ethics in Qualitative Studies
Chapter 25: Report Writing in Qualitative Research
Chapter 26: Educational Research
Chapter 27: Practical Applications of Qualitative Research

CHAPTER 21

Introduction to Qualitative Research

Roopa R Mendagudali, Amit Rao, Anusha Rashmi, Chethana K

"I want to understand the world from your point of view. I want to know what you know in the way you know it. I want to understand the meaning of your experience, to walk in your shoes, to feel things as you feel them, to explain things as you explain them. Will you become my teacher and help me understand?"
—James P. Spradley

INTRODUCTION

"Qualitative research" has gained an interdisciplinary recognition due to which (or perhaps because of it), qualitative research is not a unified field of theory and practice. On the other hand, we find a plethora of viewpoints exist on the subject, which may be sometimes absolutely opposed to one another. Researchers and practitioners in fields as diverse as anthropology, education, nursing, psychology, sociology and marketing regularly use qualitative methods to address questions about people's ways of organizing, relating to and interacting with the world. It encompasses a range of methods for data collection and analysis that are used in both academic and market research, several of which have become familiar in health care and health services research. This book aims to introduce the main qualitative methods that can be used to study health care and to argue that qualitative research can be employed appropriately and fruitfully to answer complex questions confronting researchers. These questions might include those directed to finding out about patients' experiences of health care and everyday health care practices or evaluating organizational change processes and quality improvement.

Qualitative research is a type of scientific research which seeks to understand a given research problem or topic from the perspectives of the local population it involves. Hence it is conducted in natural settings and includes a process of building a complex and holistic picture of the phenomenon of interest. It is characterized by understanding some aspect of social life and its methods which (in general) generate words, rather than numbers, as data for analysis.

The goal of Qualitative **research is to** understand a social or human problem from multiple perspectives. It generally aims to understand the experiences and attitudes of patients, the community or health care worker. It aims to answer questions about the 'what', 'how' or 'why' of a phenomenon rather than 'how many' or 'how much', which are answered by quantitative methods. It is especially effective in obtaining culturally specific information about the values, opinions, behaviors and social contexts of particular populations.

Role of Qualitative Research in Health Care

Qualitative methods which are multidimensional and multifaceted can be used in determining quality of health care or services. They offer identification of what is really important to both patients and care givers. It is used to study issues related to doctor-patient especially in general practice and primary health care; patient satisfaction, doctor-patient interaction, in addition to identifying and explaining attitudes, beliefs and behavior. It assists to identify obstacles and barriers to practice change by exploring the reasons behind certain behaviors. Qualitative studies also concentrate on factors fostering the doctor's motivation, in addition to issues related to the doctor's own health. Qualitative work can help in identifying cultural and social factors that affect health care positively or negatively making it helpful in improving service delivery. Qualitative methods can enrich research in general practice by opening up areas not amenable to quantitative methods.

Historical Aspects of QR

It is difficult to pinpoint historical changes in qualitative approaches with any clarity. But the dominant trends in the era if we look into are also not limited by chronological boundaries. Qualitative research has its roots in philosophy and human sciences since early 20th century. Qualitative research methods were first used by sociologists and anthropologists. It existed much earlier in its nonstructural form as a method of inquiry. During 1920 and 1930 qualitative research was implemented as a more focused approach compared to the old unsystematic and journalistic style. Since 1960 a steady growth started in qualitative research with development of grounded theory and new publications in ethnography. Increased number of books, articles and papers on qualitative research and researchers, health-related professionals, has moved to a more qualitative paradigm since past 2 decades.

Need for Qualitative Designs

The distinctive advantage of qualitative research is its inductive and flexible nature of qualitative methods. This offers qualitative methods in **identifying and exploring** items in a conceptual domain of the given problem, **describing** each item in detail (who, what, where, why, and how) about problem under study. Social and behavioral researchers are often interested in **explaining** why or how individuals do (or don't do) certain things, how social systems function or the relationship between two or more processes. Qualitative methods can be an important part of evaluative efforts such as program evaluation as they can provide detailed insights into preferences and thought processes of potential consumers.

When little is known or present understanding is inadequate about the given problem and wants to explore more from participants about their experiences (beliefs, motivations, opinions), qualitative research can be used. It gives opportunity to understand phenomena deeply and in detail, making sense of complex situations or social processes and further helps to construct a hypothesis/theory from the data. Following are the ways how one can apply qualitative methods in research.

As a Formative Tools

To generate hypothesis and design questionnaire for, e.g., to assess community needs assessment for BCC strategy or to design questionnaire on elderly health.

Along with Quantitative Methods as Mixed Methods

When a research question under study remains answered, e.g., health seeking behavior of elderly and why difference in preferences for health care.

To Fill the Gap in the Knowledge, Unanswered

By quantitative methods, e.g., drug abuse in adolescent girls.

Definition of Qualitative Research

There are about as many definitions depending upon the different basis of research
- **Some authors highlight the research purpose and focus:** "Qualitative researchers are interested in understanding the meaning people have constructed, that is, how people make sense of their world and the experiences they have in the world."
- **The authors who emphasize on an epistemological stance:** State it as "[Qualitative research is] research using methods such as participant observation or case studies which result in a narrative, descriptive account of a setting or practice. Sociologists using these methods typically reject positivism and adopt a form of interpretive sociology."

Other definitions focus on the process and context of data collection:
"**Qualitative research** is a situated activity that locates the observer in the world. It consists of a set of interpretive, material practices that makes the world visible. These practices transform the world. They turn the world into a series of representations, including field notes, interviews, conversations, photographs, recordings, and memos to the self. At this level, qualitative research involves an interpretive, naturalistic approach to the world. This means that qualitative researchers study things in their natural settings, attempting to make sense of or to interpret, phenomena in terms of the meanings people bring to them (Denzin & Lincoln)."

While we do not disagree with the above definitions, we do not find them particularly useful in an applied research context.

Nkwi Nyamongo and Ryan preferred the **simpler and more functional definition**: "*Qualitative research involves any research that uses data that do not indicate ordinal values.*" For these authors, the defining criterion is the type of data generated and/or used.

In short, qualitative research involves collecting and/or working with text, images, or sounds. The advantage of this definition is that it is an outcome-oriented definition which avoids (typically inaccurate) generalizations and the unnecessary (and, for the most part, inaccurate) dichotomous positioning of qualitative research with respect to its quantitative counterpart. It also allows for the inclusion of many different kinds of data collection and analysis techniques, as well as the diversity of theoretical and epistemological frameworks that are associated with qualitative research.

Assumptions Underlying Qualitative Methods

The goal of qualitative research is to uncover and discover patterns or theories that help explain a phenomenon of interest; and determinations of accuracy involve verifying the information with informants or "triangulating" among different sources of information (e.g., collecting information from different sources). While doing this process the assumptions we consider are:
1. Multiple realities exist in any given situation or problem under study. These are the multiple perspectives: the researcher's, the participant's or voices of informants (i.e., subjects) are included in the study; and the reader or audience interpreting the results;
2. The research is context-bound;
3. The researcher clearly recognizes and acknowledges the value of the research;
4. The interaction of researcher with the participants and actively working together will minimize the gap between the researcher and participants;
5. The basis of qualitative research is inductive forms of logic;
6. Different categories of interest emerge from the study participants rather than being recognized by the researcher in prior;

Difference Between a Qualitative Research and Quantitative Research in Provided Below (Table 1)

Table 1: Qualitative research differs from the quantitative approach.

	Qualitative research	Quantitative research
Definitions	It is a subjective approach used to describe life experiences and give meaning to them	A formal, objective method used to describe, test relationships, and examine cause and effect relationships
Goals	To gain insight; explore the depth, richness, and complexity inherent in the phenomenon	To test relationships, describe, examine cause and effect relations
Characteristics	• Focus: complex and broad, presents a holistic picture • Dialectic approach, involves complex reasoning goes between inductive and • Deductive and Is reflective and interpretive (i.e., sensitive to researcher's biographies/social identities) • Develops theory • Relies on the researcher as key instrument in data collection. • Emphasis on views, perceptions and interpretations of participants [viewpoints from within the social group-emic perspectives] • Studies motivations, intentions and reasons • Data collection: communication and observation • Question format: open ended • Data format: textual • Basic element of analysis: words, individual interpretation, shared interpretation • Each qualitative study is unique in nature	• Focus: concise and narrow • Logistic approach involves deductive reasoning • Reductionist approach • Tests theory • To confirm a hypothesis about a phenomenon • Relies on control Instruments • Emphasis on viewpoints from outside, i.e., perspectives of observer or researcher-etic perspectives] • Data collection: questionnaire based and measurement tools • Studies actions • Question format: close open ended • Data format: numerical • Basic element of analysis: numbers • Generalization is possible
General framework	• Flexible framework: participants responses influence/modify further course of enquiry to explore a phenomenon. Involves an emergent and evolving design rather than tightly prefigured design • Study design is iterative. Data collection and response questions are adjusted to what is learnt during the initial part of the study • Semi structured methods (Interviews, observation and discussion)	• Stable/rigid framework: participant responses do not influence further questions. • Study design subject to statistical assumptions and conditions • Structured methods of data collection and analysis (survey, questionnaires)
Analytical objectives	• To describe variation • To describe and explore a relationship • Describe individual exposure and group norms	• To quantify variation • To predict causal relationship • To describe characteristics of a population

Philosophical Underpinning in Qualitative Research

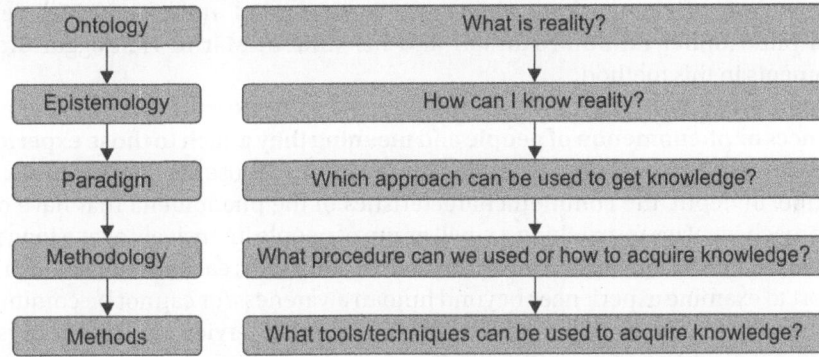

Three philosophical terms are central to our understanding of qualitative research
1. Interpretivism
2. Constructivism
3. Naturalism

Interpretivism

- Deals with how social world is **understood, experienced and interpreted**.
- Here the phenomenon **occurs naturally** and the researcher **just uncovers them**.
- The **person/individual is central** in this approach.
- This approach is underpinned by **two assumptions**
   a. **Multiple valid realities exist**
   b. **Subjectivity is the key to understanding.**

Constructivism

- Deals with **constructing reality** by subjectively engaging with the objects within the world.
- Most importantly, reality is **constructed incrementally** based on a **cluster of ideas derived from experiences, language and concepts forming a theory**
- The **person/individual is central** in this approach.
- **Example:** If we were to understand how an obese person perceive their self-image we need to construct a picture of reality by gaining knowledge regarding his family history, norms, beliefs, genetics, nutrition, occupation, exercise, hobbies and limitations to find answers.

Naturalism

- To understand the **participant holistically**, there is a need to **study them in their natural setting** where their cultural and social contexts are preserved.
- **Setting (social/cultural) is central** in this approach.

Types of Qualitative Research in Health Care

- **Phenomenology**
- **Grounded theory**
- **Ethnography**
- **Narrative research**
- **Case study**
- **Action research**

Phenomenology

- Phenomenology originated from philosophy was founded in the early 20th century by German philosopher Edmund Husserl and his student Martin Heideggar did further developments in this method.
- It is type of qualitative research with the purpose to **understand the essence of lived experiences or phenomenon of people** and **meaning they attach to those experiences i.e,** subjective experiences and understanding the structure of those lived experiences. It is used to describe, in depth, the common characteristics of the phenomena that have occurred. This approach involves researching a small group of people intensively over a long period of time and examines uniqueness of individual's lived situations; each person has own reality. It puts effort to examine experiences beyond human awareness/or cannot be communicated. The primary data collection method is through in-depth interviews and seeks persons who understand the study and are willing to express inner feelings and describe experiences, giving sense of wholeness. No clearly defined steps need to be followed to avoid limiting creativity of researcher.

Following questions are of help in development of research question:
- What does existence of feeling or experience indicate concerning the phenomenon to be explored?
- What are necessary & sufficient constituents of feeling or experience?
- What is the nature of the human being?

Example: Motherhood as a phenomenon, a study to synthesize commonalities of collective experiences and perceptions to motherhood can be done using this type. This type can also be used to evaluate chronic pain suffering in cancer patients, evaluate the levels of satisfaction with services and assess quality of life.

Types of Phenomenology

Descriptive and Hermeneutic or interpretive phenomenology or constructivist approach.
- In **Descriptive phenomenology**, the researcher focuses on understanding and describing the lived experiences of the phenomenon. The researcher is detached and objective in his interpretations and uses brackets to hold pre conceived notions in abeyance.
- In **Hermeneutic phenomenology,** the researcher goes beyond just describing the phenomenon to uncover the meanings that are not explicitly evident. The researcher is an integral part of such study and acts as a tool to make interpretations and no bracketing needed.
- **Data collection** method is through in-depth interviews (sometimes documents and observations), written experiences of phenomenon, direct observation, audio or videotape. Unit of analysis is individuals who have had similar experiences of the phenomenon. Data analysis includes identification of significant meaning elements, textual description (what was experienced), structural description (how was it experienced), and description of 'essence' of experience. Findings described from subject's point-of-view will be reported. Researcher identifies themes and structural explanation of findings is developed. One **criticism** to this type of study is **risk of bias** due to researcher's pre conceived notions distorting his interpretations.

Grounded Theory

- Grounded theory has origin in sociology and was propagated by Barney Glaser and Anselm Strauss. It is used to conceptualize phenomenon using research which is not seen as a descriptive method. Grounded theory is a systematic procedure of data analysis, typically associated with qualitative research that allows researchers to develop a theory that explains a specific phenomenon. The name grounded theory comes from its ability to induce a theory grounded in the reality of study participants.

- The **purpose of** grounded theory is to discover or generate theory in the context of the social process being studied. Used to examine **social and psychological structures** that exist in **natural setting** and seeks to **establish a theory when none exists**. Grounded theory involves formulation, testing, & redevelopment of propositions until a theory is developed.
- The **data is generated from the ground** to establish a theory and usually **conducted in natural settings**. Owing to the absence of a theory, there are **no pre conceived ideas** needing to be proved or disproved in this approach.
- The primary data collection method is through interviews of approximately 20-30 participants or until data achieves saturation. As there is usually **no pre conceived sampling frame** and **data is collected until data saturation** (when no new data emerges) is achieved. Data is usually collected from **case histories observation, record review and interviews.**
- Data is **concurrently analyzed** by comparing with other participant's narrative. The **unit of analysis** is a specific phenomenon or incident, not individual behaviors. The steps of analysis occur simultaneously a constant comparative analysis, theoretical sampling, theoretical coding and theoretical saturation are the unique feature of Grounded theory research. The results of the grounded theory analysis are supplemented with flow charts or framework diagrams of the major constructs. Even quotations from the participants are also used as supportive capacity to substantiate the findings. Strauss and Corbin highlights that "the value of the grounded theory lies not only in its ability to generate a theory but also to ground that theory in the data."
- **Example:** to examine experiences of a new illness or effect of a new drug.

Ethnography

- Ethnography was developed in the 19th-20th centuries and used by anthropologists to explore the culture specific knowledge and behaviors.
- **The purpose** in health sciences research is to study health behavior of a group of people to gain a larger understanding of their lives or specific aspects of their lives and to evaluate the extent to which people are influenced by behavior of groups and cultural patterns they live in. Ethnography is utilized to describe, analyze and interpret a culture's characteristics on health and related behavior.
- A culture sharing group can be any group of individuals who share a common social experience, location or other social characteristic of interest; meanings, customs or experiences. It is a naturalist approach where the researcher studies an intact cultural group in a natural setting over a specific period of time. Depending on the aim the scope of ethnography can be broad or narrow. The study of more general cultural groups is termed as macro-ethnography, whereas micro-ethnography focuses on more narrowly defined cultures.
- In health care, ethnography has been used in topics related to health beliefs and practices, allowing these issues to be viewed in the context in which they occur and therefore helping to broaden the understanding of behaviors related to health and illness.
- The primary data collection method is through observation over an extended period of time. It would also be appropriate to gain entrance to culture; immerse self in culture; acquire informants; gather data through direct observation and interaction with subjects (interviews), using audio visual records and document reviews. The reporting includes detailed description of characteristics of culture with emic (views of participants) and etic (views of researcher) perspectives.

- Ethnography aids in understanding why certain diseases are more prevalent in certain groups through rich, deep and holistic data on a particular setting/cultural group. It discovers culture of health care like reality about the role of nurses in acute medical care, protective role of family members in caring for hospitalized relatives. It also provides insight into current policies and working practices.
- Ethnography like other qualitative methods is time consuming and labor-intensive method. The researcher in the natural setting is always an outsider and his interpretations are subject to debate. Ethnography carries risk of Hawthorne effect, i.e., participants change their behaviour when they are being observed.

Example: Study on rape victims in crisis shelter, study of children in foster care, study of ethnic/tribal groups.

Narrative Research

- Narrative research is a type of study where the intention of the researcher is to have verbal recounting of life events in the form of a narration or story. It focuses on exploring the life of an individual and is ideally suited to tell the stories of individual experiences.
- The purpose is to use 'story telling' as a method in communicating an individual's experience to the large audience. The origins of narrative inquiry extend to humanities including anthropology, literature, psychology, education, history and sociology.
- The philosophy of this type of research draws from interpretivist and constructivist approach. Narrative research encompasses the study of individual experiences and learning the significance of those experiences.
- The process of data collection include mainly interviews, field notes, letters, photographs, diaries and documents collected and discussions which are transformed from, by and/or about participants into literary story format (creative nonfiction) from one or more individuals.

Types of Narrative Research

- **Restitution narrative:** Participants discuss how they got well from their illness. The term 'restitution narrative' describes the hope to be returned to a premorbid condition of health as soon as possible when we fall in illness or accidental impairment and it is expected that miracle of restitutions happen with use of modern medicine though wide range of illness and disability still don't have cure. In such scenario the restitution narrative fails. This study attempts to create space between health and illness.
- **Chaos narrative:** Chaos narratives imagine a world where life can never get better, i.e. the opposite of restitution. This study attempts to create space of the failed restitution, within which to explore the iatrogenic and disabling effects on bodies and minds living in a society that has come to expect not to suffer when illness or disability is incurable and chronic. Here chronically ill individuals discuss their suffering. Stories are chaotic as the events are recounted as the person experiences them. Hence, they lack any narrative order. Chaos stories are anxiety provoking and because of this anxiety they are hard to hear. The storyteller does not see him or herself as being in control of events, but instead are swept along by a series of unpredictable events.
- **Quest narrative:** The participants suffering brings knowledge which is then shared with the audience and willing to educate others.
  - **Data analysis includes** "re-storying of stories" and developing themes usually in chronological order of events. Narrative research is a valuable approach in health care research, to gain deeper insight into patient's experiences. The individual experiences can be of therapeutic use to the participants.

Case Study

- Case studies are believed to have originated in 1829 by Frederic Le Play. Case studies are rooted in several disciplines, including science, education, medicine, and law. Case studies are **retrospective investigation into a written case or an event.**
- **The purpose of the case studies is the description and in-depth analysis of the case(s) or issues illustrated by the case(s),** explores in-depth the experience of a single entity or phenomenon bounded by time and activity (one person, family, group, community, institution, a program, event, or any social group).
- Case studies are to be used when the researcher wants to focus on how and why given phenomenon occurs and to further understand the phenomenon ('the case') and case studies can also be used if the boundaries between the context and phenomena are not clear. The behavior of the case is to be observed, not manipulated in this method.
- A variety of data collection procedures over a sustained period of time have been used in the case studies like a descriptive record of an individual's experiences, field notes, journals, logs, one to one interviews, direct observation and historical documentation and/or behaviors kept by an outside observer.

  Example: Study of a highly successful school in slums, study on a highly successful intervention in rural areas producing good outcomes with minimal resources.

Types of Case Study

- **Intrinsic case study**: It is typically undertaken to learn about a unique phenomenon. The researcher should define the uniqueness of the phenomenon, which distinguishes it from all others.

  Example: Symptom distress in children with cancer.
- **Instrumental case study**: uses a particular case (some of which may be better than others) to gain a broader appreciation of an issue or phenomenon. It seeks deeper understanding on a particular issue to give a focused analysis.
- **Collective case study**: It is instrumental case study extended to include several cases with phenomena under study. It seeks to study multiple cases simultaneously or sequentially in an attempt to generate a still broader appreciation of a particular issue.
  - Case study is an objective study especially suited for sensitive topics producing emotional pain, embarrassment or trauma to participants, inaccessible situations and when methods are considered unethical for other study methods.
  - Repeated reviewing and sorting of the voluminous and detail-rich data are integral to the analysis. Data will need to be organized and coded to allow the key issues, as themes and cross-case themes.

Action Research

- In the 1940s, Action research became popular and Kurt Lewin (1946) was influential in spreading action research by helping social workers in improving their practice.

  Action research is a value-based, action-oriented research, such as in participatory action research (PAR).
- In this design, mixing the value commitments of different traditions (e.g., bias-free from quantitative and bias-laden from qualitative), the use of diverse methods, and a focus on action solutions is accepted. It should also be stressed that action research is concerned with the actual practices.
- It seeks action to improve the quality of care by implementing sustainable change in practice and study the effects of the action that was taken. It combines involvement and improvement.

- It involves learning about the real, material, concrete, particular practices of particular people in particular places. The solutions are sought in one particular problem in one particular hospital or health care setting. The implementation of solutions occurs as an actual part of the research process without any delay.
- The study starts with the research question, data collection to find the issue, develop interventions to overcome the issue. Then plan a proposed change/action, implement the change and find the effect of these interventions. It is the method where **research and action go hand in hand**. There is no goal of trying to generalize the findings of the study, as is the case in quantitative research studies.

Participatory Action Research

It is a special kind of community-based action research in which there is collaboration between the study participants and the researcher in all steps of the study: determining the problem, the research methods to use, the analysis of data, and how the study results will be used. The participants and the researcher are co-researchers throughout the research. According to Kelly, PAR provides an opportunity for involving a community "in the development and assessment of a health program". In particular, PAR attempts to help people investigate and change their social and educational realities by changing some of the practices which constitute their lived realities. In education, PAR can be used as means for professional development, improving curricula or problem solving in a variety of work situations.

Historical Research

- Historical research is the "systematic collection, critical evaluation, and interpretation of historical evidence". The purpose is to describe and examine events of the past and interpreting them in the light of the present and anticipate potential future effects.
- The data is usually collected from primary and secondary sources. The primary source mainly includes diaries, firsthand information and writings. The secondary sources are textbooks, newspapers, second or third-hand accounts of historical events and medical/legal documents. For this an inventory of sources—archives, private libraries, papers need to be developed.
- An attempt is made to reconstruct what happened during a certain period of time as completely and accurately as much as possible. There is no manipulation or control of variables as in experimental research. Hence the analysis must be carried out from synthesis from all data, reconcile conflicting evidence.
- The means of presentation of report are in the form of narratives like biography, developmental perspectives in chronology or issue paper. The ideas are interpreted in terms of the historical context and significance. The written report describes 'what happened', 'how it happened', 'why it happened', its significance and implications to current clinical practice.

Components of Qualitative Research

A good research design, is one in which the components synchronize each other, promotes efficient and successful functioning as a flawed design leads to poor operational failure. According to Maxwell a good research design has five components, each of which addresses a different set of issues that are essential to the coherence of a study. They need not be necessarily ordered or sequential. How they need to be presented depends upon the research philosophy and theoretical framework of the study, the methods chosen and the general assumptions underpinning the study. The components are **Goals, Conceptual context, theoretical framework), Research questions, Methods and Validity.**

Goals

They describe the central research problem being addressed but avoid describing any anticipated outcomes. They address "What issues need to be clarified and what practices will it influence? Why do you want to conduct it, and why should we care about the results? Why is the study worth doing? Find an unanswered question to which the answer is worth knowing."

They help to decide on other designs to ensure study is worth doing. They are crucial to justifying the study. They need to be empirically answerable by the study. One should frame research questions to serve the purpose of the study.

Conceptual Context (Theoretical Framework)

It is the design of concepts, assumptions, expectations, beliefs and theories that supports and informs the research. It explains the main things to be studied in either graphical or in narrative form. The framework addresses:

"What do you think is going on with the phenomena you plan to study? What theories, findings, and conceptual frameworks relating to these phenomena will guide or inform your study and what literature, preliminary research and personal experience will you draw on?"

Four main sources to construct the theoretical framework: prior experience, researchers' technical knowledge, research background and personal experiences; existing theory and research; the results of any pilot studies or preliminary research.

Research Questions

Research questions (RQ) address "What do you want to understand by doing this study, specifically? What do you not know about the phenomena you are studying that you want to learn? What questions will your research attempt to answer and how are these questions related to one another?"

Qualitative designs generally lack an accompanying hypothesis or set of assumptions. The findings are emergent and unpredictable. More specific research questions are generally the result of an interactive design process rather than in the beginning. **RQs** help to focus the study (relationship to purposes and conceptual context); give the guidance on how to conduct it (relationship to methods and validity). **Hypothesis** are statement of ideas generally formulated after the researcher has begun the study, they are grounded in the data and are developed and tested in interaction with it. They treat data as fallible evidence about the phenomena, to be used critically to develop or test ideas about the existence and nature of the phenomena.

Methods

The **methods** are the means to answering the research questions. This is "What will you actually do in conducting this study? What approaches and techniques will you use to collect and analyze your data and how do these constitute an integrated strategy?"

It includes **research relationship** with the people under study, **site selection and sampling decisions**, **data collection methods** and the data analysis techniques. This facilitates an understanding of the processes that led to specific outcomes, trading generalizability and comparability for internal validity and contextual and evaluative understanding.

Validity

Validity, in a strict sense–is measuring what an instrument or method should measure–is a misnomer as far as classical anthropological methods are concerned. Validity in qualitative research tries to address "How might you be wrong? What are the plausible alternative explanations and validity threats to the potential conclusions of your study, and how will you deal with these? How the data to be collected, support or challenge your ideas about what is going on? Why should we believe your results?"

Most threats to validity in the qualitative research process must be ruled out by relying on evidence collected in order to effectively argue that any alternative explanations for a phenomenon are implausible. There are two broad types of threats to validity that are often raised in relation to qualitative research: researcher bias and reactivity.

Researcher Bias

Refers to ways in which data collection or analysis are distorted by the researcher's theory, values, or preconceptions. The main concern here is understanding how a particular researcher's values influence the conduct and conclusions of the study. *Variance* is the difference between researchers in the values and expectations that they bring to the study. However, validity in qualitative research is the result not of indifference, but of integrity (personal communication).

Reactivity

It is Researcher variability which becomes an unwanted cause of variability in the outcome variables. Though, eliminating the ***actual*** influence of the researcher is impossible, and the goal in a qualitative study is not to eliminate this influence but to understand it and to use it productively.

Qualitative studies generally rely on the integration of data from a variety of methods and sources of information, a general principle well-known as triangulation. This strategy reduces the risk that, conclusions will reflect only the systematic biases or limitations of a specific method and allows to gain a better assessment of the validity and generality of the explanations that are developed.

Rigor or Quality of QR Study Design

In quantitative research internal validity, generalizability, reliability, and objectivity, are used to judge the quality of research. However, qualitative researchers speak of trustworthiness, which simply poses the question 'Can the findings to be trusted?' Several definitions and criteria of trustworthiness exist but the best-known criteria are credibility, transferability, dependability and confirmability as defined by Lincoln and Guba and reflexivity by Sim and Sharp.

Credibility

It is evaluating the truth value or internal validity of qualitative research. Credibility establishes whether the research findings represent plausible information drawn from the participants' original data and is a correct interpretation of the participants' original views. Prolonged engagement with participants and in interviews along with the persistent observation of characteristics and elements that are most relevant to the problem or issue under study and member check, i.e., feedback from the participants are required to ensure credibility in qualitative research. Triangulation as earlier mentioned aims to enhance the process of qualitative research by using multiple approaches is using different data sources, investigators and methods of data collection is one more strategy to assure credibility in research.

Transferability or Applicability

Transferability is concerned with the aspect of applicability, i.e., the degree to which the results of qualitative research can be transferred or applicable to other contexts or settings with other respondents (external validity of qualitative research). To ensure this the researcher has to provide a 'thick description' of the participants and the research process, to enable the reader to assess whether your findings are transferable to their own setting.

Dependability or Consistency

The stability of findings over time. It includes participants' evaluation of the findings, interpretation and recommendations of the study such that all are supported by the data as received from participants of the study.

Confirmability

The degree to which the findings of the research study could be confirmed by other researchers. Confirmability is concerned with establishing that data and interpretations of the findings, whether they are clearly derived from the data. This can be taken care by transparently describing the research steps taken from the start of a research project to the development and reporting of the findings.

Reflexivity

The critical self-reflection about
- Oneself as researcher (own biases, preferences, preconceptions), and
- Research relationship (relationship to the respondent, and how the relationship affects participant's answers to questions).

Therefore, the interviews, observations, focus group discussions and all analytical data need to be supplemented with reflexive notes by the researcher. Reflexive notes also included the researcher's subjective responses to the setting and the relationship with the interviewees. This will help in avoiding the impact on research decisions in all phases of qualitative studies.

Critiques

The critique of qualitative research requires the use of different standards and criteria than are used for quantitative research. The different philosophical underpinnings of the various qualitative research methods generate discrete ways of reasoning and distinct terminology; however, there are also many similarities within these methods. The great diversity of available qualitative methods further make evaluation or critical appraisal difficult especially for them who are less familiar with these methods.

- **Qualitative research is too** impressionistic and **subjective:** qualitative findings rely too much on the researcher's views and also upon the close personal relationships with the people studied.
- Qualitative research asserts that a phenomenon is more than the sum of its parts, and must therefore be studied in a holistic manner, i.e., phenomenon cannot be isolated into multiple variables that can be studied independently but studied as whole.

A qualitative study is always unstructured and **difficult to replicate**
- **Difficult to maintain rigor in qualitative studies as it is** more difficult to maintain, assess and demonstrate and problems of generalization exists. It is often suggested that the scope of the findings of qualitative investigations is restricted.
- **Lack of transparency**: It is sometimes difficult to establish from qualitative research what the researcher actually did and how he or she arrived at the study's conclusions.
- **Sometimes not as well understood and accepted as quantitative research within the scientific community.**
- **Qualitative research is** time consuming.
- The large volume of data and carrying out analysis is a hectic procedure.
- Findings of qualitative **research** can be more difficult to characterize in a visual way.

Although **Qualitative research is** blamed for these limitations, in some cases such as health, qualitative data may be the only way to approach and solve a problem. Mugenda and Mugenda point out that qualitative research is advantageous in that it permits research to go beyond the statistical results usually reported in quantitative research. Denzin has argued that, in many cases, qualitative researchers are in a position to produce what he calls *moderatum* generalizations – that is, ones in which aspects of the focus of enquiry (a group of participants) 'can be seen to be instances of a broader set of recognizable features.' In addition, Williams (2000) argues that not only is it the case that qualitative researchers can make generalizations but that in fact they often do make them as generalization is desirable and unavoidable but there are limits to these generalizing possibilities.

KEY POINTS

- Qualitative research aims at understanding a social or human problem from multiple perspectives.
- As qualitative methods are multidimensional and multifaceted, in health care they can be used in assessing quality of health care or services.
- Three philosophical background central to QR: Interpretivism, Constructivism, and Naturalism.
- Various approaches can be utilized to conduct QR: Phenomenology, Grounded theory, Ethnography, Narrative research, Case study and Action research.
- A good QR design should have 5 components: Goals, Conceptual context, Research questions, Methods and Validity.
- Qualitative researchers speak of trustworthiness or rigor in QR study design in following terms: credibility, transferability, dependability and confirmability.

BIBLIOGRAPHY

1. Denzin N, Lincoln Y. The SAGE Handbook of Qualitative Research. 5th ed. SAGE Publications Inc; 2018.
2. Eshlaghy, Abbas, Chitsaz, Shahrzad, Karimian, Leila, Charkhchi, Roxaneh. A Classification of Qualitative Research Methods. Resear J. Int. Stud. 2011;20(20):106-23.
3. Sofaer S. Qualitative methods: what are they and why use them? Health Serv Res. 1999 ;34(5.2):1101-18.
4. Denzin N, Lincoln Y. Handbook of qualitative research. 3rd edition. SAGE Publications Inc; 2005.
5. Al-Busaidi ZQ. Qualitative research and its uses in health care. Sultan Qaboos Univ Med J2008;8(1):11-9.
6. Patton M. Qualitative research and evaluation methods.3rd ed. Thousand Oaks, CA: Sage; 2002.
7. Merriam S. Qualitative research: A guide to design and implementation. San Francisco, CA: Jossey-Bass; 2009.
8. Parkinson G, Drislane R. Qualitative research. Online dictionary of the social sciences. Retrieved from http://bitbucket.icaap.org/dict.pl
9. Nkwi P, Nyamongo I, Ryan G. Field research into socio-cultural issues: Methodological guidelines. Yaounde, Cameroon, Africa: International Center for Applied Social Sciences, Research, and Training/UNFPA; 2001.
10. Creswell JW. Research design: Qualitative, quantitative and mixed methods approaches. 3rd edition. SAGE Publications Inc; 2009.
11. Mack N, Woodsong C, Kathleen M. Qualitative Research Methods: A Data Collector's Field Guide. North Carolina: Family Health International; 2005.
12. Mason J. Qualitative Researching. 2nd edition. SAGE Publications Inc; 2002.
13. Saldana J. Fundamentals of qualitative research. Oxford university press; 2011.
14. Ross T. EBOOK: A Survival Guide for Health Research Methods. McGraw-Hill Education (UK); 2012.
15. Creswell JW, Poth CN. Qualitative inquiry and research design: Choosing among five approaches. Sage publications; 2016.
16. Polit DF, Beck CT. Nursing Research: Generating and Assessing Evidence for Nursing Practice. Lippincott Williams & Wilkins; 2008.
17. Moustakas C. Phenomenological research methods. Sage publications; 1994.

18. Glaser BG, Strauss AL. The discovery of grounded theory: Strategies for qualitative research. Routledge; 2017.
19. Strauss A, Corbin J. Basics of qualitative research. Sage publications; 1990.
20. Savage M. Revisiting classic qualitative studies. Historical Social Research/ Qualitative Social Research. 2005;30(1):118-39.
21. Pinnegar S, Daynes JG. Locating narrative inquiry historically. Handbook of narrative inquiry: Mapping a methodology. Sage Publications; 2007.
22. McCormack B, Illman A, Culling J, Ryan A, O'Neill S. 'Removing the chaos from the narrative': Preparing clinical leaders for practice development. Educ Action Res. 2002;10(3):335-52. DOI: 10.1080/09650790200200190
23. Crowe S, Cresswell K, Robertson A, Huby G, Avery A, Sheikh A. The case study approach. BMC Med Res Methodol. 2011;11:100.
24. Kemmis S, Wilkinson M. Participatory action research and the study of practice. In Action research in practice; 2002.
25. Kelly PJ. Practical suggestions for community interventions using participatory action research. Public Health Nurs. 2005;22(1):65-73.
26. Nieswiadomy RM. Foundations of Nursing Research. 6th edition. Boston: Pearson; 2012.
27. Maxwell JA, Loomis D. Mixed method design: An alternative approach. In: Tashakkori A, Teddlie C (Eds). Handbook of mixed methods in social and behavioural research; SAGE publications Inc; 2002.
28. Lincoln YS, Guba EG. Naturalistic inquiry. California: Sage Publications; 1985.
29. Korstjens I, Moser A. Series: Practical guidance to qualitative research. Part 4: Trustworthiness and publishing. Eur J Gen Pract. 2018;24(1):120-4.
30. Tracy SJ. Qualitative quality: Eight 'big-tent' criteria for excellent qualitative research. Qual Inq. 2010;16:837-51.
31. Mugenda OM, Mugenda AG. Research Methods, Quantitative and Qualitative approaches. Kenya: Acts Press; 1999.
32. Williams M. Interpretivism and Generalisation. Sociology. 2000;34(2):209-24.

22 CHAPTER

Types of Qualitative Research

Hethal Rathod (Waghela), Abhishek V Raut, Amol Dongre, Swetha Rajeshwari, Amit Rao, Anusha Rashmi, Revathi

FOCUS GROUP DISCUSSION

Hetal Rathod (Waghela), Swetha Rajeshwari, Anusha Rashmi, Revathi TM

Not everything that can be counted counts. Not everything that counts can be counted.
—*William Bruce Cameron*

INTRODUCTION

The most popular and widely used qualitative methods in the field of education, demography, and public health are interviews which can be group interviews or focus group interviews. These explore the different perspectives of the participants on a particular topic or a program which are based on constructivist paradigm.

Originally called as focus group interviews, focus group discussions (FGDs) is a technique of qualitative research which is constantly evolving in different disciplines with different approaches to FGDs in terms of research questions, interview guide questioning style, the role of moderator and approach to the data analysis.

Focus group is a group discussion where group interaction is used as a source of data to explore a research topic, here the researcher has to actively encourage the discussion among the participants and pay attention to the group interaction. Thus, it explores the group norms, group expectations and group consensus. They not only explore what people think they also explore why they think so.

Need for FGD

Focus groups, as a method of data gathering, fit under a methodological umbrella concerned with how people make meaning from their experiences in the world. The researcher would be interested in participants' ideas, interpretations, feelings and also the circumstances through which meaning has been derived. It is aimed to record, understand and explain the meanings, beliefs and cultures that influence the participants' feelings, attitudes and behaviors. It is thus of particular importance for exploratory research on poorly understood or ill-defined topics. Another purpose of focus group research is to further strengthen and confirm preliminary data from studies that possibly used other research tools, i.e., an explanatory design study.

Group Size, Number of Focus Groups and Method of Sampling

After choosing the method of choice for addressing the research question, the next step in focus group discussion would be to decide the number of focus groups and sampling for selection of the participants. The size of the group depends on the topic and the context. The optimal size of a focus group would be between six and twelve participants, though it is advocated to have not more than 8 participants to keep the moderation easy, listen to the individual voices, seek clarifications, transcribe and analyze the data. It is the group dynamics and richness of the discussion that is important than the number of participants in the group that is more important.

The number of focus group discussion for a given research question is decided on several factors and there is no magic number, the deciding factor rather depends on the number and kinds of comparisons one would want to make. Though the underlying principle remains saturation of data, others like ethical issues, pragmatic reasons such as feasibility and availability of funding are few other factors to be considered.

Since the purpose of qualitative research is to build an understanding, the type of sampling that is preferred is nonprobability to suit the research question and the phenomenon of interest. The two most commonly used sampling techniques for focus groups are purposive and theoretical sampling.

Theoretical sampling as described by Glaser & Strauss is a *process of data collection for generating theory whereby the analyst jointly collects, codes and analyses the data making decisions about what data to collect next and where, in order to develop theory as it emerges"*. In other words, decisions about focus group composition serve to further elucidate concepts that emerge during the focus groups themselves and is not decided in advance. This is an inductive and iterative strategy in which composition and membership in a focus group may change as the research progresses.

While, Purposive sampling anticipates the use of selected criteria in making comparisons once the data have been generated. It starts with a purpose in mind and the sample is thus selected to include people of interest who are knowledgeable, vocal, experienced and willing to participate and exclude those who do not suit the purpose.

Though there is no hard and fast rule, Usually, a Focus group discussion should run from one to one and half hour. A focus group is meant to delve deeply into an issue or group understanding about a phenomenon. However, there is a point of exhaustion for both participants and focus group facilitators, so it is not recommended to extend a session more than two hours.

Steps in Carrying out FGD

1. Decide how you will carry out the project
2. Predict problem areas
3. Decide what you will need to carry out the project
4. Make a project timetable
5. Decide on the details of the project
6. Review the plan
7. Prepare a question guide/discussion guide (with open ended questions)
8. Decide a plan to do analysis

Process in Conducting FGD

It is important to decide on the moderator and note taker who are knowledgeable, trained to facilitate the discussion and are comfortable with the group members. The participants should be in the comfort zone to talk and express freely.

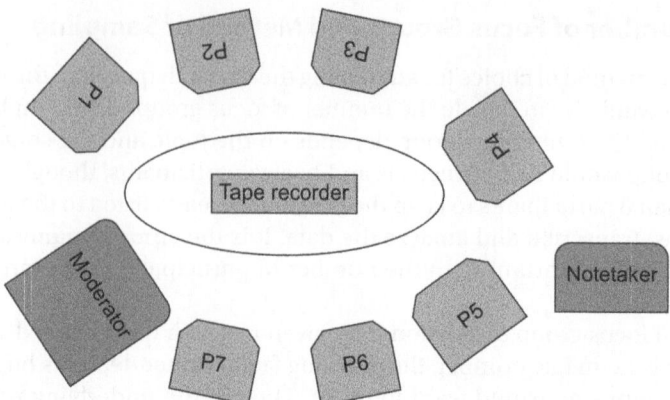

Fig. 1: FGD seating plan (P = participants).

The venue for the discussion should be accessible, comfortable and acceptable for the participants, moderators and note taker for smooth conduct of the FGD. The time and date should also be convenient to the participants.

The researcher should take care of the seating arrangements, refreshments, drinking water and remunerations (if any). The seating should be nonhierarchical, preferable in a circle so as to facilitate mutual interaction and better eye contact among the participants (P) **(Fig. 1)**.

The session should begin with a briefing on the purpose of the research, introduction to the topic followed by icebreaker, self-introductions and some warm up questions. The moderator should set few ground rules such as respect everyone's opinion and there is no right and wrong answers.

The moderator should have the interview guide or question guide with open ended questions. It is better to avoid yes or no questions. Three types of focus group questions that can be sequenced in the topic are, open ended questions, specific questions probing for clarification and an exit question. The moderator should be aware of the participants who are talking and those who are not.

Observer should record the body language, nonverbal reactions, group dynamics by drawing an interaction map or assist with a video recording and audio recording. Note down questions asked and main responses/discussion points. He/she should alert the facilitator to problems and keep a check on quality of discussion and give feedback to the moderator/facilitator.

Interaction Map/Sociogram

It is a visual diagram to depict the interpersonal lines of communications to analyze preferences within a group. It helps to understand the group dynamics and context in which the consensus is building.

All the participants and their seating arrangement is drawn on a paper and arrows are drawn each time the conversation moves from one person to another person **(Fig. 2)**. It is further verified by referring to the audiotape, group transcript or videotape

Few Pointers

1. Avoid questions having answers yes/no
2. Questions are easily understood by the respondents
3. Use simple language
4. Be sure the meaning of the question is clear

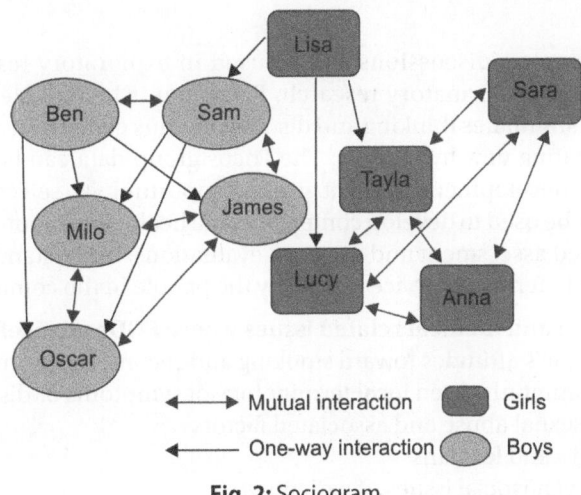

Fig. 2: Sociogram.

5. Keep questions short
6. Avoid several parts to each question
7. Limit a single focus group to two or three main ideas
8. Nonthreatening or embarrassing

Real Life Examples

Focus group discussions used for understanding the reasons for hesitancy in COVID Vaccination in the community to understand the perceptions, questions, suggestions and rumors within the community against COVID 19 vaccination. The information generated would be useful to develop tailored messages to develop health information messages and engaging the community promoting COVID 19 vaccination. A strategy of vaccinating the local leaders within the community, right in front of the general public invoked trust towards the vaccine. This worked well among the few resistant communities.

Analysis

Analysis of qualitative data from FGD can be difficult and time consuming, therefore it is important to reserve enough time for this part. A good ground work on conceptualizing the study well before collecting the data will make this process easier. Analysis essentially involves the following steps:
1. **Transcription:** It is a detailed written document of the entire FGD. Depending on the research proposal and plan of analysis, transcription can be either verbatim or with dialect.
2. **Coding:** Codes are the labels that summarize the short phrases of text, that are easy to sort and structure the data.
3. **Reviewing the memos:** This helps in refining the ideas, coding, be able to decide on the next sample.
4. **Analyzing and interpreting the data:** generate categories, themes from the codes, then interpreting in a theoretical way.
5. **Establishing validity and reliability:** Through consensus, coherence, triangulation and reflexivity. Conducting a respondent check on the findings could be done to validate the results. Being consistent and transparent while accounting for personal and research biases during data collection and analysis.

Advantages

As mentioned, focus group discussions can be used in exploratory research, explanatory research and as well as confirmatory research. Participants being able to build upon one another's comments, stimulates thinking and discussion, thus generate new ideas for research and may aid in generating new hypothesis. The Focus group data can be used as one of the steps in questionnaire development, where it gives an opportunity to select the local words and phrases. It can further be used to develop context specific health education materials. They can also be used to do need assessment and program evaluations, understanding the operational issues of the program in terms of service uptake by the people in the community.

A wide range of health and medical related issues where FGDs are useful:
- To understand people's attitudes toward smoking and second-hand Smoke
- Identification of commonly-used local terminology of symptoms or diseases
- Understanding of sexual abuse and associated factors
- Health needs of gays and lesbians
- Identification of psychosocial issues of patients
- In relation to health services, focus groups have also been used to explore issues, such as professional responses to changing management arrangements, developing ways to improve medical education and professional development.

Limitation

There is a potential for bias as the individual or group opinions might get skewed because of dominant participants or moderator. Loss of control on the group discussion is a possibility for the moderator or the participants leading to deviation from the topic and waste time. Focus groups may not be appropriate in certain situations where the research questions are directed to elicit potentially sensitive or personal information that participants might feel intimidated to share within a larger group, e.g., menstruation, domestic violence, female infanticide, etc. They are also not appropriate to measure the attitudes.

KEY POINTS

- FGDs are key in qualitative research, especially in education and public health, to gather diverse perspectives and understandings.
- They typically involve 6–12 participants, chosen through specific sampling methods like purposive or theoretical sampling, to ensure relevant and rich discussion.
- The process includes planning the discussion, facilitating an open and comfortable environment, and using open-ended questions to encourage interactive dialogue.
- FGDs are valuable for exploring new ideas and community needs, but they must be carefully managed to avoid biases and accommodate sensitive topics.

BIBLIOGRAPHY

1. COVID-19 focus group discussion guide for communities. [Internet]. [cited 2022 Feb 1]. Available from: https://www.unicef.org/media/65966/file/COVID-19%20focus%20group%20discussion%20guide%20for%20communities.pdf.
2. Dongre A, Desmukh P. Practical Guide: Qualitative Methods in Health and Educational Research.1st edition. Chennai: Notion Press; 2021.
3. Eeuwijk PV, Angehrn Z. How to Conduct a Focus Group Discussion (FGD). Methodological Manual.Base: University of Basel: 2017 [cited 2023 Apr 3]; Available from: https://www.zora.uzh.ch/id/eprint/150640.

IN-DEPTH INTERVIEWS

Abhishek V Raut, Amit Rao, Anusha Rashmi, Revathi

"You may have heard the world is made up of atoms and molecules, but it's really made up of stories. When you sit with an individual that's been here, you can give quantitative data a qualitative overlay."

—William Turner

INTRODUCTION

In-depth interview is a method of data collection in qualitative studies providing a vivid picture of participant's perspective on a research topic by conducting interviews. The participant is considered an **Expert** and the interviewer/researcher is the **student**. **In-depth interviews are one to one interview usually conducted face to face to understand** individual perspectives and Participant's feelings, opinions and experiences on the research topic. Difference between In-depth Interviews and Focus Group discussion tabulated in **Table 1**.

Guidelines for Interviewers

- Are neutral.
- Use interview guide.
- Listen attentively.
- Use follow up questions or probes based on the responses.
- Do not lead the discussion based on pre conceived notions.
- Do not express approval/disapproval to the response of the participant.
- Collect data using tape/video recorders, notes taken during the interviews.
- Expand the notes taken within 24 hours of the interview.

Steps Involved in Conducting and in-depth Interview

Before the Interview

- **Be familiar with research documents:** Familiarize with informed consent document. Understand the purpose of the study. Prepare an interview guide and be familiar with it. Choose your respondents purposively.

Table 1: Difference between in-depth interviews and focus group discussion.

	In-depth interviews	Focus group discussion
Ideal for	Elicit individual feelings, experiences and opinions on a topic Sensitive topics needing participant's privacy.	Identify group norms and their opinions Discovering variety within the population
Strength	In-depth responses are elicited Gives an interpretive perspective to different beliefs and customs and their connections and relationships to the participant	Elicit a range of norms and opinions in a short time Discussion aids participation and stimulates responses and reactions

- **Who should you interview?** This will be determined by your research objectives. Respondents for in-depth interview may be selected through direct observation or through key informants or through snow ball or during other participatory learning and action methods (e.g., social mapping, transect walk, pile sorting, etc.).

Some questions to ask yourself which usually help are:
- Why are you conducting this study?
- What do you want to learn from this research?
- What decisions will you need to make once the research is completed?
- Whose feelings, beliefs, attitudes and preferences will help you/your community to make the decisions?
- Who will be most affected by the decisions you will make?

Components of an in-Depth Interview Guide

Purpose and introduction: Interviewers should introduce themselves, the topic and the reason the research is being conducted. Emphasize the social value of the research.
- **Questions with (suggested) probes:** In an in-depth interview, the questions themselves make up the vast majority of the guide. Include a priori probes, sub-questions or follow up questions included to explore specific aspects of an issue wherever felt required.
- **Conclusion:** The interviewer ends the interview by asking if respondents have any last suggestions or comments about the topic.

Preparing an IDI Guide
- **Keep questions simple:** Think of the shortest, most direct way to ask a question. Avoid questions with multiple interpretations or a question that is really asking two questions at once.
- **Ask open-ended questions:** Questions should reveal what respondents are thinking—not what you think they are thinking. They should encourage an expansive, detailed reply.
- **Closed-ended questions are not off-limits:** Use them to narrow responses later in the guide, to bring greater focus to key questions or clarify and confirm points.
- **Ask effective probing questions:** Probes reveal greater detail by clarifying or expanding upon earlier responses.
- **Examples include:** *What else, what does that mean to you, help me understand,* etc.
- **Ask respondents to think back:** Ask respondents to "think back" to a specific event and reflect on their personal experience, what others have said" or popular opinion.
- **Minimum use of "why":** Why" puts respondents on the defensive. Can sound like an interrogation, feel inflammatory or rude, so consider alternatives. Instead of "Why do you prefer that type of program," ask "What are the major reasons, you prefer that type of program? What do you like about it?"
- **Be cautious about giving examples:** By giving examples, you risk limiting respondents' responses (they may not think beyond the example).

Practice the Interview

Role play with other researchers or study staff. Pilot interviews with people can be done to fine tune the process and improve it. These practice sessions can be done along with the data recording equipment so that there is no confusion on how to operate and manage minor glitches during the interview.

Arrangement for the Interview

Arrange the venue for the interview with emphasis on privacy of the participant. The place to conduct the interview could be a private location, Ad hoc location in the community or a location suggested by the participant. Transport of staffs and participants to the interview.

During an Interview

- **Arrive early** with the recording equipment, interview guide and the note book.
- **Explain the purpose** of the interview, **objective of the study** and anticipated risks/benefits form the study. **Anticipate questions** from the participants and clear the doubts if any.
- **Assure confidentiality** of data collected to earn trust and confidence of the participant.
- **Obtain informed consent** could be oral and tape recorded or written consent.
- **Attempt to conduct interview as per the interview guide**. However, do not forget that an in-depth interview guide is just a guide. You have the freedom to follow a respondent's train of thought and reorder the questions if it better suits the flow of the discussion. Issues may arise during the interview that could not have been anticipated and interviewers can ask additional questions to find out more about relevant issues.
- **A team including someone to help with rapporteuring may be required if:**
  - The interview is not being recorded (to take notes)
  - For safety concerns.
  - To follow cultural norms.
- Can use **separate questions for different categories** in the study (Health care workers, Pregnant women, lactating mothers, children, etc.).

Key Skills of the Interviewer

- **Rapport building** – creating a positive, relaxed and mutually respectful environment.
- **Emphasizing participant perspective** – treating participant as an expert in the topic, engaged active listening with a neutral attitude.
- **Adapting to different personalities and emotional states.**
- **Do not be judgmental. Neutral tone of the voice and body language** of the interviewer is very important.
- **Number of the interview: No predecided number, ideally should be conducted till data saturation.** Usually around 15+10 would suffice, however, even lesser are justified if data saturation was looked for in a rigorous manner and achieved.
- **Duration of the interview:**
  - Interview usually runs for 45–90 minutes. For health system research or in program settings IDIs of 10–20 minutes duration would suffice.
  - At the start of the interview, the interviewer should ask the participant the estimated time available to conduct it.
  - Conduct the interview in a manner that sufficiently covers all the topics within the available time frame.
  - Spilt the interview in two parts if getting prolonged beyond 90 minutes or there are indications of annoyance and boredom of participant.
- **Use of Follow up questions**:
  - Follow up questions are questions used to ensure complete information on a particular topic form the participant.
  - In the interviewer guide, each question will have sub-questions to shed light and provide more clarity to the response given to the main question.

- ❖ **Use of probe questions**
  - ♦ Probes are neutral questions, phrases and gestures interviewers use to encourage the participants to elaborate their answers.
  - ♦ Used when the particular response is unclear or brief or the participant is hesitant to reveal more information.
  - ♦ Example of direct probes: What do you mean when you say........? Can you tell me more?
  - ♦ Example of Indirect probes: Verbal expressions (Oh I see), Mirroring technique or repeating what he said or nodding/acknowledging what he said.
- ❖ **Do not use leading questions:**
  - ♦ Leading questions are those framed in a way as to influence the participant's response.
  - ♦ Example: Most smart people do not smoke now a day. Do you?
- ❖ **Documentation of participant's** responses
  - ♦ Documentation in the form of audio/video recording, interviewer notes and participant's behavior during the interview (e.g., distracted, emotional, reluctant, irritated or scared behavior).

After an interview

Go through the recording (audio/video) of the interview and your field notes on the same day and attempt to transcribe the interview. Reflect on the process that happened during the conduct of the IDI and what lessons do you draw for yourself to improve your facilitation skills for further IDIs. You may want to go back to respondent with transcript to confirm that whatever they wanted to convey has been captured with the true essence or do they want to modify any piece of information. One may modify/further refine the IDI guide if felt necessary for conducting further IDIs under the research work.

KEY POINTS
- In-depth interviews are one to one interview to understand individual perspectives, feelings and experiences on the research topic.
- Participant is considered an expert and the researcher/interviewer is considered a student.
- In-depth interviews are usually conducted on research topics which are sensitive in nature needing participant's privacy.
- In-depth interview guide is a prerequisite before beginning the interviews.
- Use of follow up questions and probe questions are considered crucial in increasing the yield of the interview but leading questions are usually avoided.
- Data collection process or number of participants in the study is usually decided by data saturation.

BIBLIOGRAPHY

1. Mack N, Woodsong C, Kathleen M. Qualitative Research Methods: A Data Collector's Field Guide. North Carolina: Family Health International; 2005.
2. Saldana J. Fundamentals of qualitative research. Oxford university press; 2011.

SYSTEMATIC TECHNIQUE

Amol Dongre, Swetha Rajeshwari, Anusha Rashmi

"The strength of the team is each individual member. The strength of each member is the team."
—Phil Jackson

INTRODUCTION

Systematic techniques are those methods that are qualitative in nature to begin with but use qualification or statistics to get the results, making these techniques easy to interpret and communicate. There are different types of techniques–free list, pile sort, nominal group technique (NGT) and Delphi technique.

Free lists and pile sorts are techniques that are useful in understanding the cultural domains and cognitive domain. Whereas Nominal group Technique and Delphi technique are useful for consensus building on an issue among stakeholders. It is a study of how people in a group think about lists of things that somehow go together.

Cultural domains are list of items perceived by the individual, shared across the individuals, and has an internal structure, where items are related to each other" (Borgatti, 1998) *It is a mental category like fruits, animals and illnesses, etc.*

These can be physical, observable things such as kinds of fruits, foods that are appropriate for healing or boosting immunity, symptoms of illness—or conceptual things like occupations, things you can do to help the environment and so on. The method comes from work in cognitive anthropology. It involves systematic interviewing to get lists of items that comprise a coherent cognitive domain.

Need for Systematic Techniques

In interviews, where primary questions are focused on listing items, like *"what are the traditional health practices in the community?"; "What are the traditional foods that are eaten in the community?"* These techniques can be very useful to understand the culture, values and beliefs of the community before an in-depth qualitative or quantitative research is conducted.

Free Lists

Free listing is a deceptively simple but powerful technique. It is generally used to study a cultural domain
—HR Bernard

It can rapidly explore thinking among groups of people and is suited for engaging communities and understanding shared priorities. It gathers systematic data which tends to give cultural information.

It is useful in health research to list the reasons for farmers' suicides in rural Vidarbha to problems faced by the community-based health workers. Other uses could be to explore local names of the disease, symptoms of a health condition and problems faced by staff/students in an organization, etc.

Pile sorting follows free list exercise and helps to explore the salient items inter-relationships.

Uses of Free Listing

1. To study about an unstudied community.
2. Reflects the ideas that communities or societies have specifically about, cultural contexts through themes or ideas that occur in common.
3. To understand how population defines domain.
4. Identifies the social problem and ways to approach them.

A free list can be obtained by either direct face to face interview or through coding of the transcripts of focus groups.

Steps in Conducting Free Listing

Decide on the domain to be covered or studied.

A stimulus question is developed, e.g., "please list as much as common foods in your diet as much you remember" This may produce a free list that depicts the overall health of the individual, this when used on a large scale can see overall dietary health of the community. Participants can be probed for more responses and to maximize the items.

Use of a large sample of participants of 20-30 people who are vocal and willing to participate will make an adequate sample to study the cultural domain.

Analysis

Calculate the response frequency by selecting the salient item. The most popular method to find out the cognitive salience is Smith's salience score (Smith's S value). The purpose of free listing is to identify the most prominent and representative item in the domain. It is done in two steps, first, rank items on the list inversely for each individual, then divide the rank by the number of items the individual listed to get the Salience (S). Calculate the composite salient score by dividing the sum of salience scores for each item by the number of informants.

The data analysis can be done manually or using software such as free list analysis under microsoft excel (FLAME) or ANTHROPAC package.

Strengths and Weaknesses of Free List Technique

Strengths

- It can be rapid.
- It is cost-efficient.
- It requires less training.
- It can be a good source for baseline data before conducting another research.
- It targets common perceptions and can be used to compare different group or cultures.
- Analysis is simple and easy to interpret and results are quantifiable.

Weaknesses

- It is a not a standalone method.
- Researchers need to be familiar with the culture and language of the respondents.

Pile Sorting

It is a technique to understand the structure of a cultural or cognitive domain, once the salient free list items for a given cognitive domain or cultural domain are obtained. The relationship between these items can be studied by a proximity method called pile sorting. It links human thought processes and culture and assesses the way people conceive of and think about the world.

Steps

Select the list of salient items from the free list exercise.

The participants are given the set of items and asked to divide them by groups (similar items together), they can place as many cards as they want in a group.

Then, they explain the criteria used for sorting in a particular way and will name each group.

For analysis, we can use ANTHROPAC software, which reads the data and converts them into an item-by-item similarity matrix.

Strengths

It might offer direction for future qualitative research. The technique can encourage participant\ community discussion.

It is good for breaking the ice and initiating the discussion about sensitive issues.

Study participants are forced to think analytically and lead them to initiate change from within.

Weakness

It might not give you all the information you want or raise some questions which would require further follow up interviews.

KEY POINTS

- These techniques are useful to understand the complexity of a particular topic in the community.
- Systematic techniques mix qualitative and quantitative methods to study cultural beliefs and reach group consensus in fields like education and public health.
- Free listing involves asking people to list items related to a specific topic, like health practices, to understand what's important in their culture.
- Pile sorting is used after free listing, where people group similar items together, showing how they think and categorize information in their culture.
- Findings from these techniques need to be triangulated with other methods.

BIBLIOGRAPHY

1. Bernard HR, Wutich A, Ryan GW. Analysing qualitative data: Systematic approaches. 2nd edition. New Delhi: SAGE publications; 2017.
2. Bernard HR. Qualitative Data, Quantitative Analysis. CAM Journal. 1996;8(1):9–11.
3. Dongre A, Deshmukh P. Practical guide: Qualitative Methods in Health and Educational Research, 1st edition. Chennai: Notion Press; 2021.
4. Keddem S, Barg FK, Frasso R. Practical Guidance for Studies Using Free listing Interviews. Preventing Chronic Disease. 2021;18.
5. Quinlan MB. The Freelisting Method. Handbook of Research Methods in Health Social Sciences. 2017;1–16.

CHAPTER 23

Sampling in Qualitative Research

Saritha Nair, Maria Nelliyanil, Anusha Rashmi, Sunhitha Velamala

SAMPLING METHODS

Saritha Nair, Maria Nelliyanil, Anusha Rashmi, Sunhitha Velamala

"Not everything that can be counted counts, and not everything that counts can be counted."
—*William Bruce Cameron*

INTRODUCTION

The process of sampling involves principles and procedures that are used to identify, choose, and gain access to relevant data sources from which we can generate data using the chosen methods. These data sources will belong to or relate to a relevant wider population or universe, and the sampling strategy should be able to link these sources that are selected meaningfully with that wider context. 'Sampling' is most commonly associated with a logic that is derived from the laws of statistics and probability and is often used for quantitative surveys. In qualitative research, the logic of probability is rarely employed—yet, its strong association with the term 'sampling' means that alternative logic is not well understood or less visibly practiced. However, qualitative research frequently demands a very alternative logic of sampling and selection. Sampling and selection—appropriately conceived and executed–are vitally important strategic elements of qualitative research that have direct implications for whether and how generalization is consequently possible.

It is not necessary to collect data from everyone in a community to get valid findings even if we have the resources to do so. In qualitative research, we select a sample from the population. How and who to select depends on the objectives of the research and the characteristics of the study population (for example, diversity and size).

In this module, we will focus on how researchers can come to a conclusion about the procedures of sampling and the principles by which selection should be governed.

The Purpose of Sampling in Qualitative Enquiry

What is the wider universe or population from which the researcher wishes to sample?
  What is the nature of the researcher's interest in this universe or population?
  What work does the researcher expect the sample to do?

To address the research questions, the work we want the sample to do is to help provide us with the data that we will need. There are two related elements here. First, by tapping appropriate data sources; the sample should provide useful and meaningful empirical contexts, illustrations or scenarios. However, this is not just an empirical matter–data sources mean different things in the context of different theoretical and epistemological approaches. Therefore, what is useful and meaningful needs to be seen in the context of how well it will allow in generating data and ideas that will advance the understanding and these are always theoretically informed. The theoretical and empirical considerations that come into play while making decisions regarding sampling, hinge upon the question of what we consider as the nature and significance of the wider universe or population from which our sample is drawn.

When we take a sample from a wider universe selection, we must have a clear rationale for the choices we make. Thus, it is important to have a consensus in the beginning on what basis and in what way the data that is generated from the sample signifies the wider population or universe in which we are interested. Most of the work we put in the process of sampling and selecting is to help us establish an appropriate relationship between the sample or selection on one hand and the wider population to which we see it as related on the other.

The decisions about the nature of our interest in a wider population or universe will help in making more meaningful and sensible sampling choices. Whichever applies, must feed directly into the sampling strategy. It is these features that we want to be represented or encapsulated in the sample. Or, more interpretively, the researcher will be able to say something theoretically about these features based on data analyses derived from the sample that is selected. Therefore, we need to work out the answer to the question of what we want the sample to do in the context of the particular project that we have in mind and its theoretical and empirical referents.

Nonrandom Sampling

Nonrandom sampling is known by other names such as nonprobability sampling. The goal of the research is to obtain insights into events, phenomena or individuals rather than to generalize a population as we usually see in qualitative research. In qualitative research, the researcher purposefully selects settings, individuals or groups, thus helping to optimize the understanding of the phenomenon. Thus, the most used method of sampling in qualitative research is purposeful sampling. In purposeful sampling, individuals, groups and settings are selected based on "Information-rich" areas/people. The ones listed below are the common designs for nonrandom sampling. These designs differ in whether they are implemented before data collection or after the data collection has started. How appropriate each of the designs is will depend on the research purpose, objective, and question.

Maximum Variation Sampling

In maximum variation sampling, a wide range of individuals, groups or settings is selected purposefully so that all or most types of individuals, groups or settings will be selected for the research. Thus, allowing the presentation of multiple perspectives of individuals that exemplify the complexity of the world.

Homogenous Sampling

In homogenous sampling, individuals, groups or settings are selected because they all possess similar attributes or characteristics. The selection of participants for the study may be based on specific characteristics or membership in a unit or sub-group. This approach is often used to select focus groups.

Critical Case Sampling

In this method, individuals, groups or settings are selected to bring to the fore the phenomenon of interest so that the researcher can have a better understanding of the phenomenon than would have been understood without including these critical cases.

Theory-based Sampling

In this method of sampling, individuals, groups or settings are selected because they help the qualitative researcher to develop a theory. This method of sampling is also used to expand a theory.

Snowball Sampling

This method is also known as network sampling and is usually done after data collection has started. In Snowball sampling, participants who have already been selected for the study are asked to recruit other participants.

Extreme Case Sampling

In this method of sampling, a case that has one or more extreme characteristics or that is an outlier is selected for the study. The method is useful when we need to select extreme cases and then compare them. For example, in a study of the performance of students, a researcher can select the worst and the best students in class and then compare the causes of their performances.

Typical Case Sampling

In this method, the researcher studies an individual, group or setting that is typical. For this, the researcher needs to consult several experts in the field of study so that a consensus as to what example(s) is typical of the phenomenon and should, therefore, included in the study.

Stratified Purposeful Sampling

This method of sampling is similar to stratified random sampling. In a stratified purposeful sample, the sampling frame is first divided into strata, and then from each stratum, a purposeful sample is selected. By doing this method of sampling we can facilitate comparisons among groups.

Criterion Sampling

In this method of sampling, individuals, groups or settings that meet the criteria are selected. This technique of sampling is typically used for quality assurance.

Opportunistic Sampling

In this type of sampling, the researcher capitalizes on opportunities during the collection of data to select the cases. These cases could represent negative, typical, negative, extreme or critical cases. Opportunistic sampling takes place after the study begins to take advantage of developing events. This method of sampling is useful especially when the researcher is not able or not willing to decide at the beginning of the study about what type of case will be included in the research.

Mixed Purposeful Sampling

As the name suggests, this method of sampling is conducted when more than one method of sampling is used for the research. For example, if research involves selecting two samples:

one may be selected by extreme case sampling and the other may be selected by critical case sampling method. This helps to compare the results obtained from both samples. Mixed purposeful sampling can also be helpful in data triangulation.

Convenience Sampling

In convenience sampling, individuals or groups that are available and are willing to participate in the research are selected to be part of the research. It is also referred to as "volunteer sampling" or 'accidental sampling." For example, selecting a neighbor or roommate.

Quota Sampling

In quota sampling, the researcher decides on the specific quotas or characteristics of sample members that need to be selected. For example, a researcher may want to include a certain social class or religion in the sample, thus picking quotas of each. Followed by which the researcher purposively picks the subjects to fit the identified quotas. The major limitation of this sampling design is that only those who are accessible during the time of selection have a chance of being selected.

Random Purposive Sampling

In the random purposive sampling method, the researcher chooses cases randomly from a sampling frame, which consists of a sample that is purposefully selected. In this method, the researcher first makes a list of individuals who meet the interests of the study using one of the other methods of purposive sampling and then the required numbers of individuals are selected randomly from the list. According to Miles & Huber man, random purposeful sampling "adds credibility to sample when the potential purposeful sample is too large."

Multi-stage Purposeful Random Sampling

This involves selecting a sample in two or more stages, in which the first stage is random and subsequent stages are purposive. In multi-stage random purposeful sampling, the first stage usually involves cluster sampling, whereas subsequent stages involve one of the above-mentioned purposive sampling schemes.

Multi-stage Purposeful Sampling

Multi-stage purposeful sampling also involves selecting a sample in two or more stages. What differentiates this method from multi-stage purposeful random sampling is that all stages involve the use of purposive sampling methods. Multi-stage purposeful sampling differs from mixed purposeful sampling; the former is always sequential, whereas, the latter typically involves concurrent sampling in which one sample is not a subset of other samples.

KEY POINTS

- In qualitative research, sampling methods are a vital part of the study.
- Sampling methods in qualitative research are employed to provide richly-textured information, relevant to the phenomenon under investigation.
- The main aim in qualitative research is to deeply understand specific cases or phenomena, using methods like selecting diverse groups or individuals for detailed study.
- Different sampling techniques are used for specific research needs, such as studying extreme cases for comparison, looking at typical examples, comparing different groups or combining methods for more insights.

BIBLIOGRAPHY

1. Creswell WJ. Educational Research. In: Robb C (Ed). TexTech International; 2002:11-12.
2. Mason J. Qualitative Researching. 2nd edition. London: Sage Publications; 2002.
3. Miles MHAM. Qualitative data analysis: An expanded sourcebook [Internet]. 2nd edition. USA: sage; 1994 [cited 2022 Jan 20]. Available from: https://vivauniversity.files.wordpress.com/2013/11/milesandhuberman1994.pdf
4. Omona J. Sampling in Qualitative Research: Improving the Quality of Research Outcomes in Higher Education. Makerere J High Educ. 2013;4(2):169–85.
5. Patton M. Qualitative research and evaluation methods. 3rd edition. Thousand Oaks, CA: Sage; 2002.

SAMPLE SIZE

Saritha Nair, Maria Nelliyanil, Anusha Rashmi, Sunhitha Velamala

"The goal is to turn data into information, and information into insight."
—Carly Fiorina

INTRODUCTION

It is important that sample size is ascertained for qualitative research as in quantitative research but need not be in a similar way.

Need

Sample adequacy in qualitative research is related to the fact whether the sample composition is appropriate or not. This is very important as it makes the findings trustworthy and adds quality to the research. In qualitative research sample size is small so that in-depth of case-oriented analysis can be done, which is fundamental in qualitative research.

Also in qualitative research, the selection of the sample is purposive, that is, the sample is selected in such a way that it provides richly textured information that is relevant to the research objective. That is the reason why purposive sampling which helps in selecting 'information-rich' cases is used in qualitative research as opposed to probability sampling.

Content

One of the factors that help us decide whether we have included the right number of people in our study depends on what we want to compare and to what extent the sample that we have generated will allow us to do it. Hence, it is not always possible to decide in prior regarding the sampling strategy.

An example of this in practice is found in the work of Bertaux and Bertaux-Wiame where they have claimed that the size of the sample will be dictated by the process under scrutiny. This means that we need to sample until the point of theory saturation is reached, that is, till we reach a point where we have a picture of what is going on and can also generate an appropriate explanation for the same. This point is reached when our data stops telling us anything new about the process under scrutiny, and thus we cannot anticipate when and how this point will be reached.

The concept of data saturation has been widely criticized for being ad hoc and unsystematic (it raises the question of how the researcher can demonstrate that the saturation point was reached). But two principles are very useful in guiding us regarding this; first, the sample size should help to understand the process (or whatever the study is interested in) rather than represent a population and second, the process of sample selection should be a dynamic and an ongoing practice.

This principle of understanding the process rather than representing a population must be kept clearly in mind when we are deciding how many contexts or categories of a particular type must be selected so that it will constitute a relevant range of purposes of comparison and explanation. Therefore, we should not assume that we have selected one category of a particular type as this will somehow represent all the categories of the same type. For example, if we decide that a relevant range of categories will be people of different ages selected for an interview and so we select ten people such that each of their age falls within a specified five-year period we should not slide back into the statistical or probability logic whereby we expect the one 55-year-old in the study to be representative of all 55-year-old. Instead, we need to remember that the categories that we chose to constitute a range are intended to allow generating data to explore processes, similarities and differences, to test and develop theory and explanation to account for those similarities and differences in particular contexts, rather than in making statistical comparisons between the categories themselves within the range and to infer causality on that basis.

The answers to questions about how and what to compare are based on the research questions and intellectual puzzle, but it is also likely that it may be influenced by the theories and ideas that are developed in the process of generating and analyzing data. Hence, when we begin the research, we will have some ideas about key comparisons based on existing research and theory. These will help to decide how the sample should be constituted and how large it should be so that such comparisons can be feasibly made.

Taken together, all these factors suggest that the answer to the question of how large our sample should be is that it should be large enough to make meaningful comparisons about your research questions, but not so large as to become so diffuse that a detailed and nuanced focus on something becomes impossible. In other words, there is no fixed answer, as it depends upon what meaningful sets of comparisons need to be done about the specific research project, the intellectual puzzle and its research questions and the kind of social explanation you are trying to produce. We will therefore need to keep asking ourselves: why is this or that category or group relevant? In what ways does including them in the study help in understanding the process that we wish to understand or in developing the overall kind of explanation we wish to develop? This is the logic that should drive your decisions about which categories to include as well as how many to include. Remember that qualitative research is particularly good at constituting arguments about how things work in a particular context rather than representing the full range of experience. Therefore, decisions about what exactly the range should include must be guided by a strategic logic ('How well will this range do the comparisons and help in addressing the research questions?') rather than a representational one ('It is better to include this group and that category so that everything is covered'). The key component for qualitative sampling is therefore how to focus strategically and meaningfully, rather than how to represent.

Hence, it is important to ensure that we do not simply pick the sampling categories that will support the argument and disregard those inconvenient ones that do not. Therefore, we need to set samples in a way that will help not only in developing your theory or explanation but also in testing it; and for doing this there should be a built-in mechanism. In other words, the sampling strategy should be such that we do not simply sample categories from which we will generate data that will support our analysis or explanation, but it should also show that we have rigorously looked for cases or instances that do not fit with our ideas or those that cannot be accounted for by the explanation we are developing. If we cannot find any and if we can show that you have looked in places where such negative cases are likely to occur, then our explanation is strengthened. If we can find some, then we will need to modify our explanation.

According to the model, **(Fig. 1)** we need to consider the aim of the study, specificity of the sample, theoretical background, dialogue quality and strategy for analysis to determine whether it is possible to achieve sufficient information power with fewer or more participants included in the sample. A study will need the least number of participants when the study aim is narrow if it is supported by established theory, if the interview dialogue is strong, if

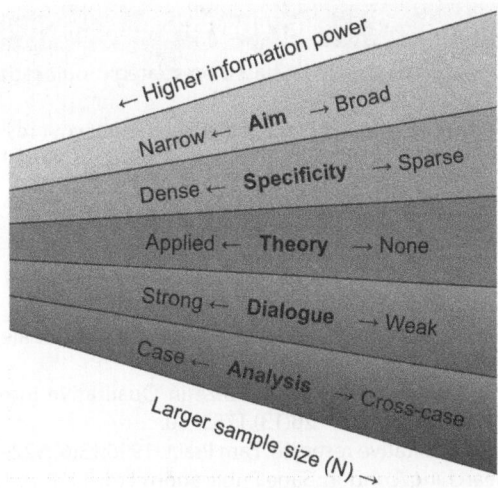

Fig. 1: Information power model.

Malterud K, Siersma VD, Guassora AD. Sample Size in Qualitative Interview Studies: Guided by Information Power. Qual Health Res. 2016;26(13):1753–60.

the combination of participants selected is highly specific to the study aim and if the analysis includes a longitudinal in-depth exploration of narratives or discourse details. On the contrary, if the study aim is broad or if it is not based on good theoretical information, if the combination of participants selected is less specific for the research question or if the interview dialogue is weak and if cross-case analysis is conducted, especially if the aim is to cover the broadest range of variations of the phenomena studied then a larger number of participants will be needed.

The dynamic interaction between the various items in the information power model involves a trade-off between conditions that need fewer versus more participants in a sample. A researcher who is well experienced, with a narrow study aim can achieve an excellent interview dialogue and will be able to do a cross-case analysis with sufficient variation of results even with a small sample size. However, a less experienced researcher with limited theoretical knowledge may need a larger group of participants to reveal something new even if the aim is well-focused and the interview dialogues are good.

Another approach that can be followed is the rule of thumb wherein if the number of units is very large, take 10 percent of the sample, if it is medium take 15–20 percent, if it is small take 20–30 percent and if it is very small take 30–50 percent of the sample.

To ensure and maintain high-quality research, qualitative researchers should be more transparent and thorough in their evaluation of sample size. It is a good practice to appraise the sample size sufficiency with a close reference to the study at hand and we need to be cautious about the use of sample size numerical guidelines, norms and principles. Although researchers might find that the sample size norms serve as useful rules of thumb, it is recommended that methodological knowledge is used to critically consider how saturation and other parameters that affect sample size sufficiency pertain to the specifics of the project.

Limitations

Estimation of the needed number of qualitative interviews or focus groups many at imes depends on the limitations of the project (e.g., budget, timing, audience availability, etc.).

KEY POINTS
■ Sample size in qualitative research should be based on strategic logic rather than a representational one. ■ It should be large enough to make meaningful comparisons about your research questions, but not so large as to become so diffuse that a detailed and nuanced focus on something becomes impossible.

BIBLIOGRAPHY

1. Bertaux D. Biography and society: The life history approach in the Social Sciences. Beverly Hills, CA: Sage Publications; 1983.
2. Luborsky MR, Rubinstein RL. Sampling in qualitative research: Rationale, issues, and methods. Res Aging. 1995;17(1):89–113.
3. Malterud K, Siersma VD, Guassora AD. Sample Size in Qualitative Interview Studies: Guided by Information Power. Qual Health Res. 2016;26(13):1753–60.
4. Marshall MN. Sampling for qualitative research. Fam Pract. 1996;13(6):522–6.
5. Mason J. Qualitative researching. London: Sage Publications Ltd; 2018. p. 120-43.
6. Patton MQ. Qualitative evaluation and research methods. 2nd edition. Newbury Park, CA: Sage; 1990.
7. Sandelowski M. One is the liveliest number: The case orientation of qualitative research. Res Nurs Health. 1996;19(6):525–9.
8. Sharples J. Assessing quality of service. Module 6. Aga Khan Foundation, Geneva; 1993.

Analysis and Ethics in Qualitative Studies

CHAPTER 24

Abhishek V Raut, Amit Rao, Anusha Rashmi, Sushantha Perduru

> "If we don't find patterns, we don't have empirical qualitative research; we have anecdotes."
> —Indi Young

ANALYSIS IN QUALITATIVE STUDIES

Qualitative research generally involves huge amounts of data in the form of audio, videos, notes that are converted into transcripts. Analysis of this data requires planning, organized working and appreciation of human behavior. It is desirable that the researcher must have a fine balance between scholarship over the concepts of the topic of concern and open-mindedness to identify varying opinions with equal appreciation. So, qualitative data analysis can be time consuming and cognitively exhausting. Computer assisted software can simplify this process especially with respect to data organization. However, the analysis and outcome of research is still ultimately dependent on the researcher's interpretation skills.

Approaches in Qualitative Data Analysis

Inductive Analysis

Theory is generated after the process of data collection and is based on the analysis from that data. There is no predetermined pattern of analysis, i.e., all the codes, categories, themes and theories emerge from the data itself. This is the preferred approach for analysis of qualitative data.

Deductive Analysis

The process of analysis is predetermined, i.e., *'a priori'* codes and categorizations will be used. Codes are generated before the analysis itself; and can be based on existing literature and/or researcher's experiences. Organization of data becomes easier with predetermined codes.

Both deductive and inductive analysis.

Stages in Qualitative Data Analysis

Stage 1: Transcribing the Data

Converting raw data which is in the form of audio, video or notes into a written record is called Transcribing the data. Data is recorded as it is spoken verbatim. All pauses, expressions, body languages are included in the written record. Transcribing can be done by:

❖ **Research assistant:** Most preferred option.

- Digital software: in research with large data.
- External transcriber: least preferred.

Stage 2: Immersion in the Data

Researchers should immerse oneself in the data by reading and re-reading the data. During the process, descriptive statements may be written about raw data to identify the similarities and differences, to organize the researcher's thoughts/observations and to ease the coding of data. These reflective notes may be written immediately after data collection/before or during the coding process. These are called **'Memos'**, which can constitute supplementary data that is to be analyzed.

Stage 3: Data Coding

It is the process of breaking sentences into meaningful units, i.e., to fragment the data into small parts. Focus is on identifying relevant words or phrases so that they can be grouped. There are **three common types of data coding:**
1. **Open coding:** Major concepts and keywords are identified.
2. **Axial coding:** Patterns are identified from the data and they are organized into categories.
3. **Selective coding:** Data is integrated to produce a theory.

Example:

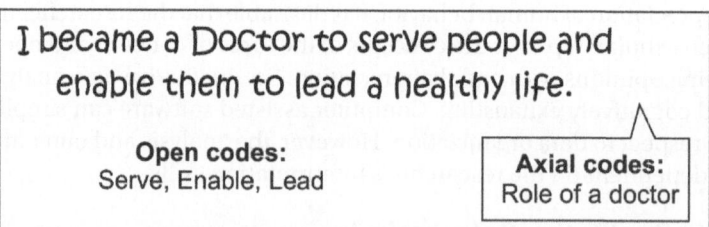

Issues with coding: Major concern with coding is its VALIDITY. This validity of interpretation can be increased either by 'Respondent validation' (researcher's interpretation is referred back to the participants for evaluation) or by comparing the codes developed by multiple researchers.

Stage 4: Data Grouping to Produce Themes

Themes: are threads of meaning in text/topic which the text is addressing. Coded data is placed in larger groups which brings out critical factors which leads to emergence of themes. There are three **levels of themes:**
- **Basic**: Prominent messages/themes are identified but not linked.
- **Organizing**: Clustering of themes to show the inter relation to each other.
- **Global**: Integrating the themes to show the global picture.

Stage 5: Formulate Theory

Themes developed may be placed to construct a theory. This can be a separate stage in itself or a part of selective coding.

Real life Example

Text	Health care should focus on people's problems and identifying strategies which are culturally acceptable, relevant and feasible. It is of no use to just build toilets in villages to stop them from the practice of open-air defecation. People still feel that toilets are not comfortable, unsanitary and difficult to maintain. There is a need to make them realize the benefits of using toilets and the harm of open-air defecation on health through sustained health education activities and build community ownership and participation
Codes	<ul><li>A focussed activity</li><li>Problems</li><li>Culturally acceptable</li><li>Relevant</li><li>Feasible</li><li>Building toilets and promoting its use</li><li>Uncomfortable, unsanitary feel and difficult to maintain</li><li>Interventions need to work</li><li>Sustained efforts needed</li><li>People made to realize benefits and harm</li><li>Community participation and ownership</li></ul>
Clustering of similar words and relationship	*Cluster one*: focused activity, problems, strategies *Cluster two*: culturally acceptable, relevant, feasible, uncomfortable, unsanitary and difficult to maintain *Cluster three*: interventions, sustained efforts, made to realize, community ownership and participation
Themes	<ul><li>Nature of health care</li><li>Acceptability of health care</li><li>Activities in health care</li></ul>
Theory	The themes describe the essence of health care as subjective phenomenon involving strategies which may not always be acceptable but needs sustained efforts to reach desired end result

Methods in Qualitative Data Analysis

There are three commonly used methods of (inductive) qualitative data analysis. They are as follows: Thematic analysis, Content analysis and Constant comparator method.

Thematic Analysis (Flowchart 1)

Themes: are threads of meaning in text/topic which the text is addressing. Common themes emerging out of interviews can be used to build a theory to explain a phenomenon. Thematic analysis is commonly used in *phenomenological studies.*

- **Researcher bias is a risk present in thematic analysis.** Pre-existing knowledge of the researcher on the subject of research can act as a source of bias in the interpretation of data and final analysis. This can be dealt with in two of the following ways:

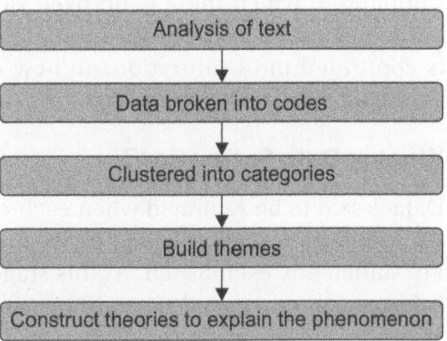

Flowchart 1: Thematic analysis.

- If the study methodology/approach accepts the researcher as a tool in the study, there is no need of Bracketing. This is the usual approach in health care research.
- If the study approach feels that it may unconsciously introduce bias and result in erroneous interpretation, then Bracketing is advised. **Bracketing of pre-existing knowledge of the researcher in data collection and analysis.** Researcher becomes a passive component which is difficult to achieve.

Content Analysis

Content analysis involves the classification of written or spoken materials into distinct categories based on shared meanings. Researchers examine qualitative data to generate explanations that either confirm or refute the research question. Here, narratives or word responses are analyzed. Content analysis is used in *Phenomenology, case studies* and *narratives*.

After saturation, descriptive paragraphs are developed in each category and looked for relationships.

Example: analyze public perception of popular health issues.

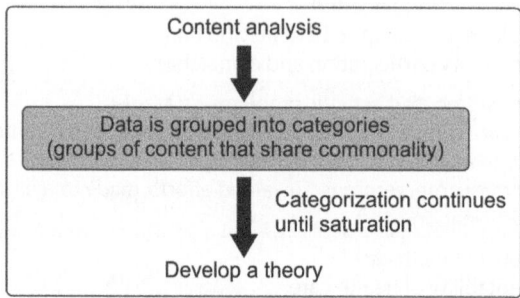

- ❖ **How does content analysis differ from thematic analysis?** As per thematic analysis, researcher examines the text paragraph by paragraph; and as per content analysis, researcher examines the whole transcript and selects topics or categories as units of meaning.

Constant Comparative Method (Flowchart 2)

This is used in *Grounded theory*. Data collection and analysis go hand in hand. Constant comparison of data from previous participants is made, to note similarities and differences. This type of analysis uses **Theoretical sampling**. This is a type of sampling in which there is no fixed sample size at the beginning of the study but data collection is continued until saturation/no new codes are emerging from further sampling.

What is Data Saturation?

Data is said to be saturated when each category is sufficiently described and links between categories are sufficiently established. At this stage, no new information emerges despite increasing sample size.

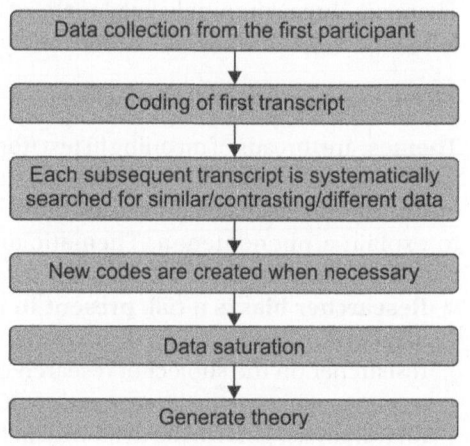

Flowchart 2: Constant comparative method.

Models of Qualitative Data Analysis

Most common models of qualitative data analysis are the three of the following: Colaizzi, Van Kaam and Giorgi.

Colaizzi Model
- ❖ Most commonly used in *Phenomenology*.
- ❖ **7 stages of analysis:**
  - Reading all the subject's descriptions.
  - Identify specific statements relating to the phenomenon under study (descriptive stage).
  - Look for meaning within statements (~ coding).
  - Organize meanings into themes and validate them against original statements (~ clustering common data).
  - Integrate findings as phenomenon's description and form a theoretical model.
  - Findings validated with original participants.
  - Changes suggested by participants incorporated into the model.

Van Kaam Model
- ❖ Characterized by **Expert validation**: Panel of expert judges to validate each stage of analysis.
- ❖ **6 stages of analysis:**
  - Expressions are listed and grouped. These groups are validated by experts.
  - Terms refined into precise descriptions. This is again validated by experts.
  - Elimination of irrelevant data.
  - Raw description of the phenomenon is established.
  - Description applied to randomly selected participants for validation.
  - Description of phenomenon is accepted as valid reality.

Giorgi Model
- ❖ Analysis is solely dependent on the judgement of the researcher. No validation steps here.
- ❖ **4 stages of analysis:**
  - Researcher reads every transcript to get an idea/context.
  - Researchers re-read each transcript individually to identify codes/themes.
  - Researchers look for relationships within themes.
  - Synthesizes themes into a consistent statement that reflects the essence of experience of participants.

Computer Assisted techniques for Qualitative Data Management (CAQDAS)

- ❖ **Functions:**
  - Storing and retrieving texts.
  - Find words, segments or phrases of data.
  - Label data.
  - Organize data.
  - Prepare diagrams.
- ❖ **Advantages:**
  - Speeds the process of data analysis.
  - Simplifies data/eases coding process especially in large data set.
  - Reduces bias.

- **Disadvantages:**
  - Reduces creativity.
  - Risk of losing context/meaning of data.
  - Can only manage data but cannot analyze.

Following is a list commonly used software and some of its salient features:

NUD.IST

This software is used for Non-numerical unstructured data indexing. The old name is NVivo. This is considered as a leading software used in content analysis. This is available in multiple languages. The **characteristic** features of this software include: (i) Searching the content for codes to create patterns or categories. This can be used in data analysis of Grounded theory.

Ethnography

This is a software that can code across different groups. Common theme identification and coding of data can be done far more rapidly than manual methods. **Limitation** of this software is that the text is limited to <40 character wide.

ATLAS.ti

This software is known to assist in text analysis and model building. With the help of ATLAS.ti, one can work with text, audio, graphs and video data. It detects segments and displays relationships and patterns. The software is good at identifying hidden phenomena. This can also be linked with SPSS in Mixed method studies.

Text Smart

This is a part of SPSS itself. The software commonly gets used in coding and characterization in open ended surveys.

Qualrus

This is a user-friendly software with simpler language and shorter learning curve. Qualrus gets disadvantageous when using large data because the process gets slow.

The General Inquirer

This was developed at HARVARD and is most commonly used in content analysis. It has large content dictionaries to recognize most modern-day languages and searches for patterns and meanings in sentences.

ETHICAL CONSIDERATIONS IN QUALITATIVE STUDIES

Codes in Ethical Research

Nurenberg Code (1947)

- Devised in response to Nazi atrocities of performing research on prison inmates against their will and knowledge.
- Principle of Informed consent arose from here.
- Ten standards were laid down on ethical consideration in research.

Declaration of Helsinki (1964)

❖ Added the importance of ethical research performed by competent experts, independent committee of reviewers and scientific justification of every study.
❖ It was updated in 2000 and 2008

Ethical Principles

Respect for Autonomy

❖ Inform in detail regarding risks and benefits of participation to every participant.
❖ Ensure that the participant has understood them.
❖ Offer the participant whether he wants to participate or not.
❖ Confidentiality: assure the participant that the data collected will be used for the research purposes and his participation in the study will not be disclosed.
❖ The participant will have the right to withdraw from the study mid-way.
❖ Respect the participant's decision not to participate.

Justice

❖ Treat every participant fairly and equally with respect to their individual rights.
❖ Participants should be selected based on suitability for the study.

Beneficence

Extent to which the research is good to the participant or society.

Nonmaleficence

Extent to which harm has been prevented to the participant or society.

KEY POINTS

- Qualitative data analysis is mostly inductive in nature.
- Qualitative data analysis involves large amount of data and its analysis is time consuming.
- Use of computer assisted software can simplify qualitative data analysis and can aid in better organizing of the data.
- Stages of qualitative data analysis involves transcribing and coding of data, grouping it into themes and formulating the theory.
- Most common methods in qualitative data analysis are thematic analysis, content analysis and constant comparative methods.
- Most common models of qualitative data analysis are Colaizzi, Van Kaam and Giorgi.

BIBLIOGRAPHY

1. Bingham A. Qualitative analysis: Deductive and inductive approaches [Internet]. Andrea J. Bingham, Ph.D.; 2023 [cited 2023 Nov 12]. Available from: https://www.andreajbingham.com/resources-tips-and-tricks/deductive-and-inductive-approaches-to-qualitative-analysis
2. Dongre A, Sankaran R. Ethical issues in qualitative research: Challenges and options. International Journal of Medical Science and Public Health. 2016;5(6):1187. doi:10.5455/ijmsph.2016.19102015179
3. Mack N, Woodsong C, Kathleen M. Qualitative Research Methods: A Data Collector's Field Guide [Internet]. North Carolina: Family Health International; 2005 [cited 2021 Oct 4]. 83-91 p. Available

from: https://www.fhi360.org/sites/default/files/media/documents/Qualitative%20Research%20Methods%20-%20A%20Data%20Collector's%20Field%20Guide.pdf.
4. Richards HM. Ethics of qualitative research: Are there special issues for health services research? Family Practice. 2002;19(2):135–9. doi:10.1093/fampra/19.2.135
5. Ross T. A Survival Guide for Health Research Methods [Internet]. New York: Mc Graw Hill House; 2012 [cited 2021 Oct 15]. 113-159 p. Available from: https://mhebooklibrary.com/doi/book/10.1036/9780335244744.

Report Writing in Qualitative Research

CHAPTER 25

Pradeep Deshmukh, Maria Nelliyanil, Roopa R Mendagudali, Amit Rao

"Stories give life to data, and data gives authority to stories."
—Wendy Newman

INTRODUCTION

Qualitative research explores complex phenomena that are encountered by health care providers, clinicians, consumers and policy makers in health care. Poorly designed studies and inadequate reporting can lead to inappropriate application of qualitative research in health care, health policy, decision-making and future research.

Requirements of Reporting Qualitative Research

- The report should be transparent
- There should be a honest presentation of the findings
- The report should be creative
- The report should be flexible
- The report needs to be focused on purpose of the research
- Follow a checklist of reporting qualitative research.

Need of the Content

Involves creative thinking, imagination and organization of thoughts. Need to keep in mind the potential readers/end-users of the report, type of written communication, purpose of the communication and reporting guidelines of the publication. Descriptive approach of reporting may suffice for most needs.

Content

Key sections of a published, qualitative research report are as follows:
- Introduction
- Aims of the study
- Review of the literature
- Methods
- Results
- Discussion
- Conclusion
- Abstract

Introduction

A good introduction provides a brief overview of the manuscript, including the research question. It needs to have justification for the research question and the rationale for using qualitative research methods. Introduction should also explain what would be the implications of understanding the phenomenon of interest. It needs to also provide background information, including relevant literature relating to the topic. If any specific educational or research terminology is used in the manuscript the same needs to be defined in the introduction.

Aims of the Study

It includes the description of the research question or the aim of the study.

Review of the Literature

Rather than offering an account of all previous research, the author should describe in detail how he or she searched the literature.

Methods

Theoretical Framework

Researchers need to clarify the theoretical frameworks underpinning their study so that the readers will be able to understand as to how the researchers explored their research questions and aims.

Theoretical frameworks in qualitative research include:
- Grounded theory, to build theories from the data;
- Ethnography, to understand the culture of groups with shared characteristics;
- Phenomenology, to describe the meaning and significance of experiences; discourse analysis, to analyze linguistic expression; and content analysis, to systematically organize data into a structured format.

Researchers need to justify and describe how the approach that they chose is suitable to answer their question.

Setting

Researchers should describe the context in which the data was collected as it helps to understand why participants would have responded in a particular way. For instance, participants might be more reserved and feel disempowered talking in a hospital setting. The presence of nonparticipants during interviews or focus groups should be reported as this can also affect the opinions expressed by participants. For example, parent interviewees might be reluctant to talk on sensitive topics if their children are present.

Participant Characteristics

Participant characteristics like basic demographic data, local culture, systems, religious faiths and socio-political circumstances should be reported so that the readers can consider the relevance of the findings and interpretations to their circumstances. This also allows readers to assess whether the perspectives of different groups were explored and compared, such as health care providers and patients.

Sample Size

The researcher needs to specify how many participants were included in the study. The criteria used for selecting the study participants needs to be mentioned and justified.

The manner in which the participants were recruited and who recruited also needs to be mentioned. A brief description regarding the people who refused to participate needs to be given. It is important to consider whether the researchers were fair in recruiting the participants, so that the research design explicitly incorporates a wide range of different perspectives so that the viewpoint of one group is never presented as if it represents the sole truth about any situation.

The process by which ethical and or research/institutional governance approval was obtained should be described and cited.

Participant Selection

Researchers should report how participants were selected, e.g., purposive, convenience, consecutive, snowball sampling. The type of purposive sampling used and the reason as to why a particular sampling strategy was chosen should be justified. The method of approaching the participants (e.g., face-to-face, telephone, mail, email) needs to be mentioned.

Data Collection

Researchers need to justify and mention the method of data collection (IDI/KII, FGD, Participant observation, etc.).

Personal Characteristics

Qualitative researchers closely engage with the participants and research process thus it is not possible to completely avoid personal bias. Instead, researchers should clarify to the readers their identity, credentials, gender, occupation, experience and training. This helps in improving the credibility of the findings as it enables the readers to assess how these factors might have influenced the researchers' observations and interpretations.

Relationship with Participants

It is necessary to describe the relationship and extent of interaction between the researcher and their participants as this may have an impact on the participants' responses and also on the researchers' understanding of the phenomena. For example, a clinician- researcher will tend to have a better understanding of patients' issues but as they are involved in patient care it may inhibit frank discussion with patient–participants when patients believe that their responses will affect their treatment. Thus, the researcher needs to identify and state their assumptions and personal interests in the research topic for transparency.

Explain how data collection tools were developed (e.g., pilot testing of interview guides). The questions and prompts that were used in data collection should be provided so that the readers can have a better understanding of the researcher's focus and the readers will be also able to assess whether participants were encouraged to openly convey their viewpoints. Researchers need to mention what efforts were taken to establish rapport with the community/respondents.

The method of recording the participants' words should be reported. Generally, audio recording and transcription are more accurate and reflect the participants' views than contemporaneous researcher notes, more so if participants have checked their own transcript for accuracy. If audio recording is not done then the reasons for the same should be provided. In addition, field notes should also maintain nonverbal expressions and contextual details and for data analysis and interpretation. Duration of the interview or focus group or nonverbal expressions should be reported as this can affect the amount of data obtained. Researchers should also clarify whether participants were recruited until data saturation, i.e., no new relevant knowledge was being obtained from new participants.

Data Analysis

An adequate account of how the findings were produced needs to be included. A description of how the themes and concepts were derived from the data should also be included. Was deductive or inductive process used? The analysis should not be limited to just those issues that the researcher thinks are important, anticipated themes, but also consider issues that participants raised, i.e., emergent themes. Qualitative researchers need to be open regarding the data analysis and provide evidence of their thinking, for example, were alternative explanations for the data considered and dismissed, and if so, why were they dismissed? It also is important that negative/deviant cases or outlying cases that did not fit with the central interpretation be presented.

Researchers should give the descriptions of coding and memoing so the readers can understand how the researchers perceived, examined and developed their understanding of the data. Researchers should mention if they used any software packages to assist with storage, searching and coding of qualitative data. Obtaining feedback from participants on the research findings will also add to the validity of the researcher's interpretations by ensuring that the participants' own perspectives and meanings are represented and not curtailed by the researchers' own agenda and knowledge.

There is a tendency for authors to overuse quotes and for papers to be dominated by a series of long quotes with little analysis or discussion. This needs to be avoided. If the research was triangulated with other quantitative or qualitative data, then the same needs to be discussed.

Results

Results interpreted in credible, innovative way. The result should start with description of the study sample: age, sex, occupation, etc., as qualitative research needs to be understood in context. It can be presented as a description of themes, text-tables or visual diagrams explaining interrelationships of concepts. The number of codes, categories and themes generated needs to be mentioned. Quotes are "raw data" and thus need to be compiled and analyzed, not just listed. Researchers need to give an explanation of how the quotes were chosen and labeled. For example, have pseudonyms been given to each respondent or are the respondents identified using codes and if so, how? It is important for the reader to be able to see that a range of participants have contributed to the data and that not all the quotes are drawn from 1 to 2 individuals.

Discussion

The findings should be presented in the context of any similar previous research and or theories. The researchers should discuss how the results of the present research will contribute to the area of interest. Transferability of the research findings to other settings needs to be discussed. Strengths and limitations of the research also should be discussed. It is a usual practice to include some discussion within the results section of qualitative research and follow with a concluding discussion. The author also should reflect on their own influence on the data, probably looking into the fact that how the researcher(s) may have introduced bias to the results. The researcher needs to critically examine their own influence on the design and development of the research, data collection and interpretation of the data.

Conclusion

The conclusion should include a summary of the main findings from the study, emphasize what the study adds to the existing knowledge and how it explains the phenomenon of interest.

Abstract

The final part of writing the report is writing the abstract for the paper. A good abstract should contain details of the background, the aim, the sample, the data collection and analysis methods and summary of the findings of the study.

> **KEY POINTS**
> - A well written report is the culmination of research.
> - The qualitative report should be transparent, creative, flexible with an honest presentation of the findings which is focused on the purpose of the research.
> - The checklist of reporting qualitative research needs to be followed.

BIBLIOGRAPHY

1. Anderson C. Presenting and evaluating qualitative research. Am J Pharm Educ. 2010;74(8):141.
2. Bluff R. Evaluating qualitative research. Br J Midwif. 1997;5(4):232-5.
3. Côté L, Turgeon J. Appraising qualitative research articles in medicine and medical education. Med Teach. 2005;27(1):71-5.
4. Elder NC, Miller WL. William L. Reading and evaluating qualitative research studies. J Fam Pract. 1995;41(3):279-85.
5. Fossey E, Harvey C, McDermott F, Davidson L. Understanding and evaluating qualitative research. Aust N Z J Psychiatry. 2002;36(6):717-32.
6. Fossey E, Harvey C, McDermott F, Davidson L. Understanding and evaluating qualitative research. Aust N Z J Psychiatry. 2002;36(6):717-32.
7. Giacomini MK, Cook DJ. Users' guides to the medical literature XXIII. Qualitative research in health care. JAMA. 2000;284(3):357-62.
8. Liamputtong P, Ezzy D. Qualitative research methods. 2nd edition. Melbourne, Victoria: Oxford University Press; 2005.
9. Malterud K. Qualitative research: Standards challenges guidelines. Lancet. 2001;358(9280):483-8.
10. Mays N, Pope C. Qualitative research in health care: assessing quality in qualitative research. BMJ. 2000;320(7226):50-2.
11. Popay J, Rogers A, Williams G. Rationale and standards for the systematic review of qualitative literature in health services research. Qual Health Res. 1998;8(3):341-51.
12. Scheff TJ. Single case analysis in the health sciences. Eur J Public Health. 1995;5(2):72-4.
13. Seale C, Silverman S. Ensuring rigour in qualitative research. Eur J Public Health. 1997;7(4):379-84.
14. Tong A, Sainsbury P, Craig J. Consolidated criteria for reporting qualitative research (COREQ): A 32-item checklist for interviews and focus groups. Int J Qual Health Care. 2007;19(6):349-57.

CHAPTER 26

Educational Research

Rashmi Kundapur, Sridevi Kulkarni, Roopa R Mendagudali, Shambhavi Ashutosh Vaidya

"The whole purpose of education is to turn mirrors into windows."
—Sydney J Harris

INTRODUCTION TO EDUCATIONAL RESEARCH

Educational research refers to a systematic attempt to gain a better understanding of the educational process, generally with a view to improving its efficiency. It is an application of the scientific method to the study of educational problems. Educational research not only plays a pivotal role in exploring novel ways to apprehend human behavior but it also assists in creating a change in behavior.

The history of educational research reflects an almost 200-year journey that began with recognition in the mid-1800s that education is a science. Integrating the historical perspective on educational research into the current approach to scientific knowledge is a major factor in determining important innovations, developments and improvements introduced in the theory and practice of education. The scientific process of deploying changes to the existing educational norms based on the results of a research peculiarly pertaining to the problems like teaching methodology, assessment interpretation techniques and others, thereby accomplishing desired outcomes in the field of education, forms the backbone of educational research.

It is often stated that there are actually two main pathways to progress in education science: 1) conducting experimental research; 2) critically capitalize and harness the intellectual acquisitions acquired through reading, reflection, intuition and generalization of practical education experience and these two means are complementary.

Though, there are varied approaches, types or paradigms in educational research, with labels implying opposite poles, such as positivist/interpretive; interventionist/noninterventionist; experimental/naturalistic; case-study, survey and qualitative, quantitative, in actual research, however, there may be overlapping or mixture of the aforementioned approaches that may be used.

Need of the Content

Research in education as in the other fields is essential for providing useful and dependable knowledge through which the process of education can be made more effective. Education has strong roots in the field like philosophy, history, economics, psychology and sociology and through it's intensive process of scientific inquiry about the philosophical, historical, economics, psychological and sociological impact on various aspects of education, that, sound theories can be established.

Education is considered as much a science as an art. As a science, it has a corpus of knowledge and as an art, education seeks to impart knowledge effectively. It needs careful research efforts to enhance teachers' effectiveness. Educational research helps to resolve numerous problems in the field of education like the problem of individual differences, expansion, buildings, discipline and so on. Solutions of such problems by trial and error or by experience from tradition and authority often yield erroneous results. There is a need for educational research because of the changing concept of education. Apart from economics and sociology other domains like psychological research also indicate that only through constant learning can a man can complete himself. If this is so, then education takes place at all ages of life, in all situations and circumstances of existence. The limits of educational research have to be extended from the formal and conventional modes of education to nonformal and innovative systems based on ecological and cybernetic models.

Levels of Educational Research

Basic or Fundamental Research

Basic research is designed to add to an organized body of scientific knowledge and does not necessarily produce results of immediate practical value. Basic research is also called pure or fundamental research as it is primarily concerned with the formulation of a theory or a contribution to the existing body of knowledge. Its major aim is to obtain and use empirical data to formulate, expand or evaluate theory. The pattern and spirit of research are similar to those of physical sciences which means a rigorous and structured type of analysis.

A meticulous sampling procedure helps to extend the findings beyond the study group or situation. Thus, basic research aids in developing theories by discovering proven generalizations or principles. The main aim of basic research is the discovery of knowledge solely for the sake of knowledge and does not focus on the application of the findings.

Applied Research

Applied research is directed at the solution of immediate, specific and practical problems. As the name indicates, it focuses mainly on solving current problems and less on knowledge contribution. Applied research also uses the scientific method of inquiry similar to that of basic research. Its methodology, however, is not as rigorous as that of basic research. Moreover, its findings are to be evaluated in terms of local applicability and not in terms of universal validity. Applied research is mainly intended to improve school practices and add to greater teacher effectiveness in a practical manner. Most of the problems faced by teachers, policy planners and administrators are solved through applied researchers.

Action Research

Action research is focused on immediate application, not on the development of theory or on general application. It has placed its emphasis on problem in a local setting. Its findings are to be evaluated in terms of local applicability, not universal validity. Its purpose is to improve school practices and, at the same time, to improve those who try to improve the practices: to combine the research processes, habits of thinking, ability to work harmoniously with others and professional spirit.

Steps in Educational Research

The steps in educational research, therefore, are more or less identical to those of scientific method. Following are the steps generally found in educational research.
1. **The research problem:** Educational research starts with the selection of a problem. Following are the fields in which one may look for problems for research.
2. **Formulation of hypothesis:** Educational research should make the use of carefully formulated hypothesis. This may be formally stated or implied.
3. **Methods to be used:** It refers to strategy followed in collecting and analyzing the data necessary for solving the problem. The methods used in the study are decided by the nature of the problem and the type of data required for answering the questions relating to the problem. The research methods are generally classified in three categories: (1) historical, (2) descriptive, and (3) experimental.
4. **Data collection:** It refers to the nature of the sample to be chosen for study selection and development of data gathering devices such as tests, questionnaires, rating scales, interviews, observations, checklists and the like.
5. **Analysis and interpretation of data:** Appropriate quantitative and quantitative techniques are to be used for processing the data collected for the study to get desired results.
6. **Reporting the results:** This is the last and important step of the research process. It is characterized by carefully formulated inferences, conclusions or generalizations. The researcher must be able report his procedures, findings and conclusions with utmost objectivity to others who may be interested in his study and its results.

Disadvantages of Scientific Approach in Education

Complexity of Subject Matter

Unlike natural science (Physics, chemistry, etc.), the subjects in social science researches are humans and their behavior. This is way more complex to study, with lot of variations, influencing factors, confounders, etc. Researchers have to consider various permutations and combinations before coming to the conclusion. Despite this, not even a singular law can be generalized across the group/generation.

Difficulties in Observation

Natural scientists study phenomena that require little subjective interpretation. Whereas Observation in social sciences is more subjective because it frequently involves interpretation on the part of the observer. Observers must make subjective interpretations when they decide that behaviors observed indicate the presence of any particular motive, value or attitude. The problem is that social scientists' own values and attitudes may influence both the observations and the assessment of the findings on which they base their conclusions.

Difficulties in Replication

Replication of results is difficult in social sciences as most of the variables are not quantifiable by specific tools. Social phenomenon is one-time events and cannot be replicated even by the same set of participants.

Interaction Between an Observer and Subjects

Mere observation of the subjects may result in variation in their behavior and thereby gives biased results. Being observed influences the regular behavior leading to changes that might not have occurred otherwise. The use of hidden cameras and tape recorders may help minimize this difficulty in some cases.

Difficulties in Control

The range of possibilities of controlled experiments on human subjects is much more limited than in natural sciences. In the latter, rigid control of experimental conditions is possible in the laboratory. Such control is not possible with human subjects. The social scientists must deal with many variables simultaneously and must work under conditions that are much less precise. They try to identify and control as many of these variables as possible, but the task is very difficult.

Problems of Measurement

The tools for measurement in social sciences are much less perfect and precise than the tools of the natural sciences. There are precision tools against which the current results can be matched or compared. Understanding of human behavior is complicated by the large number of determining variables acting independently and in interaction. The multivariate statistical devices available for analyzing data in social sciences take care of relatively few of the factors that are obviously interacting.

The above listed factors make it difficult for social science researchers to generalize any of the findings. Moreover, the observations keep changing over period of time and also from individual to individual. Despite these handicaps, education and social sciences have made great progress and their scientific status can be expected to increase scientific investigation and methodology become more systematic and rigorous in their research activities.

Real Life Example

For example, a study of the effectiveness of training teenage parents to care for their infants. The study is based on statistical and other evidence that infants of teenage mothers seemed to be exposed to more risks than other infants. The mother and children were recruited for participation in the study while the children were still in neonate period. Mothers were trained at home or in an infant nursery. A controlled group received no training. The mothers trained at home were visited at 2-weeks interval over a 12-month period. Those trained in nursery setting attended 3-days per week for 6 months, were paid minimum wage and assisted as staff in center. Results of the study suggested that the children of both group of trained mothers benefited more in terms of their health and cognitive measures than did the controlled children. Generally greater benefits were realized by the children of the mothers trained in the nursery than with the mothers trained at home.

Thus, the study shows that such researches have direct application to real world problems. Second, elements of both quantitative and qualitative approaches can be found in the study. For example, quantitative measure of weight, height, and cognitive skills were obtained in this study. However, at the start itself from the personal impressions and observations without the benefit of systematic quantitative data, the researchers were able to say that the mother in the nursery center showed some unexpected vocational aspirations to become nurses. Third, treatments and methods that are investigated are flexible and might change during the study in response to the results as they are obtained. Thus, action research is more systematic and empirical than some other approaches to innovation and change.

Conclusion

In the ever expanding educational arena, introduction of new education tools and scientific inquest of humans has led to opportunities of research in the field of education to increase its effectiveness. Selection of right kind of scientific research method and rigorous efforts helps to contribute to existing knowledge as well as finding solution to currents problems in the field of education. It takes sound knowledge of research methods for the researcher to overcome the limitations during research and help reach a conclusive result.

> **KEY POINTS**
> - It studies how to improve teaching and learning. It uses scientific methods to solve educational problems.
> - It helps make teaching more effective. It combines ideas from psychology, history, and other subjects. The aim is to solve school problems and improve learning.
> - There are various kinds, like theory-focused, problem-solving, and local issue research. Each follows steps like choosing a topic, gathering data and sharing results.
> - Studying education can be hard due to its complexity. However, it is useful, like in studies that help parents improve their children's development. Good research leads to better teaching methods.

BIBLIOGRAPHY

1. Albulescu M. Historical Perspective in Educational Research. 2016 [cited 2023 Dec 21]; Available from: https://www.academia.edu/51028946/Historical_Perspective_in_Educational_Research
2. Arandhara B, Ratul G, Sharma K, Bhuyen S. Methodology of Educational Research. Directorate of Open and Distance Learning. 2019;451.
3. Koul, L. Methodology of Educational Research. 5th edition. New Delhi, New Delhi: Vikas Publishing House. 2019; 15–25.
4. Koul L, Mukhopadhya M, Parhar M, Basanti P. Introduction to Educational Research in Distance Education: Purpose, Nature and Scope [Internet]. Indira Gandhi National Open University; 2018 [cited 2023 Dec 17]. Available from: https://egyankosh.ac.in/bitstream/123456789/41933/1/Unit-1.pdf
5. Wani SR. M.A. Edu/Research Methodology/Educational Research. Directorate of Distance Education, University of Kashmir. 2017 [cited 2023 Dec 21]; Available from: http://ddeku.edu.in/Files/2cfa4584-5afe-43ce-aa4b-ad936cc9d3be/Custom/Educational%20Research.pdf
6. Wellington J. Educational Research: Contemporary issues & Practical Approaches. Second. Bloomsbury Publishing; 2015.

27 Practical Applications of Qualitative Research

N Nakkeeran, Sridevi Kulkarni, Roopa R Mendagudali, Amit Rao

> *"The beauty of qualitative research lies in its ability to tell a complete story, to reveal the layers and dimensions of what it means to be human."*
> —Unknown

INTRODUCTION

Advancement in the medical arena has led to complexities requiring the need to explore medical science in a systematic and scientific way. Here comes the need for research methodology that aids the health professional in research and thereby expansion of their knowledge and acquisition of better skill sets. Research methods can be qualitative, quantitative and mixed/quasi.

What do you Mean by Qualitative Research?

Qualitative research is a form of inquiry that analyses information conveyed through language and behavior in natural settings. Qualitative research methods do not primarily seek to provide quantified answers to research questions. Rather the goal of qualitative research is development of concepts which help us to understand social phenomena in natural settings, giving due emphasis to the meanings, experiences and views of all the participants.

For example, a clinician runs a battery of tests to know the status of diabetic control by quantifying blood glucose levels. But it is only by in-depth inquiry/observation (qualitative means) that he can understand the cause of uncontrolled blood glucose levels.

Difference Between Qualitative and Quantitative Methods (Table 1)

Table 1 shows the overstated difference between qualitative and quantitative research methods. As stated earlier qualitative study happens in natural settings with observation and interview

Table 1: Difference between qualitative and quantitative methods.		
	Qualitative	*Quantitative*
Social theory	Structured	Action
Methods	Observation and interview	Experimental and survey
Questions	Classification	Enumeration
Reasoning	Inductive	Deductive
Sampling methods	Theoretical	Statistical
Strength	Validity	Reliability

as tools of study. Whereas quantitative research requires the means of quantification of the variables under study which can be structured questionnaire, medical equipment, etc.

Quantitative methods aim for reliability (that is, consistency on retesting) through the use of tools such as standardized questionnaires whereas qualitative methods score more highly on validity, by getting at how people really behave and what people actually mean when they describe their experiences, attitudes and behaviors.

In addition, the reasoning implicit in qualitative research is of the inductive type. That means the investigator moves from observation to hypothesis generation, whereas in quantitative research it is deductive, i.e., from hypothesis to outcome. In qualitative research, rather than starting with a research question or a hypothesis that precedes any data collection, the researcher is encouraged not to separate the stages of design, data collection and analysis, but to go backwards and forwards between the raw data and the process of conceptualization, thereby making sense of the data throughout the period of data collection.

Sampling and sample size calculation are very much applicable to qualitative studies too. Due to wide heterogeneity within qualitative research, 'sample' takes different meanings depending on the types of data, method and epistemological orientation employed in the study. The method of calculating sample size and selecting the sample is also not the same as in quantitative methods.

Strengths of Qualitative Research Methods

Practical application of qualitative research methods is derived from its unique strengths:
- Unstructured and unfolding nature of data collection process helps the investigator to collect in depth information.
- Descriptive form of data (not reduced to a disaggregated set of variables) makes it possible to document the things that are not quantifiable. For example, emotional response, severity of pain, attitude towards a health practice.
- "Research participant centered" rather than 'research process centered'.
- Transcends numerical and linguistic barriers between researcher and participants.
- Can explore sensitive areas.
- Allows scope for interpretation.
- Exploring any domain.
- Documenting any domain.
- Creating new typology.
- Identifying new vocabulary, new variables and new problems.

Using Qualitative Research Alongside of RCT

Qualitative methods can be used alongside quantitative methods. They both can be complementary to each other if used appropriately.

Use of qualitative methods-an in-depth interview of the participants enrolled in a randomised controlled trial (RCT) (quantitative method) helps to get insight into the experiences of the participants in the trial which is usually not captured by the tools used in RCT itself. This allows an understanding of the process and progress of a trial and provides evidence to intervene in the trial if necessary, including evidence for the rationale to discontinue an intervention arm of the trial.

A review of 100 articles using qualitative methods in RCT was carried out by Simon Lewis et al, 2009. The review showed that it was uncommon to use qualitative methods in RCTs. Most of the qualitative methods were used before the trial and very few used to explain the results of the trial. Even when used, the findings of qualitative study were poorly integrated in RCT results and had methodological shortcomings.

Professional Challenges for which Qualitative Research can be Used

Clinical
Finding out the reason for nonadherence to physicians advise. Improving patient's adherence to clinical recommendation. Facilitating advance directives, communicating bad news, dealing with challenges to clinical communication.

Educational
Determining what influences career choices of graduates and the post graduates. Understanding why a student course is evaluated unfavorably.

Administrative
Assessing local needs and operations when implementing new programs or when engaged in job searches. Managing disagreements with co-workers, advancing negotiations with partners or administrators. Improving professional relationships in an academic unit divided into hard working clinician teachers and overcommitted investigators.

Others
Clarifying performance expectations for patients, clinicians and students in the bottom-line-oriented health maintenance organization. Discovering what influences the behavior of the patients and health workers for quality improvement.

Triangulation
Triangulation is a research strategy that helps to enhance validity and credibility of your research findings. It can be used both in qualitative and quantitative research methods.

Triangulation uses multiple data sets, methods, theories or investigators to understand a research question.

Examples of Triangulation
- **In qualitative research:** We use different key informants of the same setting in FGDs as a source of information like parents, students, teachers of a school setting/doctors, patients and nursing staff of a hospital setting.
- **In quantitative research:** We can employ more than one data analyzer just to be sure of the right results.
- **In mixed method:** We can use qualitative and quantitative research methods one after the other.

Types of Triangulations
- **Data triangulation:** Using data on the same topic or research question from different times, spaces, and people.
- **Investigator triangulation:** Involving multiple researchers in collecting or analyzing data.
- **Theory triangulation:** Using varying theoretical perspectives in same research.
- **Methodological triangulation:** Using different methodologies to approach the same research question.

Purpose of Triangulation

To Cross-check Evidence

Having data from different sources or investigators helps us to be sure of the trustworthiness of the information. The more your data converge, or agree with each other, the more credible your results will be. Thus, increasing the credibility of the information gathered.

For a Complete Picture

Triangulation helps you get a more complete understanding of your research problem. By collecting data from different sources, you get an idea about the research question with respect to different stakeholders avoiding observation bias. Similarly, having multiple investigators or multiple methods for the same question removes the inherent flaws in them.

To Enhance Validity

Validity is about how accurate a method measures what it is supposed to measure. Since each method has its own strengths and weaknesses, you can combine complementary methods that account for each other's limitations. Thus, method triangulation helps to improve the overall validity of the study. For example, in behavioral sciences you can prepare a self-administered questionnaire for the study subjects to assess a particular behavior type and also conduct an in-depth interview or FGD's with the key informants about the same. The more the data is in line with each other, the more accurate is your research finding.

Although Triangulation is a time-consuming strategy and is not always possible because of financial/administrative/time factor reasons, it would be good if employed whenever required, as it helps to remove bias as well as improves validity and credibility.

KEY POINTS

- Research methods can be quantitative, qualitative or mixed methods.
- Qualitative studies aid in better understanding of a variety of phenomena in their natural setting.
- Strength of qualitative research lies in its unstructured, unfolding nature of data collection centered around the participant. It can explore sensitive areas and also identify new vocabularies, variables and problems.

BIBLIOGRAPHY

1. Berkwits M, Inui TS. Making use of qualitative research techniques. J Gen Intern Med. 1998;13(3):195-9.
2. Lewin S, Glenton C, & Oxman AD. Use of qualitative methods alongside randomised controlled trials of complex healthcare interventions: Methodological study. BMJ. 2009;339(7723):732–4.
3. Murtagh MJ, Thomson RG, May CR, Rapley T, Heaven BR, Graham RH., et al, Qualitative methods in a randomised controlled trial: The role of an integrated qualitative process evaluation in providing evidence to discontinue the intervention in one arm of a trial of a decision support tool. Quality & safety in health care. 2007:16(3): 224–9.
4. Nakkeeran, N. "Is sampling a misnomer in qualitative research?" Sociological Bulletin. 2016; 65(1):40–9.
5. Pope C, Mays N. Reaching the parts other methods cannot reach: An introduction to qualitative methods in health and health services research. BMJ. 1995;311(6996):42-5.
6. Puddephatt AJ. An interview with Kathy Charmaz: On constructing grounded theory. Qualitative sociology review. 2006;2(3):5-20. http://www.qualitativesociologyreview.org/ENG/archive_eng.php
7. Triangulation in Research | Guide, Types, Examples. [cited 2023 Dec 21]; Available from: https://www.scribbr.com/methodology/triangulation/ 5/9

SECTION 4

Operational Research

SECTION OUTLINE

Chapter 28: Overview of Operational Research
Chapter 29: Introduction to Health Systems Covering WHO Building Blocks
Chapter 30: Operational Research in Health Programs
Chapter 31: Role of Stakeholders and Ethical Concerns
Chapter 32: Qualitative Research in Operational Research
Chapter 33: Quasi-experimental Studies
Chapter 34: Qualitative Analysis in Operational Research
Chapter 35: Writing for Media Communication
Chapter 36: Funding Opportunities in Operational Research

CHAPTER 28

Overview of Operational Research

Shailaja S Patil, Chandrika R Doddihal, Sonu Goel

"Operational research is the art of weaving logic and mathematics into a tapestry that reveals the hidden patterns of complexity, guiding us through the labyrinth of decision-making with the thread of analytical wisdom."

INTRODUCTION

Operational research, also known as operations research or management science, is a discipline that utilizes statistical analysis and optimization techniques to improve decision-making and solve complex problems in various domains. The term "Operations Research" was first coined when British Military Management called upon a group of scientists together to apply a scientific approach to the study of military operations to win the battle. In India, Operation Research came into existence in 1949 when an Operation Research unit was established at Defense Science Laboratory to solve problems of storage, purchase and planning. In recent years, operational research has gained significant importance in the healthcare sector, where it plays a crucial role in enhancing efficiency, effectiveness, and quality of health care delivery.

Healthcare systems worldwide are confronted with various challenges like rising costs, limited resources, increasing demand and a growing emphasis on patient-centered precision care. To address these challenges, healthcare providers and policymakers are using operational research as a valuable tool to optimize processes, allocate resources efficiently, and make informed decisions. Operational research sometimes interchangeably used as "Implementation Research" in healthcare, mainly underlines the techniques to improve the delivery of healthcare services, enhance patient outcomes and support evidence-based decision-making. By embracing operational research techniques, healthcare professionals and decision-makers can navigate the complexities of the healthcare landscape and make data-driven decisions that lead to better healthcare delivery and patient care. Walley et al. (2007) observed that, "Discovering ways to increase access to and delivery of interventions is a major challenge. Typically research is divorced from implementation, which has led to a growing literature about how to get research into practice. However, OR is best prioritized, designed, implemented and replicated within national programs."

The chapter will provide an overview of key concepts and methodologies in operational research, highlighting their relevance and applicability in healthcare settings. It will discuss case studies and real-world examples that demonstrate how operational research has been successfully implemented to address various healthcare challenges globally, especially in service delivery and preventive care.

Definition

Operational Research has been defined in many ways by different agencies. WHO (2003) defines OR as "the use of systematic research techniques for program decision-making to achieve a specific outcome". It has also been defined by the Population Council as "Operations research helps policy-makers and program managers to review, redirect and restructure programs that have been in place for many years." Dictionary of Epidemiology defined it as a systematic study of the working of a system with the aim of improvement. From a health program perspective, OR is defined as the search for strategies and interventions that enhance the quality and effectiveness of the program. A global meeting held in Geneva in April 2008 to develop the framework of OR, defined the scope of OR in context to public health as "Any research producing practically usable knowledge (evidence, finding, information, etc.) which can improve program implementation (e.g., effectiveness, efficiency, quality, access, scale up, sustainability) regardless of the type of research (design, methodology, approach), falls within the boundaries of OR" The International Food Policy Research Institute (2005) considered that, "OR aims at studying the processes by which programs are implemented and interventions are delivered to intended beneficiaries. The main purpose is to identify, as early as possible in the life of a program, any shortcomings in the process that may affect the effective delivery of the intervention, and as a result, its potential impact on the expected outcomes.

Operational research is different form clinical research as clinical research focuses on studying diseases, treatments, and patient outcomes while operational research aims to optimize healthcare processes, resource allocation, and decision-making and it is different from epidemiological research as Operational research aims to improve healthcare delivery, while epidemiological research aims to understand and prevent the spread of diseases.

The distinguishing features of operational research can be summarized as below:
- It addresses specific problems within specific programs, not general health issues;
- It addresses those problems that are under control of managers, such as program systems, training, pricing and provision of information;
- It utilizes systematic data collection procedures, both qualitative and quantitative, to accumulate evidence supporting decision-making;
- It requires collaboration between managers and researchers in identification of the research problem, development of the study design, implementation of the study and analysis and interpretation of results; and
- It succeeds only if the study results are used to make program decisions; publication alone is not a valid indicator of successful OR.

Objectives

Operational research focuses on the ongoing "operations" of health programs. OR examines issues that are related to programs' supply rather than demand sides. In fact, OR is distinguished by its emphasis on current issues with supply or service delivery and its pursuit of solutions, or in the language of research, variables that may be changed through administrative action. Giving managers, administrators, and decision-makers the knowledge, they need to enhance current delivery operations and organize new ones is one of OR's key goals. OR looks for workable solutions to problematic situations and effective substitutes for inadequate operating procedures. It analyzes and diagnoses program issues and contrasts various service delivery strategies based on their effects, cost-effectiveness, acceptability among clients, and quality.

Categories of Operational Research Studies

The Population Council identifies three types of OR studies.
1. **Exploratory/diagnostic studies (problem unknown):** These studies are used to assess the nature and extent of a health or service delivery problem. They are usually retrospective or cross-sectional in design. This type of study is needed whenever there is a perceived program problem but the nature of the problem is simply unknown.
2. **Field intervention studies (program approach unknown):** These studies test novel solutions to software problems on an experimental basis. The causes of a program problem are frequently recognized, but the most effective and economical ways to solve the issue are often unknown. These studies often use an experimental or quasi-experimental study design, and they are invariably prospective and longitudinal.
3. **Studies (impact unknown):** Health programs are sometimes conducted for years without ever being evaluated. In these circumstances, evaluative studies can be a useful operational research strategy for analyzing the impact of program actions in the past or across time.

Study Designs of Operational Research

The methods of OR range from qualitative to quantitative, and the study designs from non-experimental to quasi experimental to the true experimental design. There is no single set of methods or designs unique to operations research. While OR studies may use experimental or nonexperimental designs and may include a quantitative analysis of outcome measures or a qualitative consideration of health issues, the central objective always is to obtain a better understanding of the "operations" of programs so that needed improvements can be made.

Process: OR is a process, a way of identifying and solving program problems. As currently applied in many health and development fields, operations research can be defined as a continuous process. The goal of OR is to increase the efficiency, effectiveness, and quality of services delivered by providers, and the availability, accessibility, and acceptability of services desired by user.

Steps in Operational Research

Operational research includes five basic steps:
1. **Problem identification and diagnosis:** Identifying a problematic situation by researching pertinent literature, looking at current service statistics, getting informed comments from those who are affected by the issue, and learning the most likely causes of the issue from social, economic, or health theory.
2. **Strategy selection:** Numerous solutions to the issue might be proposed, and these solutions frequently entail making an adjustment to an existing service delivery or management strategy rather than creating whole new service delivery structures.
3. **Strategy testing and evaluation:** It includes selecting appropriate study design to test the strategy and implementation of the strategy to find a solution the problem identified. It involves the process of formulating a research proposal, ethical approval, data collection and analysis.
4. **Information dissemination:** The concept of OR is to offer administrators and policymakers with information that will help them make the necessary modifications to service delivery. A dissemination strategy's main objective is to pinpoint the media outlet(s) that will allow different audience groups to be reached with study results that are most pertinent to their requirements.

5. **Information utilization:** The utilization of research results is the ultimate goal of every OR activity. The process of OR is not complete until every effort has been made to use the result of research.

Application of Operational Research in Field

- **MALAWI:** Civil society and Tuberculosis Care: An OR study was conducted by the Research on Equity and Community (REACH) Trust to explore barriers experienced by the poor in the capital city of Malawi, Lilongwe. Although TB services are free at the point of delivery, it was found that the poor incur much higher transport and opportunity costs than the nonpoor. Based on the suggestions from the community, REACH Trust then developed the intervention, "Linking Civil Society with TB Care" to bring TB services closer to the people. A main objective of this program was to reduce transport and opportunity costs incurred by the poor in the area in order to improve use of TB services through establishment of sputum collection centers at village levels and volunteers to carry them to diagnostic facility. The project was funded by the Norwegian Association of Heart and Lung Patients.
- **BURKINA FASO:** Care for PLHA: In 1990s, NGOs and Societies were providing care for people living with HIV/AIDS (PLHA). In 2005, when public hospitals also started catering to PLHA, a "therapeutic grazing" that led some patients from one sector to another according to the availability of support or aid. In response to this issue, a research project was undertaken to get a precise knowledge of actual care practices in various settings, in order to understand patients' behaviors and needs and harmonize the provision of care. The main issues that were explored and treated included: circumstances of testing and provision of counseling; access to various types of care and factors; care practices; patients' follow-up; factors of adherence to ART; prevention; caregivers' attitudes towards professional risk; collaboration and coordination between healthcare facilities.
- **INDIA:** Screening TB patients for Diabetes Mellitus: In 2007–2008, two systematic reviews showed that people with diabetes mellitus (DM) had a 2–3 times increased risk of developing TB than the general population. Subsequently WHO and the International Union Against Tuberculosis and Lung Diseases undertook real-time operational research study to identify the dual burden of diabetes and tuberculosis. A study was conducted at peripheral health institutions across India to identify the burden of Diabetes Mellitus among patients of tuberculosis. It resulted in rapid national policy decision to screen all TB patients in India for DM routinely.
- **Nicaragua:** Examining the Effectiveness of Testing and Treatment Programs for Malaria: The increasing prevalence of malaria arising after national health system decentralization and frequent natural disasters provided the rationale for an OR study on the testing and treatment of malaria in the isolated North Atlantic region of Nicaragua. As the research was planned and executed in the context of an existing program, research results were immediately translated into programmatic changes.
- **Zimbabwe:** Identifying Gaps in HIV Prevention among Orphans and Young People in Hwange District: OR was built on a study which found that girls who have been orphaned because of HIV are at greater risk of acquiring HIV themselves. The study concluded that because individuals in Zimbabwe are meeting new sexual partners in a variety of venues, it is important to incorporate HIV programs into everyday life. Several program recommendations like youth oriented preventive strategies and condom availability arose from this research.

Limitations

Operational research in healthcare, while valuable, is not without its limitations. Some of the key limitations include:
* **Complexity of healthcare systems:** Healthcare systems are inherently complex, with numerous interacting factors, making it challenging to create accurate and comprehensive strategies to test the program.
* **Data availability and quality:** In healthcare, data may be fragmented, outdated, or of varying quality, impacting the accuracy of analyses and recommendations.
* **Nonutilization of findings:** Implementing OR findings often requires changes in existing practices and may encounter resistance from stakeholders, such as healthcare professionals and administrators.
* **Time and resource constraints:** Operational research projects can be time-consuming and resource-intensive, making it challenging to conduct comprehensive studies within tight healthcare timelines and budgets.
* **Limited generalizability:** Findings from operational research studies may not always be generalizable across different healthcare settings or populations due to variations in healthcare systems and patient demographics.

Despite these limitations, operational research continues to be a valuable tool in healthcare, providing insights and solutions to enhance the efficiency and effectiveness of healthcare delivery.

KEY POINTS

- Operational research in healthcare, mainly emphasizes the techniques to improve the delivery of healthcare services, enhance patient outcomes and support evidence-based decision-making.
- It is different from clinical or epidemiological research as it deals with the process of optimization of healthcare and not with treatment or prevention of a disease.
- OR can be descriptive studies, intervention studies or evaluative studies and can utilize both qualitative and quantitative methods.
- The process of OR includes problem identification, strategy selection and testing, information dissemination and utilization.
- Complex healthcare system, data quality issues and nonutilization of research findings are the main limitations of OR.

BIBLIOGRAPHY

1. Bakiono F, Guiguimdé PW, Sanou M, Ouédraogo L, Robert A. Quality of life in persons living with HIV in Burkina Faso: A follow-up over 12 months. BMC Public Health. 2015;15:1119.
2. Fisher AA, Foreit JR, Laing J, Stoeckel J, Townsend J. Designing. HIV/AIDS intervention studies: An operations research handbook. New York: The Population Council Inc.
3. Fisher AA, Laing JE, Stoeckel JE, Townsend JW. Handbook for Family Planning Operations Research Design. 2nd edition. New York: Population Council; 1991;2.
4. Framework for Operations and Implementation Research in Health and Disease Control Programs [Internet]. Available from: http://www.theglobalfund.org/documents/me/FrameworkForOperationsResearch.pdf.
5. Garfield R. Malaria control in Nicaragua: Social and political influences on disease transmission and control activities. Lancet. 1999;354(9176):414-8. doi:10.1016/S0140-6736(99)02226-6.
6. Harries AD, Thekkur P, Mbithi I, Chakaya JM, Tweya H, Takarinda KC, et al. Real-Time Operational Research: Case Studies from the Field of Tuberculosis and Lessons Learnt. Trop Med Infect Dis. 2021;6:97. https://doi.org/10.3390/tropicalmed6020097.

7. Last JM. A Dictionary of Epidemiology. Oxford University Press Inc. 2001;4:129.
8. Loechl C, Ruel MT, Pelto G, Menon P. The Use of Operations Research as a Tool for Monitoring and Managing Food-Assisted Maternal/Child Health and Nutrition (MCHN) Programs: An Example from Haiti. FOOD CONSUMPTION AND NUTRITION DIVISION, Washington, IFPRI's Discussion Papers. 2005: 187.
9. Mahto D. Introduction to Operations Research. 2012:3-4.
10. Simwaka B, Bello G, Banda H, Chimzizi R, Squire B, Theobald S. The Malawi National Tuberculosis Programme: An equity analysis. Int J Equity Health. 2007;6:24. doi:10.1186/1475-9276-6-24.
11. Singh K, Sambisa W, Munyati S, Chandiwana B, Chingono A, Mahati S, Mashange W. PLACE in Zimbabwe: Identifying Gaps in HIV Prevention among Orphans and Young People in Hwange District, 2006.
12. Walley J, Khan M, Shah S, Witter S, Wei X. How to get research into practice: First get practice into research. Bull World Health Organ. 2007;85:424. doi:10.2471/BLT.07.042531.
13. Zachariah R, Harries AD, Ishikawa N, Rieder HL, Bissell K, Laserson K, et al. Operational research in low-income countries: What, why, and how? Lancet Infect Dis. 2009;9:711-7.

29 CHAPTER

Introduction to Health Systems Covering WHO Building Blocks

Pentapati Siva Santosh kumar, Bhavesh Modi

"Health systems are a symphony of interconnected elements; orchestrated through the WHO's six building blocks—service delivery, health workforce, health information systems, access to essential medicines, financing, and governance—harmonizing to compose a melody of robust, equitable healthcare for all."

HEALTH SYSTEM

A health system consists of all the organizations, institutions, resources and people whose primary purpose is to improve health. This includes efforts to influence determinants of health as well as more direct health-improvement activities. The health system delivers preventive, promotive, curative and rehabilitative interventions through a combination of public health actions and the pyramid of health care facilities that deliver personal health care—by both state and nonstate actors. The actions of the health system should be responsive and financially fair, while treating people respectably. A health system needs staff, funds, information, supplies, transport, communications and overall guidance and direction to function. Strengthening health systems thus means addressing key constraints in each of these areas.

Goals of the health system are as follows:
- Improving health status
- Defending against threats to health
- Providing equitable access to people-centered care
- Protecting people against the financial consequences of ill-health

Frame Works for Monitoring Health System's Performance

Over the past several years, the World Health Organization (WHO) and its partners have been working to reach a broad-based consensus on key indicators and effective methods and measures of health systems capacity, including "inputs", "processes" and "outputs", and to relate these to indicators of "outcome". The existence of multiple analytical and strategic frameworks for health systems results in considerable potential for duplication, overlap and confusion.

Existing frameworks include:
- WHO framework for health systems performance assessment
- World Bank control knobs framework
- WHO building blocks framework

Such frameworks have varying starting points, resulting in emphasis on different outcomes to be tracked. However, the choice of the strategic framework does not necessarily substantively affect the monitoring and evaluation strategy. It is beyond the scope of this book and chapter to discuss all the three frameworks in detail, so the current chapter will focus on the WHO building blocks framework.

WHO Building Blocks Framework

WHO framework that describes health systems in terms of six core components or "building blocks" (*see* **Figure 1**)
1. Service delivery
2. Health workforce
3. Health information systems
4. Access to essential medicines
5. Financing
6. Leadership/governance

Service Delivery

Overview: Good service delivery is vital to any health system. Service delivery is to deliver the safe, effective, good quality services viz., preventive, curative, palliative and rehabilitative services to those who need it, with minimum wastage. Some established requirements for effective provision include trained staff, right equipment/consumables and adequate financing. The service delivery building block is concerned with how inputs and services are organized and managed, to ensure access, quality, safety and continuity of care across health conditions, across different locations and over time.

Characteristics

- **Comprehensiveness:** A comprehensive range of services appropriate to the needs of the target population
- **Accessibility:** Services should be accessible with no undue barriers related to cost, language, culture or geography. Health services should be available close to the people, with a routine

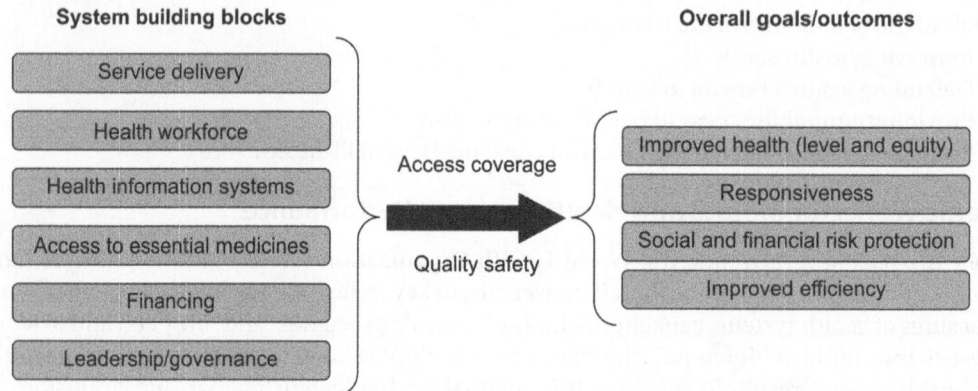

Fig. 1: WHO building blocks framework.

Source: World Health Organization. Monitoring the building blocks of health systems: A handbook of indicators and their measurement strategies [Internet]. Geneva: World Health Organization; 2010. Available from: https://apps.who.int/iris/handle/10665/258734.

Six building blocks of the WHO building blocks framework:

point of entry to the service network at primary care level (not at the specialist or hospital level).
- **Coverage:** All the people in a defined target population are to be covered, i.e., the sick and the healthy, all income groups and all social groups
- **Continuity:** Service provision to be planned in a way to provide with continuity of care across the network of services, health conditions, levels of care, and over the life-cycle.
- **Quality:** Services should be of high quality, i.e., effective, safe and centered on patients needs.
- **Person-centeredness:** Users should perceive services to be responsive and acceptable to them
- **Coordination:** Local area health service networks are actively coordinated, across types of provider, types of care, levels of service delivery, and for both routine and emergency preparedness.
- **Accountability and efficiency:** Health services are well managed so as to achieve the core elements described above (with priority towards those who need them, when and where needed) with a minimum wastage of resources.
- **Examples of indicators:** No. of health facilities/beds/OPD visits/laboratory tests/vaccination coverage per 10,000 population.

Health Workforce

Health workers are all people engaged in actions whose primary intent is to protect and improve health. This includes private as well as public sector health workers; unpaid and paid workers; lay and professional cadres. Overall, there is a strong positive correlation between health workforce density and service coverage and health outcomes. In any country, a "well-performing" health workforce is one which is available, competent, responsive and productive. To achieve this, actions are needed to manage dynamic labor markets that address entry into and exits from the health workforce, and improve the distribution and performance of existing health workers. In simple words, sufficient numbers of staff with fair distribution without any imbalances in terms of Urban/Rural/Tribal, Public/Private is needed.

Health Information Systems

A well-functioning health information system is the one which ensures production, analysis, dissemination and use of reliable and timely information on health determinants, health systems performance and health status. It is vital for day-to-day decisions and also for policy directives.

To achieve the well-functioning status, health information system must:
- Generate population and facility based data: From census, household surveys, civil registration data, public health surveillance, medical records, data on health services and health system resources (e.g., human resources, health infrastructure and financing);
- Have the capacity to detect, investigate, communicate and contain events that threaten public health security at the place they occur, and as soon as they occur
- Have the capacity to synthesize information and promote the availability and application of this knowledge.

Some examples of health information system are Civil Registration System (CRS), HMIS, IDSP, NFHS, DLHS, others with the use of technology (NIKSHAY, eVIN, electronic health records), etc.,

Access to Essential Medicines

According to the WHO framework for health systems, a well-functioning health system ensures equitable access to essential medical products, vaccines and technologies of assured quality, safety, efficacy and cost-effectiveness, and their scientifically sound and cost-effective use. To achieve these objectives, the following are needed:

- National policies, standards, guidelines and regulations that support policy;
- Information on prices, the status of international trade agreements and the capacity to set and negotiate prices;
- Reliable manufacturing practices when they exist in-country and quality assessment of priority products;
- Procurement, supply and storage, and distribution systems that minimize leakage and other waste; and
- Support for rational use of medicines, commodities and equipment, through guidelines and strategies to assure adherence, reduce resistance, maximize patient safety and training.

Monitoring access to essential medicines is closely intertwined with at least two other building blocks: service delivery and governance.

Financing

A good health financing system raises adequate funds for health, in ways that ensure people can use needed services, and are protected from financial catastrophe or impoverishment associated with having to pay for them. Like all aspects of health system strengthening, changes in health financing must be tailored to the history, institutions and traditions of each country. Most systems involve a mix of public and private financing and public and private provision, and there is no one template for action.

Important principles to guide the approach to financing include:

- Raising additional funds where health needs are high, revenues are insufficient, and where accountability mechanisms can ensure transparent and effective use of resources.
- Reducing reliance on out-of-pocket payments where they are high, by moving towards prepayment systems involving pooling of financial risks across population groups (taxation and the various forms of health insurance are all forms of prepayment).
- Taking additional steps, where needed, to improve social protection by ensuring the poor and other vulnerable groups have access to needed services, and that paying for care does not result in financial catastrophe.
- Improving efficiency of resource use by focusing on the appropriate mix of activities and interventions to fund and inputs to purchase, aligning provider payment methods with organizational arrangements for service providers and other incentives for efficient service provision and use including contracting, strengthening financial and other relationships with the private sector and addressing fragmentation of financing arrangements for different types of services.
- Promoting transparency and accountability in health financing systems.
- Improving generation of information on the health financing system and its policy use.

Leadership and Governance

The leadership and governance of health systems, also called stewardship, is arguably the most complex but critical building block of any health system. It is about the role of the government in health and its relation to other actors whose activities impact on health. This involves overseeing and guiding the whole health system, private as well as public, in order to protect the public interest. It requires both political and technical action, because it involves reconciling competing demands for limited resources, in changing circumstances, for example, with rising expectations, more pluralistic societies, decentralization or a growing private sector. There is increased attention to corruption, and calls for a more human rights-based approach to health. There is no blueprint for effective health leadership and governance. While ultimately it is the responsibility of government, this does not mean all leadership and governance functions have to be carried out by central ministries of health. Accountability is an intrinsic aspect of governance that concerns the management of relationships between various stakeholders in health, including individuals, households, communities, firms, governments, nongovernmental organizations, private firms and other entities that have the responsibility to finance, monitor, deliver and use health services. Accountability involves, in particular:

- Delegation or an understanding (either implicit or explicit) of how services are supplied;
- Financing to ensure that adequate resources are available to deliver essential services;
- Performance around the actual supply of services;
- Receipt of relevant information to evaluate or monitor performance;
- Enforcement, such as imposition of sanctions or the provision of rewards for performance.

KEY POINTS

- Organizations and people working together to improve overall health and provide equitable, quality care.
- Various models, especially the WHO's building blocks, guide the monitoring and improvement of health systems.
- Core components focuses on service delivery, workforce, information, medicines, financing, and governance to ensure effective health care.
- Accountability and efficiency is essential for coordinating resources and stakeholders to deliver health services effectively and equitably.

BIBLIOGRAPHY

1. Anello E. Ethical infrastructure for good governance in the public pharmaceutical sector. Geneva, World Health Organization; 2006.
2. Arndt C, Oman C. Uses and abuses of governance indicators. Paris, Organisation for Economic Co-operation and Development, 2006 (OECD Development Centre Studies) (http://www.oecd.org/dataoecd/21/16/40037762.pdf, accessed April 9, 2010).
3. Bloom G, Standing H, Joshi A. Institutional arrangements and health service delivery in low-income countries. Brighton, Institute of Development Studies, 2006 (unpublished).
4. Bloom G, Standing H, Joshi A. Institutional context of health services. In: Peters DH, Seharty E, Siadat B, Vujivic M, Janovsky K (Eds) Implementing health services strategies in low and middle income countries: from evidence to learning and doing. Washington DC, World Bank; 2009.
5. Declaration of Alma Ata, 1978; Universal Declaration on Human Rights 1948; WHO Gender Policy 2002. The Right to Health and other human rights instruments institutionalise in law many aspects of Primary Health Care.
6. This is an expanded version of the definition given in the World health report 2000 Health Systems: Improving Performance.
7. WHO Country Presence 2005: CCS s provide the medium-term strategic framework for WHO's work at country level.
8. World Health Organization: Everybody's business: Strengthening health systems to improve health outcomes. WHO's Framework for Action. Geneva: World Health Organization; 2007.
9. World Health Organization: Monitoring the building blocks of health systems: A handbook of indicators and their measurement strategies. World Health Organization; 2010.

Operational Research in Health Programs

CHAPTER 30

Sumit Malhotra, Saranya R, Bhavesh Modi

"Operational research in health programs is the alchemy of transforming data into insights, ingeniously blending analytical methods with real-world health challenges to optimize interventions and elevate the efficacy of healthcare delivery."

INTRODUCTION

Operational research (OR) provides decision-makers with information to enable them to improve the performance of their programs. Operational research helps to identify solutions to problems that limit program quality, efficiency and effectiveness, or to determine which alternative service delivery strategy would yield the best outcomes. In simple terms, it is described as "the science of better". OR is defined as "Any research producing practical usable knowledge (such as evidence, findings, information) which can improve program implementation (e.g., effectiveness, efficiency, quality, access, scale-up, and sustainability) regardless of the type of research (design, methodology and approach)"

Operational research focuses on factors which are under the control of programs. It seeks to improve the number and quality of services and program outputs and outcomes by optimizing program inputs (e.g., personnel and supplies) and processes (e.g., training, supervision and promotion of services). Operational research can also determine cost-effective and sustainable ways to build service delivery capacity, test financing alternatives and make advocacy and communication strategies and tools more effective. For example, a study to increase condom use among patients on antiretroviral (ARV) treatment might experiment with changes in provider training or client counseling and measure the impact on the number of condoms distributed or frequency of consistent condom use.

The use of operational research is started in military and industrial modeling, in which it is defines as "the application of analytic methods to help make better decisions". OR is also used in commercial sectors, e.g., better designing of waiting lines at Disney theme parks.

What is Implementation Research?

The scientific inquiry into questions concerning implementation—the act of carrying an intention into effect, which in health research can be policies, programs, or individual practices (collectively called interventions).

Defining the Research Domain (Fig. 1)

To improve health systems, three domains of research can be defined using their primary characteristics: the focus of the research, the users of the research outputs, and the utility of

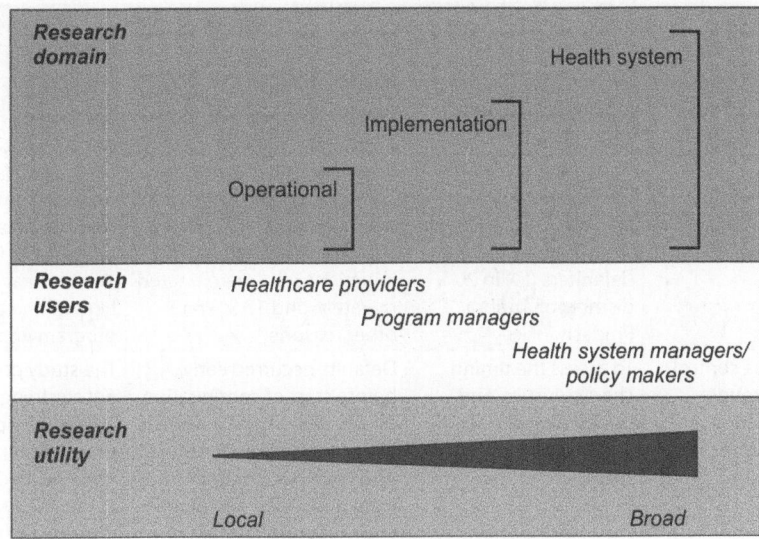

Fig. 1: Defining research domains.

the research outputs. Operational research focuses on operational issues of specific health programs, whereas the focus of implementation research is on implementation strategies for specific products or services and health system research focuses on the issues affecting some or all of the building blocks of a health system. The users of the research outputs (published results, findings, methodologies, etc.) fall broadly into three groups with operational research being predominantly, but not exclusively, of use to healthcare providers; implementation research predominantly of use to managers of programs scaling up an intervention; and research on the health system as a whole (or one of its building blocks) of most use to those who manage or need to make policy for the health system. The importance of how amenable the research is to adaptation and use in other contexts or locations—also varies across the three domains. Operational research tends to address a local problem, taking into account the particular context in which it occurs. It aims to develop solutions to current operational problems of specific health programs or specific service delivery components of the health system, e.g., a health district or a hospital.

A wide range of study designs and research methods are used, ranging from descriptive and analytical studies to operational experiments and the use of mathematical modeling. The research often starts with exploratory studies to better define the problem and its determinants, and to identify potential solutions that can subsequently be tested under operational conditions. Few examples of operations research study in India tabulated in **Table 1**.

Why Operational Research

- ❖ Improve program outcomes in relation to medical care or prevention
  Examples:
  - Voluntary counseling, HIV testing and adjunctive cotrimoxazole reduced mortality in TB patients in Thyolo, Malawi, which has led to Country-wide expansion of HIV testing and cotrimoxazole for TB patients.
  - Payment for ARV drugs are associated with higher rate of patients lost to follow up than those offered free of charge therapy in Nairobi, Kenya. Around 58% higher risk of loss to

Table 1: Few examples of operations research studies from India.

Authors (ref.)	Type of study	Objective	Results	Programme/policy relevance
Babu et al.	Cross-sectional	To evaluate reasons for treatment noninitiation in smear-positive pulmonary TB patients diagnosed and reported as initial defaulters (ID) in 20 districts of Andhra Pradesh	Of 1,304 reported ID, 619 (47.5%) had been placed on treatment. Out of total confirmed (685) ID, 51% were untraceable, 22% had died before treatment initiation, 5.5% were treated privately, and 13.5% had other reasons	Inadequate documentation of referrals, delays in treatment initiation, and registration along with deficiencies in address documentation were highlighted areas for program improvement
Jha et al.	Case control (through record reviews)	To assess the timing, characteristics, and risk factors for default among re-treatment TB cases	Defaults occurred early, before start of continuation phase. Being male, previous history of default during ATT, previous treatment from nonRNTCP providers or DOT at public health facility were key risk factors identified.	The study pointed out to strengthen efforts to improve pretreatment counseling, retrieval mechanisms of interrupters and to increase the proportion of patients treated by community DOT providers
Varkey et al.	Non-equivalent control quasi-experimental	To investigate the feasibility, acceptability, and cost of a new, more comprehensive model of maternity care that encouraged husbands' participation in their wives' antenatal and postpartum care in Employee State Insurance Corporation (ESIC) dispensaries in Delhi	Significant changes were noted in family planning knowledge and behaviors of both men and women in intervention group. Significant higher client-provider discussions occurred during maternity care in the intervention group. The marginal cost of implementing the intervention per dispensary per year was Rs 50,000 (approx. US$ 1,000)	On the basis of the results, the model was scaled in all the ESIC dispensaries in Delhi
Tripathy et al.	Cluster randomized trial	To assess the effect of community mobilization through participatory women's group in improving birth outcomes in underserved tribal clusters of Jharkhand and Orissa	Neonatal Mortality Rate (NMR) was 32% lower in intervention clusters after adjustments	The study underscored the importance of involving women groups as an alternative to just having health worker led interventions for improving NMR
Patel et al.	Economic analysis	To ascertain the efficiency of zinc and copper supplementation in the treatment of acute diarrhea under 5 years	The study demonstrated lower cost of treating acute diarrhea, lower cost per unit health and incremental cost effectiveness ratio	Cost savings as evidenced by the study makes a stronger case for micronutrients supplementation as an adjunct therapy to ORS management

follow up was associated with payment for ART; ART dose dilutions by patients who had to pay for ART. Detrimental effect of payment-based therapy on outcomes, service began free of charge in hospital
- ❖ Assess feasibility of new strategies or interventions in specific settings or population
  Examples:
  - *HIV treatment in a conflict setting (Democratic Republic of Congo):* Provided knowledge and contingency planning for sustaining comprehensive HIV/AIDS care, including antiretroviral therapy in chronic conflict settings
  - *Descriptive report of a rural model of antiretroviral treatment:* A decentralized, simplified model of antiretroviral therapy delivery based on nurses was feasible in rural South Africa, which has led to policy change in allowing nonphysician clinicians to administer antiretroviral therapy
- ❖ Advocate for policy change
  Examples:
  - High prevalence of lipoatrophy among patients on Stavudine containing first line ART in Rwanda, showed that lipoatrophy was an important complication of WHO recommended first line ART regimens. It has highlighted the urgent need for access to more affordable and less toxic ART regimens in Africa (Van Griensven et al.).
  - Multicentre studies of drug resistance and efficacy in falciparum malaria showed high levels of drug resistance in falciparum malaria and ineffective national regimens, led to a shift in national and international policy on use of more effective antimalarial treatment

What is the Source of Data?

In operational research, mostly secondary data is used from routine data monitoring system. Many distinguished OR scientists in public health strongly believe in secondary data analysis as retrospective record reviews, utilizing data that is already generated in the programs. Such data in the field often are not used to its maximum potential and much problem identification and gaps can be found out by reviewing the program reports and data sets.

Example:
The global public health decision including in India to switch over from three sputum smear examination to two smears in diagnosing pulmonary tuberculosis stemmed from laboratory register records reviewed retrospectively looking for additional gains by performing third smear over second in these patients.

Researcher can also collect primary data, i.e., real time operational research.

Example:
Incorrect Registration of New and Recurrent TB in Malawi: In 1999, the National TB Programme (NTP) in Malawi became concerned about the declining numbers of patients registered nationally as 'recurrent TB'. NTP was concerned that patients with recurrent TB were being misregistered as having new TB. All patients in the hospital registered with new TB were interviewed using a structured questionnaire, and they were asked whether they had ever had previous TB and treatment: if this was the case, the patient was recorded as having recurrent TB. At the end of each regional supervision, the data were analyzed and discussed. The study confirmed the NTP hypothesis that a substantial number of patients with recurrent TB were misregistered as having new TB. This had important programmatic implications.

Themes of OR

Lack of Knowledge

- **Example:** Lack of knowledge about patients lost to follow up
- **Objective:** Achieve an 85% treatment completion (TB) or excellent retention on therapy (ART, asthma and smoking cessation tool)
- **Constraint:** High loss to follow up rates (30%) from therapy and treatment completion is 70%
- **Research question:** Why are people lost? (payment/side effects/transport costs to clinic/unreported death)
- Answer the question and find solutions to decreasing losses from the therapy.

Lack of a Tool or Intervention

- **Example:** Lack of tool to screen severely ill TB patients at diagnosis
- **Objective:** 90% reduction in TB deaths by 2025 when compared to 2015 by early identification of severely ill TB patients
- **Constraints:** Criteria for assessing severe illness requires clinical, laboratory and radiological assessment. Not possible to cover all TB patients (Lack of screening tool)
- **Research question:** How feasible it is for paramedical TB program staff to use a simple screening tool based on severe undernutrition (BMI), respiratory insufficiency (RR, SpO2) and performance status (inability to stand)?
- Answer the question and find solutions to screen and refer severely ill patients

Inefficient Use of a Tool or Intervention

- **Example:** Inefficient use of a tool—sputum smears for diagnosing PTB
- **Objectives of NTP:** High quality sputum smear diagnosis using three sputum smears per patient
- **Constraints:** Three smears per patients are demanding for the laboratory technicians (Shortage and high caseload)
- **Research question:** Are two smears as efficient as three smears for diagnosing smear-positive pulmonary TB
- Research questions are generated by identifying constraints/challenges of implementation
  The answers to these questions should have direct, practical relevance to solving these problems and improving healthcare delivery.

Scope of Operational Research with Example (Table 2)

HIV prevention and circumcision: In 1980s, there was low prevalence of male circumcision in the parts of sub-Saharan Africa most affected by the epidemic. A review of 28 observational studies in African countries concluded that circumcised men had about a 44 percent lower risk of HIV infection compared to noncircumcised men. As all were observational study, it showed an weaker association and there was a need for experimental studies.
- Trials were performed:
  - In South Africa, Orange Farm, 3,000 men aged 18–24; circumcised men 60 % less likely to acquire HIV than the uncircumcised men
  - In Uganda's Rakai District, 4,996 men aged 15–49, circumcision reduced the risk by 51 %
  - In Kenya, Kisumu, 2,784 men aged 18–24; risk was reduced by 59 %. An ongoing follow-up study found that this protective effect was sustained over 42 months, reducing men's chances of becoming infected with HIV by 64%

Chapter 30: Operational Research in Health Programs

Table 2: Scope of OR with examples:

Identifying the problem

Despite patients offered ARVs, opportunistic Infections like diarrhea and pneumonia were high amongst them
Why are HIV positive clients experiencing poorer health outcomes?
Problem of adherence to regimens

Considering the reasons

Poor communication between clients and staff
Low-income clients do not have enough money for transportation – refill their prescriptions
Clients cannot afford to miss their work to come to clinic
Perceived stigma
Frequent drug stock outs

Testing the solutions

Drug stock outs-
Staff in service training to improve drug forecasting
Developing clinic-based performance standards that inform the basis for problem solving among staff
Which solution solves problem best?

Contemplation: Access

Low coverage
Failure to scale-up
Equity issues such as not reaching the poor, those living in remote areas, the marginalized, women, children, adolescents
Not reaching those who are stigmatized
Insufficient staffing - may need to look at task shifting approaches, e.g., use of community workers

Contemplation: Quality issues

Poor quality of services and target groups avoiding the service
Poor diagnostic and dispensing services
Other technical problems
Poor information/education/communication (IEC) programs
No job aids or poor use of them
Poor referral systems

Contemplation: Managerial issues

Poor adherence to policy recommendations
Poor record-keeping and reporting, M&E
Poor information dissemination
Interaction or competition with other interventions for other diseases
Marketing and advocacy

Contemplation: Delivery system at community/individual level

Levels of household income that influence affordability
Stigma
Other participation barriers
Perceptions and misperceptions

- Circumcision introduction framework

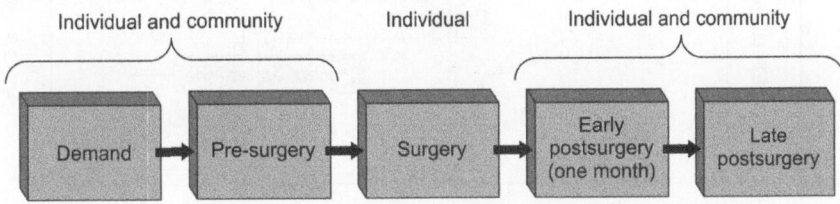

❖ System model for medical male circumcision:

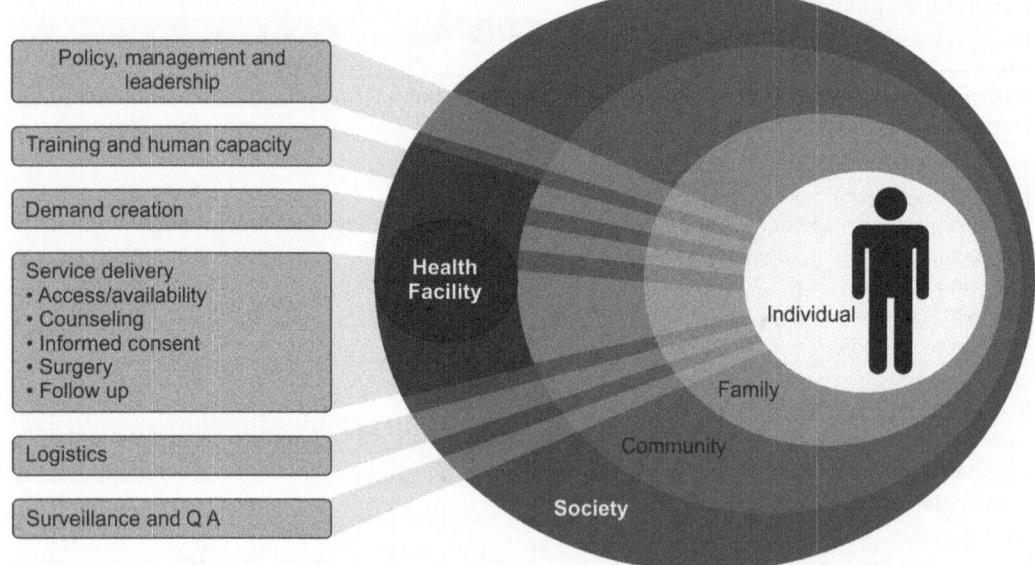

Key Operational Research Issues

❖ What are the most effective and cost-effective ways of integrating male circumcision services into existing HIV programs?
❖ Which messages are most effective in conveying to clients and their partners that male circumcision is an additional HIV prevention option, and not a replacement for correct, consistent condom use and other risk-reduction measures?
❖ What are the most effective and cost-effective approaches to training and supervising staff to provide male circumcision services?
❖ What are the most effective and cost-effective ways to maintain and monitor the safety of the procedure in different resource-constrained settings?
❖ What are the most effective strategies for including private-sector providers in programs that offer male circumcision for HIV prevention?
❖ What is the feasibility and the cost of training clinical officers and nurses to provide safe, high-quality male circumcision services?
❖ What is the impact on access and safety of offering male circumcision through outreach services?
❖ Proven interventions lose impact in health systems:

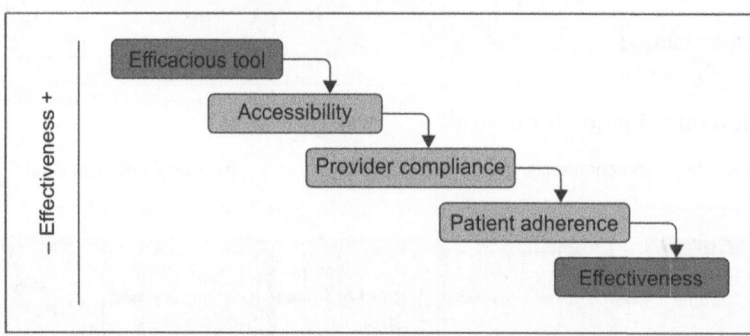

❖ Implementation of intervention–interacting domains

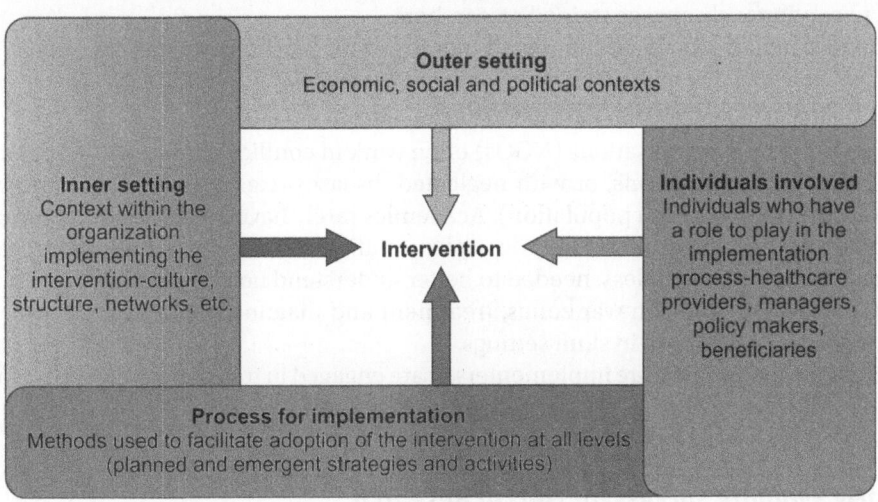

Enabling Factors for Operational Research

Direct Program Relevance

❖ Research question must be relevant to programme implementation and connected to health service delivery. Coordination mechanism to provide clear strategy about setting of research priorities.
❖ OR addresses those problems that are under control of managers, such as program systems, training, pricing and provision of information.

Partnerships

❖ **Paradigm shift:** A "partnership model" that promotes better involvement, co-ownership and responsibility of program staff with researchers. It will help in identification of the research problem, development of the study design, implementation of the study and analysis and interpretation of results. Thus, build funding and resources for operational research into a national program.
❖ Collaboration with partners is the best way to introduce these new implementation strategies into the health system and facilitate their full scale implementation, evaluation and modification as required.

Build Research Capacity/Time

❖ Starting from research question-protocol development, including ethics approval-secure funding-implementation, collection of data, cleaning of data-data analysis and interpretation-paper writing, submission, peer review to re-writing- "The Hard Work" to translate findings into policy and practice.
❖ Sufficient program capacity exists to host workshops, present, and discuss research findings, and ensure their translation into policy and practice.
❖ Program staff have access to scientific literature through subscribed journals or the internet.
❖ Sufficient numbers of program staff are available with the capacity to do operational research, write up manuscripts, and publish relevant research.

Retain and Engage Trained Researchers
- Plan to continuously engage trained researchers.
- Retain researchers who have completed training or those who have Masters or PhD.

Role of Nongovernmental Organizations
- Nongovernmental organisations (NGOs) often work in conflict settings, with marginalized and vulnerable populations, or with neglected diseases (e.g., prisoners, commercial sex workers and hard to reach population). Academics rarely have access to such settings, and national programs might decide they do not have sufficient resources to study them. Research in these areas is, nevertheless, needed to better understand how to manage questions such as mental health issues in war zones, treatment and diagnosis of neglected diseases, or offering of HIV/AIDS care in slum settings.
- By mandate, many NGOs are implementers or are engaged in translating research into policy and practice.
- Many NGOs are well resourced.

Regularly Evaluate Success (or Not) of Research
- Have research activities completed and publishes?
- Has it influenced policy/practice?
- Provide feedback and disseminate
- OR succeeds only if the study results are used to make program decisions; publication alone is not a valid indicator of successful OR.

Challenges
- One challenge is that foreign academic institutions often have the funding, time, and mandate for research and thus the associated power in decisions about what gets done. Local institutions should also be supported with money and staff for operational research, thus allowing them the necessary independence to make decisions, take responsibility, and establish partnerships that are more equal in resources and decision-making power.
- Many health programs and health system managers do not see operational research as a priority, and it is sometimes perceived as a waste of time and resources, distracting from the need for operational action on the basis of "common sense". Such attitudes tend to soften with exposure to properly executed operational research that delivers practical results, but quality operational research does not come easily, given the general lack of research capacity and research funding at the operational level. Several global health initiatives offer additional funding for operational research but most of these funds are not taken up at country and program level because of the lack of appreciation for this type of research and insufficient local research capacity.
- Capacity and time for research activities, such as writing study protocols or dealing with peer review are often lacking within most program settings but are essential to see research to completion.
- NGOs are sometimes not the appropriate entities for designing or implementing research. They might lack the institutional support, culture, and skills for interacting with national programs and decision makers. NGO focus might be on solving localized, short-term problems, they might have had little exposure to systems thinking and they might lack the training and capacity to do rigorous research. Hence, this challenge can be overcome by collaborating with trained researchers.

Creating Opportunities

- There are various ways in which these opportunities could be created. First, small grants could be offered to pursue locally applied research. Second, junior and senior operational research fellowships could be created for colleagues in low-income countries with active mentoring by international researchers, institutions, or NGOs.
- Bureaucracy should be kept to a minimum with the main focus on deliverable outcomes that would include publications with specific benefits to programs and communities.
- Attention must also be paid to the problem of poor access to up-to-date scientific literature, and despite laudable initiatives, this remains a barrier in low-income countries. Free and open access for all articles of interest to low-income countries is urgently needed.

KEY POINTS

- Operational research enhances program performance by solving problems and optimizing resources for better healthcare outcomes.
- OR focuses on specific program issues, while implementation research looks at broader strategies for health service delivery.
- Key benefits of OR are it improves care quality, tests new strategies, and informs policy changes based on practical evidence.
- OR utilizes existing data to explore issues like knowledge gaps and tool efficiency to improve service delivery.
- OR faces challenges like capacity and perception, but offers opportunities through partnerships, capacity building, and targeted funding.

BIBLIOGRAPHY

1. Caleb-Varkey L, Mishra A, Ottolenghi E, Huntington D, Leila CV, Das A, et al. Involving men in maternity care in India. Reprod Health [Internet]. 2004 Jan 1 [cited 2024 Jan 16]; Available from: https://knowledgecommons.popcouncil.org/departments_sbsr-rh/420
2. Culbert H, Tu D, O'Brien DP, Ellman T, Mills C, Ford N, et al. HIV treatment in a conflict setting: outcomes and experiences from Bukavu, Democratic Republic of the Congo. PLoS Med [Internet]. 2007 May [cited 2023 Sep 2];4(5):0794–8. Available from: https://pubmed.ncbi.nlm.nih.gov/17535100/
3. ENN. Operational research in low-income countries: What, why, and how? Field Exchange 42, -. Field Exchange 42 [Internet]. 2012 [cited 2023 Sep 2];18. Available from: www.ennonline.net/fex/42/operational
4. Guthmann JP, Checchi F, Van Den Broek I, Balkan S, Van Herp M, Comte E, et al. Assessing antimalarial efficacy in a time of change to artemisinin-based combination therapies: the role of Médecins Sans Frontières. PLoS Med [Internet]. 2008 Aug [cited 2023 Sep 2];5(8):1191–9. Available from: https://pubmed.ncbi.nlm.nih.gov/18684011/
5. Harries AD, Thekkur P, Mbithi I, Chakaya JM, Tweya H, Takarinda KC, et al. Real-Time Operational Research: Case Studies from the Field of Tuberculosis and Lessons Learnt. Trop Med Infect Dis [Internet]. 2021 Jun 1 [cited 2023 Sep 2];6(2). Available from: /pmc/articles/PMC8293385/
6. Jha UM, Satyanarayana S, Dewan PK, Chadha S, Wares F, Sahu S, et al. Risk Factors for Treatment Default among Re-Treatment Tuberculosis Patients in India, 2006. PLoS One [Internet]. 2010 Jan 25 [cited 2024 Jan 16];5(1):e8873. Available from: https://journals.plos.org/plosone/article?id=10.1371/journal.pone.0008873
7. Malhotra S, Zodpey SP. Operations research in public health. Indian J Public Health [Internet]. 2010 Jul [cited 2023 Sep 2];54(3):145–50. Available from: https://pubmed.ncbi.nlm.nih.gov/21245584/
8. Patel AB, Dhande LA, Rawat MS. Economic evaluation of zinc and copper use in treating acute diarrhea in children: A randomized controlled trial. Cost Effectiveness and Resource Allocation [Internet]. 2003

Aug 29 [cited 2024 Jan 16];1(1):1–10. Available from: https://resource-allocation.biomedcentral.com/articles/10.1186/1478-7547-1-7
9. Remme JHF, Adam T, Becerra-Posada F, D'Arcangues C, Devlin M, Gardner C, et al. Defining Research to Improve Health Systems. PLoS Med [Internet]. 2010 Nov [cited 2023 Aug 29];7(11):e1001000. Available from: https://journals.plos.org/plosmedicine/article?id=10.1371/journal.pmed.1001000
10. Sai Babu B, Satyanarayana AVV, Venkateshwaralu G, Ramakrishna U, Vikram P, Sahu S, et al. Initial default among diagnosed sputum smear-positive pulmonary tuberculosis patients in Andhra Pradesh, India.
11. Tripathy P, Nair N, Barnett S, Mahapatra R, Borghi J, Rath S, et al. Effect of a participatory intervention with women's groups on birth outcomes and maternal depression in Jharkhand and Orissa, India: A cluster-randomised controlled trial. Lancet [Internet]. 2010 [cited 2024 Jan 16];375(9721):1182–92. Available from: https://pubmed.ncbi.nlm.nih.gov/20207411/
12. Zachariah R, Harries AD, Ishikawa N, Rieder HL, Bissell K, Laserson K, et al. Operational research in low-income countries: what, why, and how? Lancet Infect Dis [Internet]. 2009 Nov 1 [cited 2023 Sep 2];9(11):711–7. Available from: http://www.thelancet.com/article/S1473309909702294/fulltext
13. Zachariah R, Spielmann MPL, Chinji C, Gomani P, Arendt V, Hargreaves NJ, et al. Voluntary counselling, HIV testing and adjunctive cotrimoxazole reduces mortality in tuberculosis patients in Thyolo, Malawi. AIDS [Internet]. 2003 May 2 [cited 2023 Sep 2];17(7):1053–61. Available from: https://pubmed.ncbi.nlm.nih.gov/12700456/

Role of Stakeholders and Ethical Concerns

CHAPTER 31

Pentapati Siva Santosh kumar, Anwita Khaitan, Anil Jacob Purty

> *"Ethical operational research requires transparency, accountability, and a commitment to the well-being of both individuals and communities."*

STAKEHOLDERS IN OPERATIONAL RESEARCH

Stakeholders' knowledge regarding their roles and responsibilities in the conduct of biomedical research is crucial in determining the soundness of the methodology followed and, hence, the validity of the findings. The stakeholders must also know how to apply the principles of community engagement, especially if a vulnerable population is involved in the study. Further, each stakeholder must be aware of the ethical concerns that may arise during their commitment to the project at hand and how to deal with them in a manner that is in harmony with the principles of ethical research as per national guidelines.

As is well known, a harmonious equilibrium among the various stakeholders is crucial to the smooth conduct of a large-scale study. These stakeholders include—but are not limited to—study team members (right from the principal investigator to the data collector), the study participants themselves, partner agencies providing logistical support, members of various bodies safeguarding the rights of the study participants (e.g., Institute Ethics Committees' members), members of scientific and technical advisory bodies, funding agencies (governmental or nongovernmental), and political decision-makers **(Fig. 1)**.

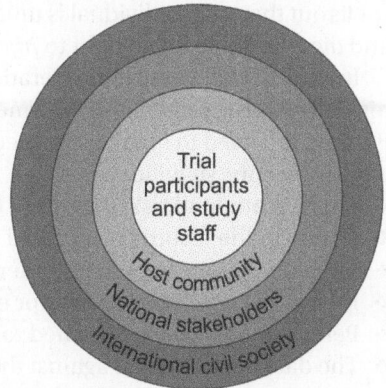

Fig. 1: Graphical representation of the important stakeholders in an operational research study.

Study Participants and Study Staff

At the heart of any operational research study lies in its participants. Along with them, we can also include the study team members at the study site, whose members directly interact with the study participants. We also have the other study team members in the inner circle and, in some instances, the partner agencies since they might provide on-the-ground support.

Host Community

Our next stakeholder group of import comprises the host community members. This includes the individuals living in the study area (but not the study's actual participants), the local leaders, and community-based organizations that serve or represent them directly. This may include traditional healers, local radio, and other community structures (including community advisory boards).

National Stakeholders and International Civil Society

These collectives include anyone and everyone who has a role to play in the political, scientific, and social enterprise for health development in the larger national community. Some important members who must be on board are national and (when applicable) international ethical review committees and regulatory bodies, political decision-makers including officials in the Ministry of Health and Family Welfare (MoHFW), nongovernmental organizations (NGOs), financial donors, as well as media organizations.

Ethical Considerations in Operational Research

Broadly, eight to ten ethical principles are to be considered during the planning and conduct of any study, including an operational research study. These can be read in detail from the references below. The following considerations are the most important when looking through the lens of operational research.

Respect for Persons

Just as in our day-to-day dealings in the real world, the principle of respect for persons holds steady and strong in the controlled environment of a research study as well.

When we talk about respect for persons while conducting research, we are mainly focused on actively protecting the autonomy of the participants—The principle of autonomy explicitly spells out that each individual is unique and free, has the right and capacity to decide, has value and dignity, and has the right to *informed consent*.

In the specific context of operational research, some critical points on autonomy must be highlighted. The principle of informed consent does not apply to publicly available information. Further, the need to obtain informed consent from participants for using their records may be waived in some specific scenarios:

- There is minimal risk of harm to the individuals.
- Access to the records is essential to achieve the objectives of the research.
- There is a public benefit to undertaking the research.
- Informed consent is logically or economically impracticable.
- Permission has been obtained to use the data from the custodian of the records.
- The data are protected against those not involved in the research.

In such cases, the request for waiver of informed consent must be explicitly made in the research proposal submitted to the ethics committee, accompanied by a rationale on why informed consent is not needed/not possible.

Further, permission to use relevant records, where applicable, must be sought from the custodian of the records (or a nominee).

We are also concerned with protecting the vulnerable members of the participant group from any such harm during the study, which would not have occurred had that individual not been a participant in the study. Hence, special provisions must be in place for those whose decision–making capacity is impaired or diminished, whether due to physical or social factors.

Beneficence/Nonmaleficence

The protection of the study participants is the essential responsibility of the researcher. Researchers must protect each research participant's physical, mental and social well-being, minimize physical and social risks, maximize the possible benefits, and retain the community perspective.

Justice/Nonexploitation

This principle calls for *fairness in the conduct of research* in both letter and spirit.
- The research must ensure a fair distribution of risks and benefits.
- Further, research should only be done in a community that is likely to benefit from the results.
- There should also be equitable recruitment of research participants and the provision of special protection for vulnerable groups.
- Further, rules of data confidentiality and anonymity (as applicable) must be strictly followed. This can be ensured by removing personal information and linking the data to the participant. If names or other personal identifiers have been used, they must be removed from the research database when data collection is completed and before the analysis starts. Records with private information must be maintained securely, and access to the data must be limited to the relevant authorized personnel only. Records of personal data and research findings must then be kept separately (logically and physically under lock and key or password secured) and linked only by bar code. Records must only be maintained if they are needed but usually for a minimum of five years, depending on the ethics committee and funder requirements. There are certain exceptional situations where confidentiality may be breached. For example, to link data from a laboratory database to that in the electronic tuberculosis register. To identify a possible participant before tracing, it is possible to request their participation.

Approval From the Institutional Ethics Committee

The research proposal must be submitted to the Institute Ethics Committee/Institutional Review Board for approval before the research is undertaken.

Depending on the geographical location of the study site(s), the researcher's employer and the research partners, the proposal may have to be submitted to one or more ethics committees. The research can only start when the various institutions' ethics committees have approved the study. Hence, the month(s) for ethical approval must be taken into account when the project work plan is being developed. A Gantt chart may be used to prepare the entire study timeline.

It must be stated that even when an ethics committee has approved a research proposal, the responsibility for good ethical practice ultimately lies in the hands of the researcher.

Dissemination of Findings of the Research Study

At the end of a study (and sometimes even at intermediate stages), it is of paramount importance to inform the broader scientific community of the findings of the study, as well as any new learnings regarding methods of conducting operational research, if any. Dissemination of findings is an essential step, and some would argue that skipping this step is unethical, The disseminated research findings should outline the broad roles of stakeholders in biomedical research. Notably, the findings must be disseminated even if they are negative (e.g., failure to reject the null hypothesis). Once findings are disseminated on public platforms (such as peer-reviewed journals), the broad community can reap the rewards of the results, and the research community may avoid unnecessary future expenses by repeating a similar study.

The study team members must make an active effort to inform the study participants of the study's findings when, for instance, a modifiable risk factor is identified that may be hazardous to the participant and/or others. The significance of the results should be explained in simple, straightforward terms, a clear recommendation for the following appropriate action should be made, and an effort must be made to ensure that the recommendation is followed. Such information must be provided in a balanced manner with a sensitivity to the possible anxiety such news may bring with it. Proper counseling may be needed in certain scenarios.

KEY POINTS

- Stakeholders in operational research must understand their ethical roles and responsibilities, including the need for informed consent and data protection.
- Research must adhere to ethical principles, with proposals requiring approval from relevant ethics committees.
- Findings should be transparently shared with the scientific community and participants, especially when it affects their health and well-being.

BIBLIOGRAPHY

1. Bagepally BS, Rao RR, Vijayaprabha R, Saravanan M. NIeCer 102: Ethics Review of Health Research. Multifaculty. New Delhi: ICMR-National Institute of Epidemiology; [date unknown]. Available from: https://onlinecourses.swayam2.ac.in/aic22_ge22/preview&#8203
2. Desmond Tutu TB Centre, Department of Paediatrics and Child Health, Faculty of Medicine and Health Sciences, Stellenbosch University, International Union Against Tuberculosis and Lung Disease. Operational Research to Improve Health Services: A guide for proposal development. Cape Town: University of Stellenbosch - Desmond Tutu TB Centre; 2013. Available from: www0.sun.ac.za/dttc.
3. Indian Council of Medical Research. National Ethical Guidelines for Biomedical and Health Research Involving Human Participants. New Delhi: ICMR; 2017. Available from: https://main.icmr.nic.in/guidelines

Qualitative Research in Operational Research

CHAPTER 32

Rashmi Kundapur, Suthanthira Kannan

> *"Qualitative research in operational research is the art of listening to the whispers of human experience, transforming subjective narratives into objective insights that illuminate the nuanced complexities of operational challenges."*

INTRODUCTION

Qualitative research has been a significant cornerstone of the social sciences and humanities for decades and has recently been increasingly recognized for its value in the healthcare field. In operational research in health, qualitative research provides invaluable insights into the human factors that affect health systems. This chapter explores the role of qualitative research in operational research in health.

- **Operational research in health:** Operational research is an analytical approach that aims to make health service provision more efficient and effective. It uses statistical and mathematical models to analyze complex situations, providing objective information to support decision-making. In healthcare, operational research can optimize scheduling, inventory management, resource allocation, and overall patient outcomes.
- **Role of qualitative research in operational research:** Unlike quantitative research, which primarily focuses on numerical data, qualitative research explores people's experiences, attitudes, and behaviors. In the context of operational research, qualitative techniques can elucidate the context in which health services operate and the human behaviors that impact these services.

Qualitative research provides rich, descriptive data that allows researchers to understand the 'why' and 'how' of observed phenomena. This information is crucial in shaping interventions, developing strategies, and improving health services' efficiency and effectiveness.

Common Qualitative Research Techniques in Health Operational Research

- **Interviews and focus groups:** These techniques involve direct communication with individuals or groups. They can reveal deep insights about personal experiences, perceptions, and suggestions for improvements within the health services context.
- **Observational studies:** These studies involve observing interactions in a natural setting to understand behaviors, relationships, and environmental factors affecting health service delivery.
- **Document analysis:** Reviewing documents such as patient records, internal reports, and policy documents can provide contextual information that aids operational efficiency.

Integration of Qualitative and Quantitative Methods

The integration of qualitative and quantitative research methods, known as mixed-methods research, can provide a holistic understanding of health operations. Quantitative data can provide hard evidence about efficiency and effectiveness, while qualitative data can offer insight into the experiences and perceptions of those involved. This holistic understanding can guide the design and implementation of interventions and inform policy development.

Challenges and Solutions in Implementing Qualitative Research

The implementation of qualitative research in operational research in health can pose challenges. These may include issues of objectivity, difficulties in data interpretation, and challenges in ensuring validity and reliability. Solutions can involve careful study design, rigorous data analysis, and the use of strategies to ensure trustworthiness, such as triangulation and member checking.

Theories

Decision Theory in Qualitative Health OR

Incorporating decision theory into qualitative health OR is a means to improve the accuracy and relevance of the decision-making process. By understanding the qualitative aspects of a healthcare decision—like patient preferences, ethical considerations, or systemic biases—we can create decision-making models that better reflect the complexity of real-life healthcare settings.

For example, qualitative research can help to understand a patient's decision-making process, their perceptions of risk, and their value judgements. These insights can be incorporated into decision analysis models, leading to more patient-centered healthcare. Similarly, on an organizational level, qualitative research can help to illuminate the factors that influence a health system's strategic decisions, such as how to allocate resources, which can also be modeled and analyzed.

Game Theory in Qualitative Health OR

Game theory, which studies strategic interactions among rational decision-makers, can also be enriched by qualitative insights. In a healthcare context, game theory can be used to understand and predict the outcomes of interactions between various stakeholders—like healthcare providers, patients, insurers, and regulators.

Qualitative research can provide in-depth understandings of the strategies these players use, their preferences and payoffs, and the nature of their interactions. This can lead to the development of more nuanced and accurate game-theoretical models. For instance, qualitative insights could inform the design of a game-theoretical model that predicts how healthcare providers might respond to a new reimbursement policy.

Implementation Outcomes

Definitions, *see* **Table 1**.

Conclusion

The Future of Qualitative Research in Operational Research in Health: With the growing recognition of the value of human factors in healthcare, the use of qualitative research in operational research is likely to increase. Continued innovation in qualitative research

Table 1: Implementation outcomes definitions.

Implementation outcome	Working definition*	Related terms**
Acceptability	The perception among stakeholders (e.g., consumers, providers, managers, policy-makers) that an intervention is agreeable	Related factors (e.g., comfort, relative advantage and credibility)
Adoption	The intention, initial decision, or action to try to employ a new intervention	Uptake, utilization, intention to try
Appropriateness	The perceived fit or relevance of the intervention in a particular setting or for a particular target audience (e.g., provider or consumer) or issue	Relevance, perceived fit, compatibility, perceived usefulness or suitability
Feasibility	The extent to which an intervention can be carried out in a particular setting or organization	Practicality, actual fit, utility and trialability

*,** *Source:* Proctor et al 2011; Peters, Adams, Alonge et al, 2013.

methodologies and increased integration with quantitative approaches promises a richer understanding of health operations. This knowledge will underpin improvements in health service efficiency and effectiveness, ultimately benefiting patients and the healthcare system as a whole.

In conclusion, qualitative research plays an essential role in operational research in health, offering invaluable insights into human behaviors, perceptions, and experiences. It allows for a more comprehensive understanding of health service operations and can significantly inform decision-making processes.

KEY POINTS

- Provides insights into human factors affecting health systems, elucidating the 'why' and 'how' behind phenomena and improving intervention strategies.
- Employs methods like interviews, observational studies, and document analysis to gather rich, descriptive data on experiences and behaviors within health services.
- Combines with quantitative data for a holistic understanding of health operations, aiding in designing effective interventions and policies.
- Incorporates theories like decision and game theory for nuanced decision-making models, with growing recognition and innovation promising deeper insights and enhanced healthcare efficiency.

BIBLIOGRAPHY

1. Crowe S, Brown KM, Tregay J, Wray J, Knowles R, Ridout D, et al. Combining qualitative and quantitative operational research methods to inform quality improvement in pathways that span multiple settings. BMJ Qual Saf. 2017;26:641-52.
2. Dixon-Woods M. Interpreting change: The role of qualitative research in evaluating interventions in chronic respiratory disease. Chronic Respir Dis. 2007;4:127-8.
3. Herbert R, Higgs J. Complementary research paradigms. Aust J Physiother. 2004;50(2):63-4.
4. Kirsch L. Quantitative Techniques for Hospital Planning and Control. Health Serv Res. 1974;9:246-8.
5. Ngamvithayapong-Yanai J. The role of qualitative research in ending TB. Public Health Action. 2016;6(4):209.
6. Nicolson P. Qualitative research, psychology and mental health: Analysing subjectivity. J Ment Health. 1995;4:337-46.
7. Sofaer S. Qualitative methods: What are they and why use them? Health Serv Res. 1999;34(5 Pt 2):1101-18.

Quasi-experimental Studies

Ashwini Lonimath, Sumit Malhotra, Sonu Goel

"If we knew what it was, we were doing, it would not be called as research, would it?"
—*Albert Einstein*

INTRODUCTION

Research in the social and natural sciences often seeks to establish causal relationships between variables. In traditional experimental research, researchers manipulate an independent variable to observe its effect on a dependent variable while controlling for other factors. However, in many real-world situations, conducting a classical experiment with full control over variables and random assignment is either impractical or ethically problematic. This is where *quasi-experimental studies* come into play.

Quasi-experimental studies provide a valuable alternative to traditional experiments by allowing researchers to investigate causality in settings where randomization is difficult or impossible.

Defining Quasi-experimental Studies: Quasi-experimental studies share similarities with traditional experiments but differ in terms of the researcher's level of control and manipulation of variables that is they aim to evaluate interventions but lack randomization. While they fall short of the ideal conditions of a randomized controlled trial (RCT), they remain a powerful tool for investigating causal relationships (causality between an intervention and an outcome).

Characteristics of Quasi-experimental Studies

- ❖ **Lack of randomization:** Unlike true experiments, quasi-experiments do not involve random assignment of subjects to groups. Instead, pre-existing groups or naturally occurring conditions are used.
- ❖ **Controlled variable manipulation:** Researchers still manipulate one or more independent variables to examine their impact on a dependent variable. However, this manipulation is constrained by the circumstances.
- ❖ **Non-equivalent groups:** Quasi-experiments often deal with nonequivalent groups, meaning that participants in different conditions may not be equivalent at the outset. Researchers must account for these differences statistically.
- ❖ **Time series analysis:** Some quasi-experimental designs involve the analysis of data collected over time, allowing researchers to assess changes or interventions' effects across multiple points.

- **Real-world context:** Quasi-experimental studies are often conducted in real-world settings, making them highly relevant to practical applications and policy decisions. Characteristics of true experiments and quasi-experimental depicted in **Table 1**.

Table 1: Characteristics of true experiments and quasi-experimental.

Sl. No	Characteristics	True experiment	Quasi-experiment
1.	Includes manipulated independent variables	Yes	Yes
2.	Includes a comparison	Yes	Yes
3.	A high degree of control over the experimental situation (most notably a random assignment)	Yes	

The Role of Quasi-experimental Studies

Quasi-experimental studies are employed in various fields, including psychology, education, public health, economics, and sociology, to answer research questions where strict experimentation is challenging. They are particularly valuable when:
- Ethical concerns prevent random assignment.
- Researchers want to assess the impact of interventions or policies that naturally occur.
- The research context involves pre-existing groups, such as different schools, hospitals, or communities.
- Researchers aim to understand the long-term effects of an intervention or treatment.

Types of Quasi-experimental Studies

Post-test Only Design

This design has no control/comparison group. Gives descriptive and demographic information. It is a design with challenges and threats to validity exists such as selection, history, maturity, mortality **(Fig. 1)**:

Examples:
- Acceptors/non-acceptors of vasectomy in a district.
- Characteristics and experiences of adolescents that attended AFC versus that did not.

Experimental group $\xrightarrow{\text{Time}}$ X O_1

Fig. 1: Post-test only design.

Post-test Design

There is no control group in this design. One earlier measurement before intervention is present. It Is the most common type of quasi-experimental study design used by the researchers. There might be possible threats to validity **(Fig. 2)**.

Example: Increasing the accessibility, acceptability and use of the IUDs in Gujarat, India.

Experimental group $\xrightarrow{\text{Time}}$ O_1 X O_2

Fig. 2: Pretest - Post-test design.

Specific Objectives

- Increasing awareness and correct knowledge of the IUD among men and women in the reproductive age group.
- Enhance the acceptability of IUD among providers.
- Increase use of the IUD by making services more accessible, and providing services of higher quality.
- Estimate the cost of scaling up of the intervention in larger areas.

Research Questions Addressed

- Does reorientation of providers and providing supportive supervision stimulate them to use the balanced counseling approach (BCS) and to offer the IUD as a safe, long-acting contraceptive?
- Does reorientation training help in improving the quality of counseling and services?
- Does improved community-based BCC about the IUD increase interest and intention to use the IUD as a contraceptive method?
- Does provision of accurate information on the IUD reduce the myths and misconceptions about IUD use?
- Does the increased awareness and knowledge of the IUD and increased accessibility to services result in its increased use?
- Is the intervention feasible, sustainable and economically viable in the Indian context?

Study Design and Intervention Package

$$O_1 \quad X+Y+Z \quad O_2$$
$$\underline{\qquad 9\ Months \qquad}$$

Where,
- X is strengthening counseling and technical skills of the providers for insertion and removal of the IUD
- Y is the BCC effort to educate potential users about the IUD as a safe and long-acting contraceptive method
- Z is strengthening the provision of IUD services in selected sub-centers, PHCs and VMC centers
- O_1 is IUD service statistics over a 9-month period before the intervention and data from the baseline survey of currently married men and women
- O_2 is IUD service statistics during nine months after the intervention and data from the endline survey of currently married men and women.

An experimental pre and post survey design with no control group was used. The intervention was implemented for a period of nine months. The figure below illustrates the design and the package of interventions.

- **Dependent variables:** The key dependent variable considered for the study was use of the IUD among clients.
- **Process variables:** However, given the short intervention period available (9 months) and that behavior change is a continuous process and passes through a series of stages (e.g., precontemplation, contemplation, preparation, action and maintenance (Prochaska et al 1992)), a major increase in the adoption of the IUD was not expected, but instead changes in process variables were anticipated, such as increased positive perception and knowledge of the IUD at the community level and a decrease in myths about the device. Because of this, some process variables were also assessed:
    - Increased knowledge of IUD and its mode of functioning, and the duration for which IUD could prevent pregnancy among clients
    - Decrease in myths surrounding the IUD among clients
    - Improved knowledge about benefits and side effects of the IUD
    - Change in knowledge of the providers towards the IUD and its effectiveness
    - Increase in technical knowledge and counseling skills of providers about IUD and quality of services

Proportion of providers who used teaching aids/IEC materials to make counseling more effective. Change in Knowledge among health care providers depicts in **Table 2 and Figs. 3 and 4**

Table 2: Change in knowledge among health care providers.		
percentage aware or knew that	Baseline	Endline
It is a very effective family planning method	48.7	71.4*
It protects from pregnancy up to 10 years	78.9	96.1**
How IUD works	84.2	87.0
It should not be inserted in woman having an STI/abnormal discharge	40.8	67.5**
First follow up should be done after 3–6 weeks of IUD insertion	50	80.5**
IUD does not have hormonal side effects	19.7	24.7
IUD does not interfere during sex	23.7	13.0
Number of HCPs	76	77
*p<0.05, **p<0.01		

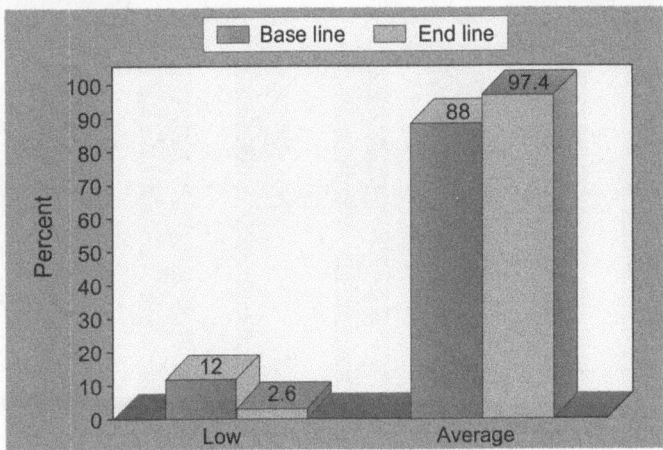

Fig. 3: Level of IUD knowledge among HCPs.

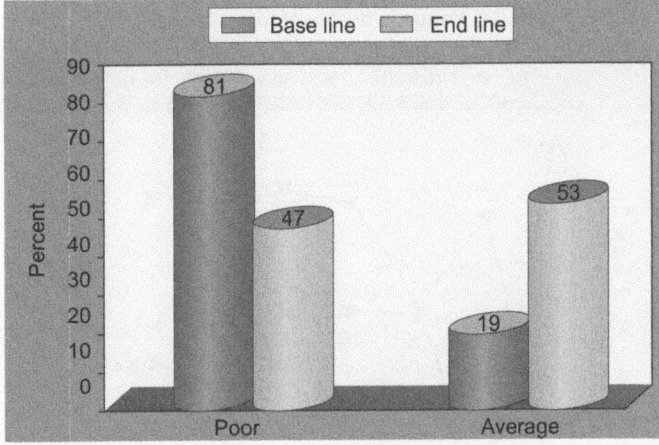

Fig. 4: Level of counseling skills among HCPs.

Change in level of knowledge among women and their husbands is represented in **Table 3**, whereas change in quality of IUD services is represented in **Figure 5**. IUD insertion rate in urban and rural populations is present in **Figs. 6 and 7**. Economic analysis is tabulated in **Table 4**.

Table 3: Change in level of knowledge among women and their husbands.

Level of knowledge	Urban %		Rural %		Total %	
	Baseline	Endline	Baseline	Endline	Baseline	Endline
Women						
Average	24.7	55.6**	13.3	44.4**	19	53**
Poor	75.3	46.1**	86.7	53.9**	81	47**
N	449	450	445	430	894	880
Husbands						
Average	4.9	23.9**	3.8	22.2**	4.4	23.3**
Poor	95.1	76.1**	96.2	77.8**	95.6	76.8**
N	223	235	212	217	435	452
**p<0.01						

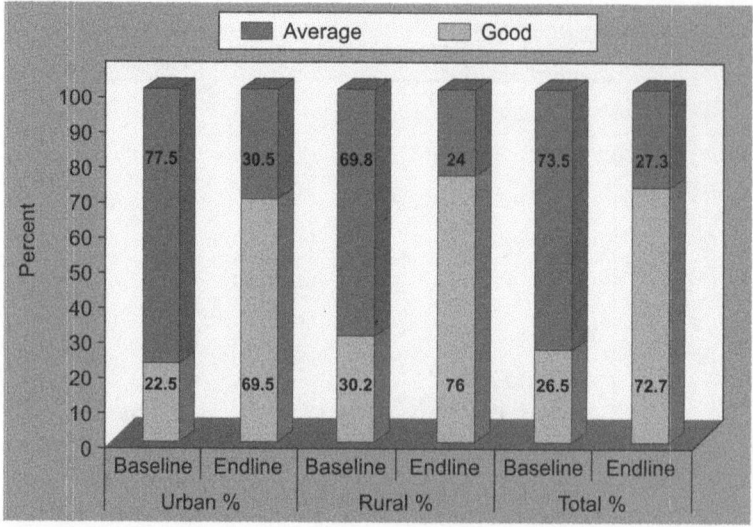

Fig. 5: Change in quality of IUD services.

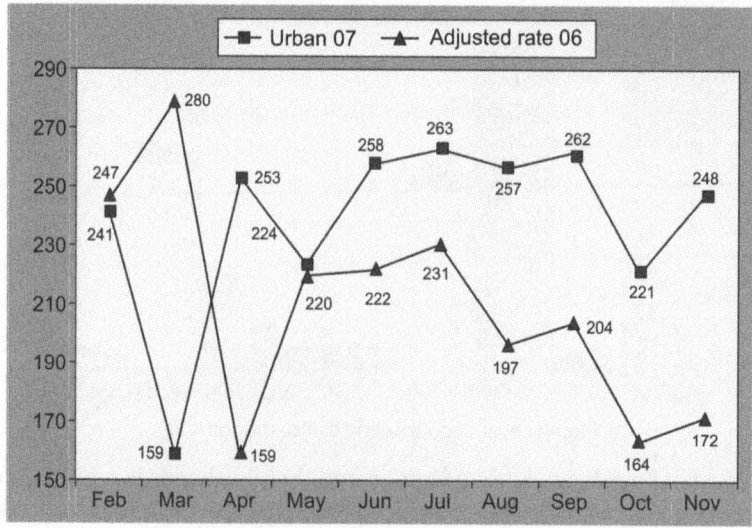

Fig. 6: IUD insertion rate in urban areas 2006-07.

Table 4 : Economic analysis.		
Cost items	Amount (in INR)	Amount (in Dollars)
A. Training		
Off-site training of paramedical workers	20,480	512
Off-site training of doctors	5,110	128
Off-site training of private practitioners	5,110	128
Off-site refresher training of paramedical workers	1,000	25
Travel cost of council staff during training (2 visits)	40,000	1,000
B. Trainer Fees		
Professional fees for external expert (13 days)	13,000	325
Professional fee of FRONTIERS staff (8 days)	19,386	485
C. Development of IEC materials		
Cost of development and printing IEC materials*	47,752	1,194
D. Cost of Supervisory Visits		
Travel cost for supervisory visit (5 visits)	100,000	2,500
Total cost	251,838	6,296

*IEC materials were developed for the entire district and the approximate costs for development and printing of these IEC materials in the study area were considered for economic analysis.

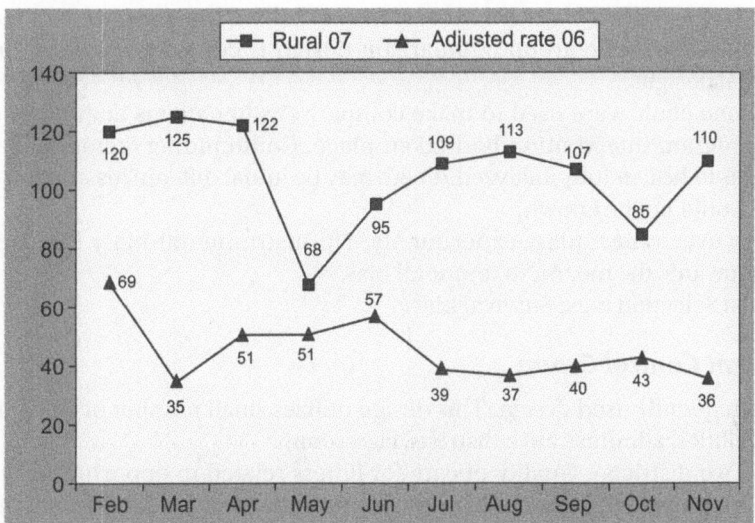

Fig. 7: IUD insertion rate in rural areas 2006–07.

The total cost of the intervention amounted for up to Rs 120,452. Routine service statistics showed that there were 886 new IUD users due to the intervention, giving a cost per new IUD user of Rs 135 ($3.37) during scale up. As the study was implemented in 41 health centers, Rs 2,938 ($73.5) would be the estimated unit cost to introduce the IUD services in an additional center.

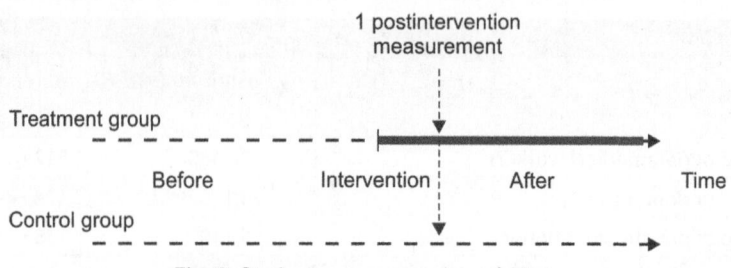

Fig. 8: Static-group comparison design.

Static-group Comparison (Fig. 8)

The static-group comparison design is a quasi-experimental research approach that involves measuring the outcome of interest only once, following the exposure of a nonrandomly selected group of participants to a specific treatment or intervention. This group is then compared to a control group. The primary aim of this design is to assess the impact of the treatment or intervention, which can encompass various factors such as medical treatments, training programs, policy changes, environmental events, and more.

This design exhibits three key features:
- Participants are not subjected to random assignment, making it a quasi-experimental approach.
- Both the treatment and control groups are assessed simultaneously.
- There are no measurements taken prior to the intervention.
- It represents an improvement over the one-group post-test-only design, which relies solely on a single postintervention measurement without the presence of a control group. Consequently, the static-group comparison design is considered better among quasi-experimental designs.
- Patients at one clinic were used to make comparisons to patients at another clinic where a special program intervention had taken place. Confounding factors of selection and mortality has to be carefully analyzed. There may be initial differences and the extent of the difference would not be known.
- Advantages over other quasi-experiments: No instrumental bias; Not susceptible to regression towards the mean; No temporal bias.
  Limitations: Selection bias; Survival bias.

Nonequivalent Control Group

It is the most frequently used design. This design utilizes small number of collective units like health care facilities, administrative districts, classrooms.
- **Example:** Two districts—Quality of care for illness related to opportunistic infections in PLHA can be improved; Training in and use of standard case management guidelines for provider; Facilities are available for inclusion.
- Randomly assign some caregivers in each facility to experimental and control groups. Use providers in the first facility as the experimental group and providers in the other as the comparison group. Use the design-nonequivalent control group
- **Limitations:** There might be Selection bias and lack of randomization. Compare pretest of both O1 and O3; Selection effects or major differences between intervention and comparison groups that might help explain differences (or lack of differences) in the post test O2 and O4.

Time Series Design (Fig. 9)

This design involves repeated measurement observations before and after the program intervention. It has multiple observations allow to determine trend. Often it may happen that there is no access to control/comparison group. It provides universal access to intervention. There will be regular access to regularly collected information (monthly service statistics). It is considered as superior to just one time measurement prepostest design. But however, threats to validity remain.

Example: Mass media campaign—condom use, **(Figs. 10–13)**. Antismoking campaigns, etc.

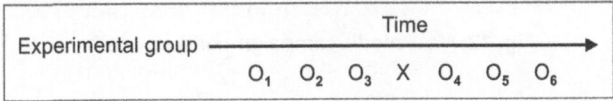

Fig. 9: Time series design.

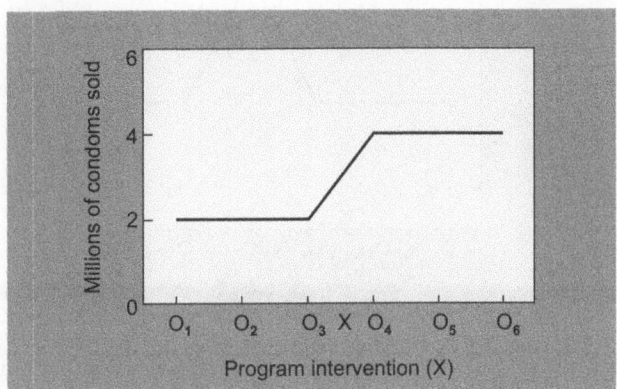

Fig. 10: Mass media campaign-condom use-1.

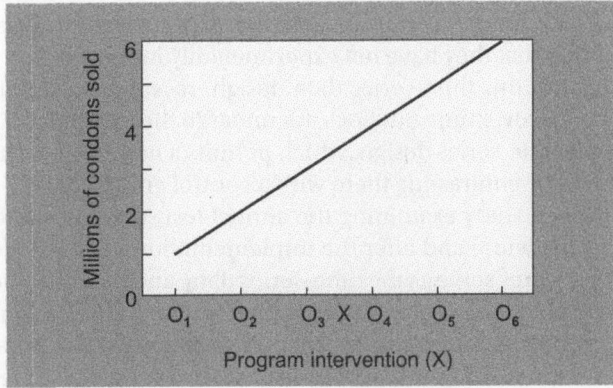

Fig. 11: Mass media campaign-condom use-2.

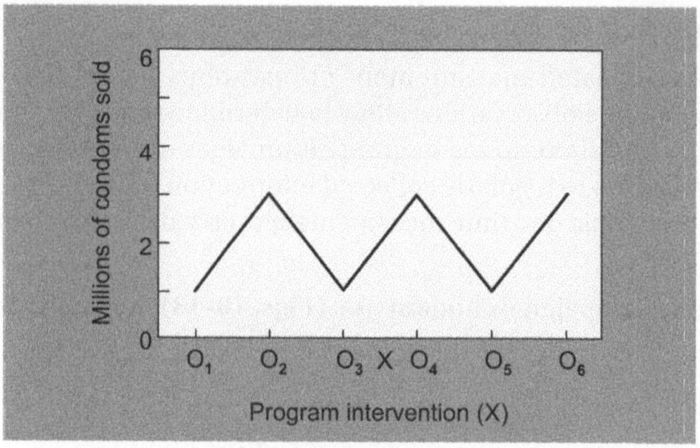

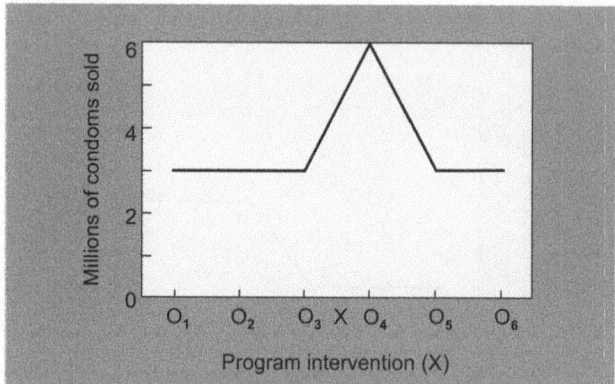

Fig. 12: Mass media campaign-condom use-3.

Fig. 13: Mass media campaign-condom use-3.

Time Series Data

In this research design, investigators repeatedly observe a single group of subjects both before and after applying an intervention. This method can be employed within a controlled experimental environment, but it's also adaptable to more real-world scenarios where data is routinely collected on a group of subjects, and researchers want to assess the impact of a treatment or intervention that they have not experimentally introduced.

To enhance the rigor of this time-series data design, researchers can introduce a control group that is also observed over time but does not undergo the treatment. This arrangement is referred to as a multiple time-series design, which permits a more comprehensive assessment of the treatment's effects by contrasting them with a control group's data.

For instance, consider a study examining the annual test scores of students at a particular school over several years before and after the implementation of an extended school day. In this case, the yearly test scores serve as the time-series data, and the shift to an extended school day is a naturally occurring, quasi-experimental intervention. This design offers advantages over a single pretest/posttest design because it allows researchers to explore long-term effects. **Others examples:** Frequency (number of sterilization acceptors) **(Fig. 14)**; Percentage (prevalence rates of disease over time); Average measure (median desired family size)

Month	Number	
January	120	
February	110	
March	130	Average January–April = 116
April	105	
May	1,120	
June	30	
July	45	
August	15	
September	30	Average June–December = 55
October	60	
November	90	
December	115	
Total	**2,050**	

Fig. 14: Number of male sterilizations per month.

Time series design with nonequivalent control group
The researcher also has an option of keeping a control group concurrent to an experimental group, thus employing a time series with nonequivalent control group design. Since the control group is not chosen through random technique, hence, the term nonequivalent is employed.
❖ Group 1 - O1 O2 O3 O4 O5 X O6 O7 O8 O9 O10
❖ Group 2 - O1 O2 O3 O4 O5 X O6 O7 O8 O9 O10
Example: Effect of strict drunk driving law on decreasing traffic fatalities

Challenges and Considerations

While quasi-experimental studies offer valuable insights, they also come with challenges. Researchers must carefully address issues like selection bias, statistical controls, and the validity of their findings.

Quasi-experimental studies serve as a bridge between purely observational research and randomized experiments, offering a practical and ethical way to investigate causal relationships in complex real-world settings.

Trials in public health

Cluster Randomized Trials

Cluster randomized trials (CRTs) differ from individually randomized trials in that the unit of randomization is something other than the individual participant or patient. CRTs are in common use in areas such as education and public health research; they are particularly well suited to testing differences in a method or approach to patient care (as opposed to evaluating the physiological effects of an intervention). For instance, when intervention targets for clusters like health care units rather than individuals.

Clusters can be geographical clusters like administrative blocks, villages, arbitrary geographic zones; Institutional clusters like schools, offices, hospitals, clinics, factories; and smaller clusters such as households. The possible reasons for choosing cluster randomization may be as some interventions by their nature have to be implemented at the cluster level, may not be, acceptable to local communities or logistically very complex. There might be risk of contamination between treatment groups. These also help to capture the indirect effects of interventions. But, CRT's are statistically less efficient that individual randomized trials.

Within cluster correlation **(Fig. 15)**. People within a cluster tend to be more alike than people in different clusters. This is called intracluster correlation (ICC).
- Implications of ICC
- Sample size – The more the correlation the bigger the sample size.
- Randomization methods also need to be taken into consideration.
- Conduct –logistics and contamination.
- For analysis use regression techniques which account for clustering.

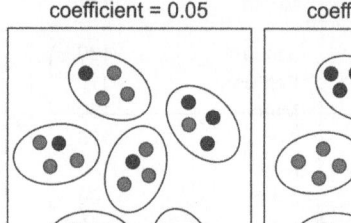
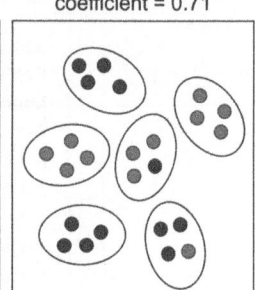

Fig. 15: Intracluster correlation.

Problems with CRT

Contamination: The most compelling reason to randomize at the cluster level rather than at the individual level is the potential for contamination, whereby participants within a cluster are likely to be treated similarly and hence exhibit similar outcomes.

When contamination occurs during a clinical trial, it dilutes the observed differences between comparators and can affect the reliability and validity of the study. Contamination can occur:
- Between intervention and control arm
- Between intervention and wider population
- Between control and wider population selection bias occurs when:
- Small number of clusters are involved
- Lack of allocation concealment
- Drop out of clusters

Step wedge designs **(Fig. 16)**

An alternative approach to randomization in CRTs is stepped-wedge randomization. In stepped-wedge designs, the clusters are randomized into several groups or waves that defines when the intervention begins, and all clusters start the trial in a controlled condition. Groups of

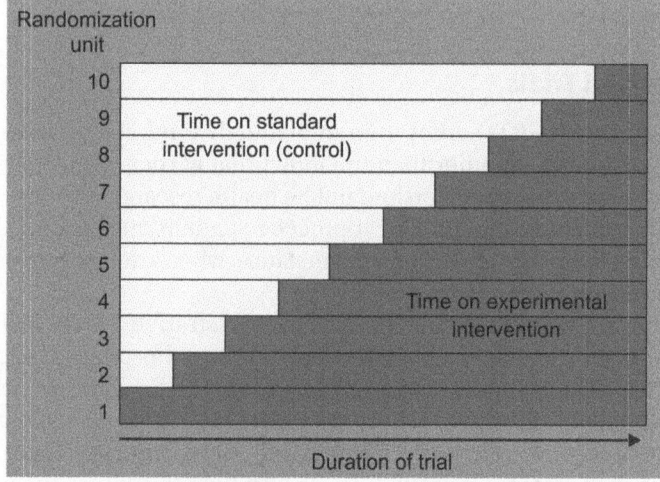

Fig. 16: Rationale for step wedge designs.

clusters cross over to the intervention condition on a staggered schedule, and all groups receive the intervention before the end of the trial.

Most appropriate situation for a stepped wedge design is one in which the experimental intervention is anticipated to be beneficial. But Practical considerations mean that it cannot be widely implemented immediately.

Advantages

Sometimes, it is impractical or impossible to roll out the intervention to all participants at the same time. Stepped-wedge randomization overcomes this problem by introducing the intervention to groups of clusters at different times. Moreover, because all sites in a stepped-wedge trial will eventually receive the intervention, these designs may be more appealing to the broader community and thus lead to greater study participation, especially in trials of interventions that seem particularly promising.

The choice to employ a stepped-wedge CRT design should primarily depend on its ability to outperform other trial designs in addressing the research question. There are instances where a stepped-wedge design becomes the sole practical avenue for collecting necessary data. Nonetheless, it is crucial to carefully weigh the practical, ethical, and analytical complexities involved. Stepped-wedge designs should be reserved for cases where no other robust study design is viable and capable of addressing the research inquiry adequately.

KEY POINTS

- Quasi-experimental studies allow for causal research in real-world settings where full control and randomization are not possible.
- They involve nonrandomized groups and manipulate variables to a limited extent, focusing on real-world applications and policy implications.
- Various designs like post-test only, pretest-posttest, and static-group comparison address different research needs with inherent strengths and limitations.
- Challenges include addressing selection bias and ensuring the validity of findings, often employing statistical controls for reliability.
- Quasi-experiments bridge the gap between observational studies and randomized trials, offering practical ways to study causal relationships in complex settings.

BIBLIOGRAPHY

1. A brief history of the cluster randomized trial design [Internet]. The James Lind Library. 2015 [cited 2023 Sep 14]. Available from: https://www.jameslindlibrary.org/articles/a-brief-history-of-the-cluster-randomized-trial-design/
2. Campbell DT, Stanley J. Experimental and Quasi-Experimental Designs for Research. 1st edition. Cengage Learning; 1963.
3. Choueiry G. Static-group comparison design: An introduction [Internet]. Quantifyinghealth.com. [cited 2023 Sep 13]. Available from: https://quantifyinghealth.com/static-group-comparison-design/
4. Cluster randomized trials [Internet]. Rethinking Clinical Trials. 2022 [cited 2023 Sep 14]. Available from: https://rethinkingclinicaltrials.org/chapters/design/experimental-designs-and-randomization-schemes/cluster-randomized-trials/
5. Gujarat IME, Kishor V, Pratibha D, Itare PBP, Khan ME, Kar S, et al. Increasing the accessibilityIncreasing the accessibility, acceptability and use of the IUD in, acceptability and use of the IUD in [Internet]. Popcouncil.org. [cited 2023 Sep 13]. Available from: https://knowledgecommons.popcouncil.org/cgi/viewcontent.cgi?article=1417&context=departments_sbsr-rh
6. Krishnan P. A review of the non-equivalent control group post-test-only design. Nurse Res. 2019;26(2):37-40. doi:10.7748/nr.2018.e1582

Qualitative Analysis in Operational Research

Sathiabalan M, Jeyashree Kathiresan

"Qualitative research can illuminate the whys and hows behind complex realities."
—*Robert K. Yin*

INTRODUCTION

Decision-making in complex problems. OR is a process used in identifying and studying possible solutions to program problems. OR may be programmatic or action research. It looks for causes and possible solutions to problems affecting service delivery. This is used to study factors under the control of managers.

Types of OR Studies

1. Diagnostic/exploratory (descriptive) studies
2. Intervention
3. Evaluation
4. Cost-effectiveness studies

The methods of OR range from the qualitative to the quantitative, and the study designs from the nonexperimental to the true experimental. There is no single set of methods or designs unique to operations research.

Tools and Techniques on OR Studies

Operations research uses any suitable tools or techniques available. The common frequently used tools/techniques are mathematical procedures, cost analysis, electronic computation. However, operations researchers have given special importance to the development and the use of techniques like linear programming, game theory, decision theory, queuing theory, inventory models and simulation. In addition to the above techniques, some other common tools are nonlinear programming, integer programming, dynamic programming, sequencing theory, Markov process, network scheduling (PERT/CPM), symbolic models, information theory, and value theory. There are many other operations research tools/techniques also exist. The brief explanations of some of the above techniques/tools are as follows:

Linear Programming

This is a constrained optimization technique, which optimizes some criteria within some constraints. In linear programming the objective function (profit, loss or return on investment) and constraints are linear. There are different methods available to solve linear programming.

Game Theory

This is used for making decisions in conflicting situations where there are one or more players/opponents. In this the motives of the players are dichotomized. The success of one player tends to be at the cost of other players and hence they are in conflict.

Decision Theory

Decision theory is concerned with making decisions under conditions of complete certainty about the future outcomes and under conditions such that we can make some probability about what will happen in the future.

Queuing Theory

This is used in situations where the queue is formed (e.g., customers waiting for service, aircrafts waiting for landing, jobs waiting for processing in the computer system, etc.). The objective here is minimizing the cost of waiting without increasing the cost of servicing.

Inventory Models

Inventory model make a decisions that minimize total inventory cost. This model successfully reduces the total cost of purchasing, carrying, and out of stock inventory.

Simulation

Simulation is a procedure that studies a problem by creating a model of the process involved in the problem and then through a series of organized trial and error solutions attempts to determine the best solution. Sometimes this is a difficult/time consuming procedure. Simulation is used when actual experimentation is not feasible or the solution of a model is not possible.

Nonlinear Programming

This is used when the objective function and the constraints are not linear in nature. Linear relationships may be applied to approximate nonlinear constraints but limited to some range, because approximation becomes poorer as the range is extended. Thus, the nonlinear programming is used to determine the approximation in which a solution lies and then the solution is obtained using linear methods.

Dynamic Programming

Dynamic programming is a method of analyzing multistage decision processes. In this each elementary decision depends on those preceding decisions and as well as external factors.

Integer Programming

If one or more variables of the problem take integral values only then dynamic programming method is used. For example, number or motor in an organization, number of passenger in an aircraft, number of generators in a power generating plant, etc.

Markov Process

Markov process permits to predict changes over time information about the behavior of a system is known. This is used in decision making in situations where the various states are defined. The probability from one state to another state is known and depends on the current state and is independent of how we have arrived at that particular state: MBA-H2040.

Case Study

A mental health service provider in the UK provided treatment to patients via several specialist workforces. Here, focus was on two: psychology and psychiatric talking therapies (PPT) and recovering independent life (RIL) teams. Waiting times to begin treatment under these services were high (e.g., for RIL team median = 55 days, interquartile range = 40–95 days), and treatment could last many years once it had begun. The trust's management team were eager to implement new procedures to help staff manage case load and hence reduce waiting times to prevent service users, here defined as patients, their families, and carers, from entering a crisis state due to diminishing health without treatment. Management believed that the reasons for delays were more complex than lack of staff, but the exact details were unclear and there was much disagreement between senior management. The implementation science intervention I detail was conducted as an OR problem structuring exercise.

A system dynamics (SD) model was constructed to aid management target their interventions. SD is a subset of system thinking—the process of understanding how things within a system influence one another within the whole. SD models can be either qualitative or quantitative. In this case, a purely qualitative model was created. **Figure 1** illustrates stock and flow notation that is commonly used in SD. The example is the concept of a simple waiting list for a (generic) treatment. It can be explained as follows. General practitioners (GPs) refer service users to a waiting list at an average daily rate, while specialist clinicians treat according to how much daily treatment capacity they have. The variable *waiting list* is represented as a rectangular stock: an accumulation of patients. The waiting list stock is either depleted or fed by rate variables, referring and treating, represented as flows (pipes with valves) entering and leaving the stock. **Figure 1** also contains two feedback loops that are illustrated by the curved lines. The first loop is related to the GP reluctance to refer to a service with a long waiting time. As the waiting list for a service increases in number, so does the average waiting time of service users and so does the pressure for GPs to consider an alternative service (lowering the daily referral rate). The second loop is related to specialist clinicians reacting to long waiting lists by creating a small amount of additional treatment capacity and increasing admission rates.

A preliminary version of the SD model was created using a series of interviews with clinicians and managers from the three services. This was followed by a group model building workshop that involved all senior management. Group model building is a structured process that aims to create a shared mental model of a problem. The workshop began with a nominal group exercise.

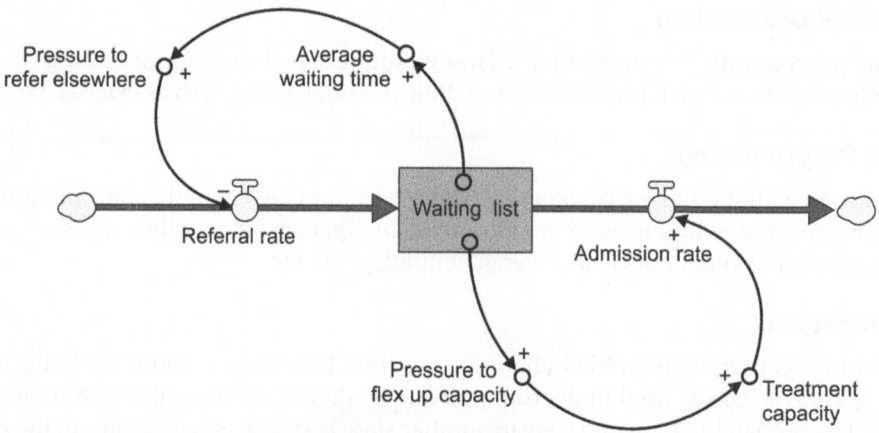

Fig. 1: Stock and flow notation.

The group were asked to individually write down what they believed were the key factors that affected patient waiting times. The group were specifically asked to focus on strategic issues as opposed to detailed process-based problems. After all individual results had been shared, the group were asked to (i) hypothesize how these factors influenced each other and (ii) propose any missing variables that may mediate influence. For example, available treatment capacity is reduced by nonclinical workload. Nonclinical workload is increased by several other factors (discussed below in results) and so on.

OR as a Tool for Prospective Evaluation

The second role of OR within implementation science is as a *prospective* evaluation tool. That is, to provide a formal assessment and appraisal of competing implementation options or choices before any actual implementation effort, commitment of resources or disinvestment takes place. Informally, this approach is often called *what-if analysis*.

Outline of Approaches

Systems modeling and simulation encompasses a wide diversity of approaches. These range across a spectrum from so-called 'soft' techniques at one end to 'hard' techniques at the other. Soft methods include problem structuring and conceptual modeling techniques such as Soft Systems Methodology, Strategic Options and Decision Analysis (SODA) and Strategic Choice Approach. These approaches are used to tackle complex and unstructured problems with multiple stakeholders and typically aim to help improve group understanding of the aims of a system, to ask questions of it, and to facilitate team consensus. Such techniques generally employ qualitative methods such as cognitive mapping and extensive interaction with stakeholders through facilitated workshops. Outline of methods commonly used in healthcare system modeling and stimulation tabulated in **Table 1**.

Examples of applications of soft methods in health include a study on improving the organization of multidisciplinary team meetings for colorectal cancer and addressing the gap between patients' and providers' expectations in NHS hospital outpatients' department.

Table 1: Outline of methods commonly used in healthcare system modeling and simulation.

Approach	Use	Examples of methods
Qualitative modeling	To build a picture of the current system and structure the problem. To inform dialogue among participants help focus and scope on key issues	Cognitive mapping, Process mapping, Soft Systems Methods (SSM), Strategic Options and Decision Analysis (SODA)
Mathematical modeling	To support stakeholders in exploring system trade-offs and evaluating different courses of action using quantitative information and outputs	Regression, Forecasting, Optimization methods, Queuing theory, Markov models, Data Envelopment Analysis (DEA)
Simulation	To test 'what-if' scenarios for service design. Determine levels of uncertainty. Provide visualizations, inform clear understanding and dialogue among stakeholders	Discrete event simulation System dynamics Monte Carlo simulation Agent based simulation Behavioral simulation

At the other end of the spectrum, hard systems modeling makes extensive use of mathematical and computer simulation methods to provide quantitative analysis and insights to problems that have a clearer structure, metrics and quantitative outputs. Mathematical methods such optimization, data envelopment analysis and queuing theory use analytical formulations to develop models that fit a problem description under a range of restrictive assumptions. In comparison, computer simulation methods such as system dynamics, Monte Carlo simulation, discrete event simulation and agent based simulation often allow for fewer assumptions to be used to capture details of the care system at the expense of more complex and time-consuming experimentation procedures and some loss of clarity and repeatability in the model.

KEY POINTS

- Operations research (OR) identifies and studies solutions to problems affecting service delivery, using a range of qualitative to quantitative methods and designs from nonexperimental to true experimental.
- Common OR tools include linear programming, game theory, decision theory, and simulation, each addressing different aspects of problem-solving and decision-making.
- OR in implementation science acts as a structuring exercise and a prospective evaluation tool, using systems modeling to assess and appraise implementation options.
- OR techniques range from 'soft' methods for complex, unstructured problems to 'hard' methods using mathematical and computer simulations for more defined issues.

BIBLIOGRAPHY

1. Craig P, Rahm-Hallberg I, Britten N, Borglin G, Meyer G, Köpke S, et al. Researching Complex Interventions in Health: The State of the Art. BMC Heal Serv Res 2016 161 [Internet]. 2016 Apr 4 [cited 2023 Nov 6];16(1):1–5. Available from: https://bmchealthservres.biomedcentral.com/articles/10.1186/s12913-016-1274-0
2. Gilbert N, Bankes S. Platforms and methods for agent-based modeling. Proc Natl Acad Sci [Internet]. 2002 May 14 [cited 2023 Nov 6];99(suppl 3):7197–8. Available from: https://www.pnas.org/doi/abs/10.1073/pnas.072079499
3. Gupta D, Denton B. Appointment scheduling in health care: Challenges and opportunities. IIE Trans. 2008;40:800–19.
4. Jun JB, Jacobson SH, Swisher JR. Application of discrete-event simulation in health care clinics: A survey. J Oper Res Soc. 1999;50(2):109–23.
5. Kotiadis K, Tako AA, Rouwette EAJA, Vasilakis C, Brennan J, Gandhi P, et al. Using a model of the performance measures in Soft Systems Methodology (SSM) to take action: A case study in health care. J Oper Res Soc. 2013;64(1):125–37.
6. Law AM. Simulation Modeling and Analysis, 5th edition. 2015 [cited 2023 Nov 6]; Available from: www.averill-law.com
7. Monks T. Operational research as implementation science: Definitions, challenges and research priorities. Implement Sci [Internet]. 2016 Jun 6 [cited 2023 Nov 6];11(1):1–10. Available from: https://implementationscience.biomedcentral.com/articles/10.1186/s13012-016-0444-0
8. Nacht M. Operations Research. Int Encycl Soc Behav Sci [Internet]. 2001 [cited 2023 Nov 6];10873–6. Available from: https://linkinghub.elsevier.com/retrieve/pii/B0080430767011839
9. Principles and Applications of Operations Research [Internet]. [cited 2023 Nov 6]. Available from: https://sites.pitt.edu/~jrclass/or/or-intro.html
10. Vidal RVV, Rosenhead J, Mingers J (Eds)., Rational Analysis for a Problematic World Revisited, Problem Structuring Methods for Complexity, Uncertainty and Conflict, Wiley, Chichester, 2001, xviii+366 pages, £ 22.50. Eur J Oper Res. 2005 Mar;161(2):582–3.

CHAPTER 35

Writing for Media Communication

Chandana H, Rashmi Kundapur, Suthanthira Kannan

> *"The most important thing in communication is hearing what isn't said."*
> —Peter Drucker

INTRODUCTION

Media writing is the process of generating information for widespread distribution through certain media venues, which included newspapers, periodicals, well-known websites, blogs, social media, and other publications. Media writing is used by many professionals from many backgrounds, but it also requires certain talents to interact with readers successfully. Specific guidelines and classifications are used in this sort of writing to give viewers particular kinds of information. Mass media is frequently used by audiences to inform, amuse, and engage in social interaction.

Dos and Don'ts of Writing in Media Communication

Dos of writing in media communication	Don'ts of writing in media communication
Be open, honest, and genuine. People can connect and relate to what is "real"	An insult need not be answered right away. As a representative of your organization, consider your reaction carefully. Moreover, avoid being impolite in your responses. Nevertheless, be sure to reply
Use a provocative phrase or engaging question to draw the readers' attention. Make readers want to read more	Do not speak robotically. People like speaking with real people, not with machines. For their post or remark, they want genuine emotion and sentiments
Be concise. The article should contain the information, not necessarily only what was shared on social media. Just enough should be written to keep readers interested	It should not lack context and create a false image. The language you use should be optimistic.
Instead of coming across as pushy, try to help individuals or find solutions to their issues	Do not use misspelt terms, you will lose all credibility.
Write with your audience in mind to make sure the information they are reading is pertinent to them. Give the populace what they want while giving your clients something worthwhile	Do not use 50 hashtags to a post. It is irritating and seems desperate. However, Hootsuite* is quick to point out that hashtags must be relevant to the content and claims that 9–11 hashtags receive the highest interaction.

Dos of writing in media communication	Don'ts of writing in media communication
Share the wonderful things your business is doing with the public. Do not be afraid to let the world know positive things about the individuals and businesses you follow because we want to read about them. Write about it in the present tense and with a sense of urgency	Don't write as you would text. When publishing on a professional site, 'C u L8r' acts impolitely
	Never overthink a post. It wo not make or ruin your business. Simply state what you are doing or the website you are referring them to in one phrase, and then move on.
	Do not indicate your political affiliation.

* Hootsuite is a social media management platform

Writing for Broadcast Media

Writing for broadcast requires a unique set of abilities from writing for print. The writer must apply all of the writing strategies they have acquired while crafting print copy, and they must hone these strategies when crafting broadcast content. Condensation is the most crucial of these methods. The writer for television or radio must learn to choose and compress content. The author has to understand that, in contrast to writing for print, brevity is valued much more highly.

The main distinction between writing for broadcast and writing for print is that writers for broadcast write for the ear, not the sight. Students must comprehend that their writing will be read out loud rather than silently. Clarity in writing thus becomes one of the writer's main objectives.

Writing for Press Release

A press release is now more crucial than ever in today's digital environment; they are now an essential part of social media marketing. It is impossible to overstate the value of press releases in disseminating critical information about a health event or other pertinent updates as social media continues to develop into a major marketing tool for companies throughout the world.

You may utilize your press releases to assure immediate and global exposure with a new, reimagined angle, and there's always the chance of becoming viral. Additionally, news releases are now accessible and readable via a variety of platforms at any time, making them a very effective and practical marketing tool.

It's crucial to stick to a prewritten framework when creating press releases. Your material will appear more organized and professional as a result. Additionally, it will captivate and keep your audience reading. A press release should begin, "For Immediate Release," and then provide the name of the press contact, date, phone number, and email. Summarize your three major themes after writing your headline. The city and state should next be mentioned, followed by your introduction paragraph. Add a quotation to maintain the credibility and interest of your news release. Next, write two to three paragraphs, add a quote, and finally, draught your concluding paragraph. A "boilerplate," or brief statement that summarizes the business or organization, should be included at the end of your press release. Following this format can help you communicate your ideas properly and prevent misunderstandings and uncertainty.

Writing for Social Media

Writing on social media calls for abilities distinct from writing for other purposes. The assumption that the information will be read and enjoyed underlies the entire premise. You are succeeding if your audience can read and comprehend the writing you have produced. A great content producer will need to have the abilities and craftsmanship to produce blogs, articles, website material, and any other writing that may draw you into this field.

According to Time magazine research from May 14, 2015, people's attention span has decreased from an average of 12 seconds to 8 seconds. People seldom have the time or attention to read a whole piece of material due to the availability of various media outlets; as a result, the content must be very captivating to keep the audience's interest. Without taxing the audience's cognitive abilities, the entire piece should be basic and easy to read. Clarifying what will keep your readers engaged to your material is the most crucial thing to think about before you start writing. You need to know your audience better.

How Media Communication Helps a Common Man?

Folk music and theatre were once performed by individuals in numerous civilizations. The use of media to spread messages to a larger audience initially emerged at that time. Then came mass media, social media, and print media. Radio, the internet, print media, and television are currently the most popular kinds of media. The media has a significant role in our lives.

For example, COVID-19 outbreak: The tracking and updating of the coronavirus epidemic through a live updates' dashboard involved the media on a global scale. The World Health Organisation (WHO) and the Centre for Disease Control and Prevention (CDC) were able to respond quickly and widely to public health messaging thanks to the media. We observed a rise in the adoption of safe health practices, such as enhanced hand washing, the wearing of face coverings, and social seclusion, for the promotion of health and hygiene practices across the world. Daily health advice was reaffirmed in the media, and telehealth was promoted as a way for individuals to get the healthcare they needed. Today's society depends heavily on mass media, which may offer a centralized platform for all public health messages, thorough healthcare education standards, and effective social distancing tactics while yet preserving social relationships. It provided equitable access to healthcare, put an end to prejudice, and remove social stigma.

KEY POINTS

- It is the process of generating information for widespread distribution through certain media venues.
- The main distinction between writing for broadcast and writing for print is that writers for broadcast write for the ear, not the sight.
- Clarity in writing is one of the writer's main objectives.
- Need to know your audience better.
- Today's society depends heavily on mass media, which may offer a centralized platform for all public health messages.

BIBLIOGRAPHY

1. 15 Dos and Don'ts of Writing for Social Media [Internet]. [cited 2023 Oct 10]. Available from: https://www.linkedin.com/pulse/15-dos-donts-writing-social-media-ashlee-stepp
2. Anwar A, Malik M, Raees V, Anwar A. Role of Mass Media and Public Health Communications in the COVID-19 Pandemic. Cureus. 12(9):e10453.

3. Khan MT. Social Media Writing: How To Write Compelling Posts [Internet]. IIM SKILLS. 2023 [cited 2023 Oct 10]. Available from: https://iimskills.com/how-to-write-social-media-posts/
4. Writing a Press Release? Here are the Do's and Don'ts [Internet]. UrbanMatter. 2021 [cited 2023 Oct 10]. Available from: https://urbanmatter.com/writing-a-press-release-here-are-the-dos-and-donts/
5. Writing for Broadcast Media. Writing for the Fashion Business. 141 [Internet]. [cited 2023 Oct 10]. Available from: https://www.academia.edu/37893504/Writing_For_Broadcast_Media

Funding Opportunities in Operational Research

CHAPTER 36

Siva Santosh Kumar Pentapati, Aditi Mohta, Deepak B Saxena

"There's no investment you can make which has a better return than research."
—*Arlen Specter*

INTRODUCTION

'Funding' refers to monetary support provided by the government or an organization for a specific purpose. One of the sources of funding is grant. "A grant is a mechanism by which an agency awards money to fund a research study or other activity, such as an educational program, service program, demonstration, or research project." It is important to learn to write a proposal for funding or grant, because it provides monetary resources to execute operational research (OR) to generate evidence for the greater good, aids in their publication and dissemination, and also helps meet professional goals of the individual in the form of appraisals or promotions.

There are two types of operational research proposals.
1. Solicited proposals on a theme or focus area, wherein the agency announces request for proposal (RFP) or request for application (RFA).
2. Unsolicited proposals, which are researcher-initiated, based on the agency's broad guidelines.

Modes of Funding in Operational Research

Modes of funding in operational research vary as per the applicant and the purpose. Research project grant may be awarded to an individual project. It may be applied by a single institution or a consortium of institutions. If it is applied by an individual, it may be granted as a fellowship. Program project grants may be awarded for several projects. Independent scientist award may be given to demonstrate certain models.

Identifying a Funding Agency

- Begin with searching databases and funding agency websites.
- Search published literature in your domain of interest for funding sources acknowledged.
- Interact with peers who are undertaking funded projects and explore who is funding them.
- Interact with potential funders and learn about their priority areas.
- Once you shortlist a few funding agencies, study the agency's mission and aims, and review other proposals funded by them and awards granted. Ask yourself if your research interest is aligned with the agency's mission.

Online Database of Funding Opportunities

The following databases list funding sources relevant for operational research.
- **ProQuest Pivot (formerly 'Community of Science'):** Funding opportunities in the United States of America (USA) and Canada.
- GrantForward (includes former Illinois Researcher Information Service, IRIS).
- InfoEd Global's SPIN Plus: Up-to-date listing of national and international government and private funding sources.
- **Foundation directory:** Funding opportunities and details about grant providers for non-profit organizations.
- Indiabioscience (www.indiabioscience.org/grants)
- INCLEN Trust International (www.inclentrust.org/inclen)
- DevNetJobs India (www.devnetjobsindia.org)
- NGO Box (www.ngobox.org/full_grant_announcement)

Funding Agencies

Government or Federal Agencies

Indian Government Agencies
- Department of Health Research (DHR), Ministry of Health & Family Welfare
- Indian Council of Medical Research (ICMR)
- Department of Biotechnology (DBT), Ministry of Science and Technology
- Department of Science and Technology (DST), Ministry of Science and Technology
- Council of Scientific and Industrial Research (CSIR)

International Federal Funding Agencies
- National Institutes of Health (NIH), USA
- Medical Research Council (MRC), United Kingdom (UK)
- National Research Council (NRC), Canada

Cooperative Agreements Between Governments
- Indo-US (ICMR-NIH, DBT-NIH)
- Indo-Australian
- Indo-German
- Indo-UK
- BRICS (Brazil, Russia, India, China, and South Africa) countries

International Organizations
- World Bank
- World Health Organization (WHO)
- United Nations Children's Fund (UNICEF)
- United Nations Population Fund (UNFPA)
- United Nations Development Programme (UNDP)

Government Development Agencies Providing Foreign Aid
- Australian Agency for International Development (AusAID)
- British Department for International Development (DFID)
- Canadian International Development Agency (CIDA)

- ❖ Danish International Development Agency (DANIDA)
- ❖ German Agency for International Cooperation (GIZ)
- ❖ Japan International Cooperation Agency (JAICA)
- ❖ Norwegian Agency for Development Cooperation (NORAD)
- ❖ Swedish International Development Cooperation Agency (SIDA)
- ❖ United States Agency for International Development (USAID)

Foundations
International Foundations

- ❖ Bill & Melinda Gates Foundation
- ❖ Ford Foundation
- ❖ MacArthur Foundation
- ❖ Rockefeller foundation
- ❖ Wellcome Trust
- ❖ Children's Investment Fund Foundation (CIFF)

Indian Foundations

- ❖ Tata Trusts
- ❖ Wipro Foundation
- ❖ Infosys Foundation
- ❖ Reliance Foundation
- ❖ Shiv Nadar Foundation

KEY POINTS

- Funding for operational research is vital for conducting studies, disseminating findings, and achieving professional growth, accessible through grants from various agencies.
- Researchers can identify suitable funding sources by exploring databases, literature, and networking, ensuring alignment with the funder's priorities and mission.
- A wide range of agencies offer funding, including government bodies, international organizations, development agencies, and foundations, each with specific focus areas and application processes.

BIBLIOGRAPHY

1. Gitlin, Laura N, Kevin J. Lyons. Successful Grant Writing: Strategies for Health and Human Service Professionals. 2nd edition; 2004.
2. Yadav C. Funding vs Financing: Difference and Comparison [Internet], 2021. Available from: https://askanydifference.com/difference-between-funding-and-financing-with-table/Accessed 28th August 2023.

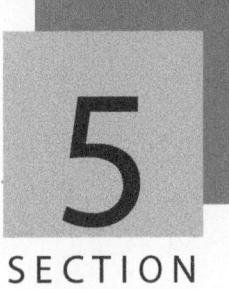

SECTION 5

Economic Evaluation and Health Technology Assessment

SECTION OUTLINE

- **Chapter 37:** Economic Evaluation and its Types
- **Chapter 38:** Concept of Cost and Cost Analysis
- **Chapter 39:** Micro and Macro Health Economics
- **Chapter 40:** Introduction to HTA and Steps in HTA Protocol Development
- **Chapter 41:** Outcome Assessment in Economic Evaluation Studies
- **Chapter 42:** Sensitivity Analysis and Modeling
- **Chapter 43:** Budget Impact Analysis
- **Chapter 44:** Drawing up the Protocol for an Economic Evaluation Study

CHAPTER 37

Economic Evaluation and its Types

Farah Naaz Fathima, Rivu Basu, Sudhir Prabhu, Chandralekha Kona

"Healthcare is not just another commodity. It is not a gift to be rationed based on the ability to pay."
— *Senator Edward Kennedy*

INTRODUCTION

In the ever-evolving landscape of healthcare, the need to make informed and effective decisions regarding resource allocation is paramount. As healthcare systems globally grapple with finite resources and an expanding array of interventions, the concept of economic evaluation has emerged as a guiding principle. This chapter endeavors to provide an in-depth exploration of economic evaluation, elucidating its core tenets, highlighting its critical role in healthcare decision-making, dissecting various types of economic evaluation studies, and examining their practical applications.

After reading this chapter, the reader will be able to:
❖ Define economic evaluation of healthcare programs.
❖ Justify the need for economic evaluation in healthcare.
❖ Explain the types of economic evaluation studies.

Definition and Need for Economic Evaluation

Economics deals with making good use of the available resources that we have. Economic evaluation of healthcare programs as defined by Drummond is the ***systematic comparison of alternative healthcare actions in terms of both their costs and consequences***. This multifaceted evaluation seeks to determine the most efficient approach to achieving desired health outcomes.

As healthcare systems confront the formidable challenge of resource scarcity, the imperative to optimize resource allocation becomes increasingly urgent. When faced with two program options in the healthcare sector, how do you decide between them? This scenario involves considering factors such as the program's objectives, anticipated benefits, and associated costs. There are instances where certain services or products come at a high price tag. In such cases, you may question whether the expense is justified, pondering whether the benefits outweigh the costs.

The realm of economic evaluation addresses this challenge by offering a structured methodology for evaluating competing healthcare interventions. By delineating the cost-effectiveness of different strategies, economic evaluation ensures that limited resources are channeled toward interventions that yield the maximum health benefits to achieve desired healthcare goals. Economic evaluation's role in enhancing economic efficiency thus becomes central in healthcare decision-making processes.

In economic evaluation two fundamental domains namely cost and consequence are compared. Costs pertain to the financial outlays associated with each course of action, while consequences refer to the outcomes or impacts that result from these actions. Essentially, you are scrutinizing the financial expenditure of each option and the outcomes it generates.

Economic evaluation is needed because markets alone do not provide efficient solutions, particularly in healthcare. However, when free markets do not exist, active decisions have to be made about which health services should be funded given the scarce resources available. Or, in other cases choice may have to be made between healthcare interventions and other public sector interventions. Resources are always scarce and they have to be used judiciously. This scarcity includes time, technology, capital and labor inputs as well as monetary budgets. The overall aim is to maximize benefits given the resources available.

Economic evaluations compare the costs and consequences of two (or more) healthcare interventions. Thus, the science of using the meagre resources for optimal utilization is economics and ways to make that analysis is Economic Evaluation. It is a way of thinking, backed up by a set of tools, which is designed to improve the value for money from investments in healthcare and welfare. It thus can be defined as a 'comparative analysis of alternative courses of action in terms of their costs and consequences'. From this definition it can be seen that evaluation involves some comparison between alternatives, which may include nothing, while the evaluation includes both the costs involved and the benefits that are derived from each of the alternatives.

Healthcare professionals are fully aware of the pressures facing the health service and initiatives relating to cost-effective prescribing. So an awareness of economics help those who are charged with making decisions, e.g., about whether to make available a new therapy or new service, or provide assistance for those trying to convince decision-makers of the relative merit and worth of their products, therapies, interventions, programs and services.

Health economic evaluation determines the efficiency of a service or activity by comparison with an alternative or alternatives, which may include no service provision. The basic framework of health economic evaluation is shown in **Figure 1**. Thus there are two components, inputs and outcomes/outputs. Once we have a basic structure of the analysis, we can start by saying that for economic evaluation, inputs are costs, in monetary terms. It is the output that differs. To give a brief overview of the outputs and the type of analysis the **Table 1** can be consulted.

Approaches to Economic Evaluation

There are two approaches of doing economic evaluations: trial-based and model-based evaluations. Both trial-based economic evaluation and model-based economic evaluation

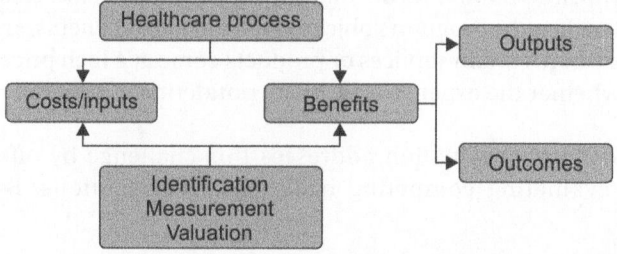

Fig. 1: Basic framework of economic evaluation.

Table 1: Types of economic evaluation.

Type of analysis	Input	Output	Example
Cost minimization	Monetary units	One intervention costs less than the other in monetary terms	Which drug/intervention costs less compared to other
Cost-benefit analysis	Cost in monetary terms	Single or multiple effects, not necessarily common to both alternatives in monetary terms	Other (nonhealth) public sector investments
Cost-effectiveness analysis	Cost in monetary terms	One single clinical or health effect of interest to both alternatives not in monetary terms but natural units	Two vaccines to reduce malaria incidence
Cost-utility analysis	Cost in monetary terms	Single or multiple effects, not necessarily common to both alternatives in DALYs averted or QALYs gained	Health sector interventions comparing interventions of two or more diseases

involve comparing alternatives and examining the cost and consequences, which are fundamental aspects of economic evaluation studies. However, the key distinction lies in how you acquire and source your data. In trial-based economic evaluation, you obtain cost and outcome data from a randomized controlled trial, whereas in model-based economic evaluation, you gather data from diverse sources and incorporate it into a developed model for analysis.

The trial-based approach entails integrating economic assessment into existing randomized controlled trials (RCTs). This approach capitalizes on the data generated by RCTs to simultaneously evaluate costs and outcomes. In other words, an economic evaluation is piggybacked on an already planned randomized controlled trial.

Conversely, the model-based approach involves constructing mathematical models that integrate data from diverse sources. A model serves as a simplified representation of reality. These models serve as predictive tools, enabling the estimation of costs and consequences under varying scenarios. Two common techniques include decision-tree model and the Markov state transition model. Data may be collated from various sources. These sources include outcomes of randomized controlled trials, surveillance data, independent small-scale surveys, published cross-sectional studies, government reports, commercial databases, and insurance reports. Essentially, any published literature could be integrated into the economic evaluation database. However, it was emphasized that the importance of maintaining data quality when incorporating these diverse sources into the analysis.

Types of Economic Evaluation Studies

Economic evaluation studies encompass a spectrum ranging from partial evaluations to complete evaluations. Partial evaluations entail an in-depth focus on either costs or outcomes, while complete evaluations encompass a holistic comparison of both costs and outcomes in two groups **(Fig. 2)**.

Partial Economic Evaluation

❖ **A cost of illness (COI) study** is conducted to comprehensively analyze the economic burden imposed by a particular disease or health condition on individuals, healthcare systems, and society as a whole. The financial impact of a specific health issue is sought to be understood through these studies, which can inform healthcare policy and resource allocation. The

	Consequences only	Costs only	Both consequences and costs
One group	Descriptive study	Cost description*	Cost outcome description*
Two groups	RCT	Cost analysis*	Full economic evaluation

* Partial economic evaluations

Fig. 2: Types of economic evaluation studies.

various types of costs typically included in a cost of illness study include direct, indirect and intangible costs.
- In a **cost outcome study,** both the cost and the consequences are examined within a single group. An example of this would ne assessing the cost of diagnosing a patient with diabetes through the training of community health workers or ASHA workers. An outcome, namely the number of diabetes cases diagnosed, is established, and an impact on costs is observed. Thus, the analysis centers around the cost per outcome.
- **Cost analysis** studies delve into intricate cost comparisons between different interventions, facilitating a nuanced understanding of cost effectiveness.

Complete Economic Evaluation

In a complete/full economic evaluation, two groups are involved, and both the costs and consequences are examined. An example of this scenario might involve two geographical areas randomly assigned to either receive an intervention or not. In both groups, the focus is on studying the outcomes. For instance, in the previously mentioned example, one area employs community health workers for diabetes diagnosis, while the other relies on the usual care approach. The outcome under scrutiny is the number of diagnosed or referred patients. This constitutes the outcome measure. In this context, costs, including training, equipment, and population-related expenses, among others, are analyzed in both groups.

The four types of complete economic evaluation studies are depicted in the **Table 1** centers. As explained earlier, economic evaluation focusses on two critical aspects: costs and consequences. In all the four types of studies, monetary units consistently serve as the measurement for costs. The four distinct types of full economic evaluation studies differ in the manner in which consequences are assessed.

Cost Minimization Study

Monetary units are employed to gauge costs, and typically, no distinction arises in terms of effectiveness. Two products are juxtaposed, both yielding identical consequences. The objective is solely to ascertain which one offers a more economical option. For instance, consider the scenario where you visit a shopping mall and purchase a dress you like. Subsequently, while browsing the internet, you encounter the exact same dress online, but at a 20% discount. In this instance, the product itself remains unchanged; only the cost differs.

It's important to note that, in practical situations, cost minimization studies are exceedingly rare since it is challenging to guarantee identical outcomes in both groups. However, a comparable example can be found in the case of a drug available as a generic brand versus any of the other commercially available brands. Even though the outcomes are identical the difference lies in the cost. This encapsulates the essence of cost minimization analysis, where costs are quantified in monetary units, two groups are compared, and both exhibit identical outcomes or consequences.

Cost Benefit Analysis

Here costs are measured in monetary units and consequences are similarly assessed in monetary units. A challenge in this context would involve the conversion of health benefits into monetary terms. An example illustrating this challenge is an occupational health intervention, where interventions such as screening or health education are employed, and the resulting improvement in health is required to be transformed into monetary units. The underlying objective here is to assess return on investments by measuring both costs and consequences into monetary units.

Cost Effectiveness Analysis

In this analysis, two groups are typically involved, with costs being quantified in monetary units, while consequences are expressed in natural units. The term "natural units" refers to the standard measurements employed in research. For example, if researching hypertension, the natural unit would be systolic blood pressure, measured in mm Hg. Similarly, in studies focused on mental health, PHQ-9 scores may be used, while investigations into cardiovascular diseases or cancer might measure outcomes in terms of deaths averted or lives saved. Therefore, in a cost effectiveness study, whatever natural unit is being measured constitutes the outcome in both groups.

In a study on cardiovascular diseases, aiming to compare the effectiveness of adherence to medication, physical activity, and dietary interventions, the outcome of interest would be the reduction in systolic blood pressure, quantified in mm Hg. The outcome or consequence is consistently assessed in accordance with the specific natural units relevant to the study.

Cost Utility Study

Here costs are quantified in monetary units, while outcomes or consequences are assessed in terms of "health utilities" and quality-adjusted life years. This represents facilities comparisons and informed decision-making between options with outcomes measured in different units.

Within a healthcare context, various health issues vie for the allocation of limited resources, each holding significant importance for individual health. Nevertheless, comparing and selecting among these diverse options, such as tuberculosis and cardiovascular disease or mental health measures like depression scores versus systolic blood pressure, can be challenging. This is precisely where cost utility analysis proves invaluable.

In cost utility analysis, all consequences are transformed into a metric known as "health utilities", from which quality-adjusted life years are computed. Utility represents a value that individuals assign to their own health, typically measured on a scale ranging from zero to one.

To recap, these are the four distinct types of economic evaluation studies you should bear in mind. You will delve into each of these in greater detail as your studies progress. At this juncture, let's summarize what you've absorbed in this session.

First, you've grasped the concept of economic evaluation and the crucial keywords to remember. Economic evaluation involves comparing two alternative courses of action in terms of costs and consequences, with both dimensions holding significance.

The second aspect covered in this session pertains to the rationale behind economic evaluation. Two vital points to underscore are the scarcity of resources and the imperative of optimizing resource allocation for the greatest benefit.

Challenges and Limitations

Despite its undeniable merits, economic evaluation encounters several challenges and limitations. Converting health outcomes into monetary terms, addressing data accuracy concerns, and accounting for evolving factors over time present formidable challenges. Additionally, the applicability of findins across diverse contexts and populations remains a concern. As economic evaluation continues to evolve, addressing these challenges becomes essential to ensuring the validity and reliability of its results.

> **KEY POINTS**
> - Economic evaluation of healthcare programs is the *systematic comparison of alternative healthcare actions in terms of both their costs and consequences*.
> - Need for economic evaluation is optimal allocation of available resource and to enable policy makers and providers to take informed decisions.
> - There are two approaches of doing economic evaluations—trial-based and model-based evaluations.
> - Partial evaluations focus on either costs or outcomes, while complete evaluations encompass a holistic comparison of both costs and outcomes in two groups.
> - Partial economic evaluations include: cost of illness (COI) study, cost outcome study and cost analysis.
> - The four types of complete economic evaluation studies are 1. cost minimization analysis 2. cost benefit analysis 3. cost effectiveness analysis 4. cost utility analysis

BIBLIOGRAPHY

1. Drummond MF, Sculpher MJ, Claxton K, Stoddart GL, Torrance GW. Methods for the Economic Evaluation of Health Care Programmes. Oxford: Oxford University Press; 2015.
2. Gold MR, Siegel JE, Russell LB, Weinstein MC (Eds). Cost-Effectiveness in Health and Medicine. Oxford: Oxford University Press; 1996.
3. Weinstein MC, Stason WB. Foundations of cost-effectiveness analysis for health and medical practices. N Engl J Med. 1977;296(13):716-21.

CHAPTER 38

Concept of Cost and Cost Analysis

Somen Saha, Kedar Mehta

"Of all the forms of inequality, injustice in healthcare is the most shocking and inhumane."
—*Martin Luther King Jr*

INTRODUCTION

Cost refers to the actual expenditure made by service provider to deliver the service. It is often confused with price (an amount which beneficiary or any other purchaser of services pays, e.g., fee paid to get ECG done), but the cost of services is different from the price of services.

Cost is defined as opportunity costs which is 'the sacrifice (of benefits) made when a given resource is consumed in a program or treatment'. Accurate measurement of costs is very important in economic evaluation and in the overall process of Health Technology Assessment.

Approaches for Costing

There are different known approaches for costing of healthcare services.

Normative costing is an exercise to estimate unit cost of service delivery by taking assumptions and expert opinions about various resources required. Here, analysts take expert opinion from various clinical and administrative experts; to arrive at a consensus about resources like staff, equipment, essential drugs and other consumables, etc., consumed in the delivery of a service.

Clinical trial data can be used to find the unit cost of the intervention either prospectively, by planning costing exercise along with clinical trial or by using trial data retrospectively. By this approach, it is easier to avail the required data but results from clinical trials cannot often be generalized to real world settings.

Pragmatic costing includes use of real-world data, i.e., how much of resources are actually being used to deliver the given service. This approach is most appropriate to estimate costs for doing HTA as well as for deciding package rates; but, is relatively the most difficult of the three approaches, especially in lower and lower middle-income countries due to lack of maintenance of records.

Perspectives in Health Economics

In health economics, perspectives refer to the viewpoint from which the costs and benefits of healthcare interventions are analyzed and interpreted. They determine whose costs and benefits are considered in an economic evaluation, shaping the scope and implications of the analysis. Perspectives can significantly influence the outcome and recommendations of health economic studies, reflecting the interests and priorities of different stakeholders within the healthcare system. Various types of perspectives are as follows:

Societal Perspective

This perspective evaluates the overall impact of healthcare interventions on society, accounting for both direct and indirect costs.

For example, a public smoking cessation campaign would be analyzed not just for its direct costs (like advertising and support programs) but also for its broader societal benefits, such as reduced healthcare expenses due to fewer smoking-related illnesses and increased productivity from a healthier workforce.

Centered Perspective

Centres on the costs and outcomes that are directly relevant to patients. Take, for instance, the introduction of a new medication for arthritis. From this perspective, the focus would be on factors like the medication's effectiveness in reducing pain, its side effects, the ease of adhering to the treatment regimen, and its impact on the patient's quality of life.

Provider/Health System Perspective

Centers the economic implications of health interventions from the viewpoint of healthcare providers. Consider the adoption of electronic health records (EHRs). Providers would evaluate the costs of implementing EHRs, the potential for improved efficiency in patient care, and the impacts on clinical practice, including time spent on documentation versus patient interaction.

Payer Perspective

Focuses on the financial implications of healthcare interventions for those footing the bill, like insurance companies or government programs. An example is the coverage decision for a new, costly cholesterol-lowering drug. Payers would analyze the drug's cost relative to its effectiveness in reducing heart disease risk and compare it with other available treatments.

Public Health Perspective

Examines the impact of health interventions on the overall health of the population. An example is the fluoridation of public water supplies. This perspective would assess the intervention's effectiveness in reducing dental caries across different population groups and its cost-effectiveness as a public health measure.

Perspective

Involves moral considerations in healthcare decisions, particularly around justice and equity. A pertinent example is the distribution of a limited supply of a life-saving drug. From this perspective, the focus would be on how to allocate the drug in a way that is considered ethically fair, taking into account factors such as patient need, prognosis, and the potential for benefit.

Types of Costs

Direct Cost

Direct costs represent the value of all goods, services, and other resources utilized in the implementation and continuation of a healthcare service or program. (e.g., costs on surgical equipment, drugs, etc.). Two types of direct costs are *direct healthcare costs* and *direct nonhealth care costs*.

Direct health care costs include costs of physician services, hospital services, drugs, etc. involved in delivery of healthcare. *Direct nonhealth care costs* are incurred in connection with health care, such as for care provided by family members and transportation to and from the site of care. In quantifying direct healthcare costs, many analysis use readily available hospital or physician *charges* (i.e., taken from price lists) rather than *true costs,* whose determination may require special analyses of resource consumption. Charges (as well as actual payments) tend to reflect provider cost-shifting and other factors that decrease the validity of using charges to represent the true costs of providing care.

Indirect Cost

Resources utilized or forgone by patients or attendants to enable them to receive service. These include the costs of lost work due to absenteeism or early retirement, impaired productivity at work (sometimes known as "presenteeism"), and lost or impaired leisure activity. Indirect costs also include the costs of premature mortality.

Overhead Costs

Resources, which are not utilized directly in providing services but are necessary to support the organization or program (e.g., electricity, etc.).

Capital Cost

The value of resources which have long useful lives, usually greater than one year (e. g., building of a hospital or OT table, etc.).

Recurrent Cost

The value of resources which are consumables and need to be replenished regularly as they have small useful lives (e.g., gloves, syringes, etc.).

Fixed Cost

The value of resource that does not vary with variation in the levels of output (e.g., rent of healthcare facility, etc.).

Variable cost

The value of resource that varies directly with variation in the levels of output (e.g., gloves, syringes etc.).

Marginal Cost

The change in the total cost if one additional unit of output is produced. Marginal cost analysis considers how outcomes change with changes in costs (e.g., relative to the standard of care or another comparator), which may provide more information about how to use resources efficiently.

Average Costs

Average cost analysis considers the total (or absolute) costs and outcomes of an intervention.

Key Concepts Related to Cost

Opportunity Cost

Value of the next best alternative choice forgone, by making decision to deliver a service (e.g., opportunity cost of providing free coronary bypass surgeries can be loss of opportunity to provide medical care as secondary prevention for 100 hypertensives for a year).

Annualization

A process to spread the cost of a capital resource over the life-time period of the same on the basis of average life expectancy of the capital resource.

Productivity Loss

Monetary loss borne due to patients' absence from work because of disease, disability or premature death.

Time Horizon

Interpretation of cost analysis must consider that the time horizon (or time-frame) of a study is likely to affect the findings regarding the relative magnitudes of costs and outcomes of a healthcare intervention. Costs and outcomes associated with a particular intervention usually do not accrue in steady streams over time. In many cases, health benefits resulting from investing in a health program are realized years after most of the spending. Any determination of the cost effectiveness of a particular health program can vary widely depending on the time horizon (e.g., 5, 10, 15, or 20 years since inception of the program) of the analysis.

Costing Methodologies

Different methodologies are used for determining costing. Here, we will learn three costing methodologies—Top-down, Bottom-up and mixed method.

Top-down Method

Top down costing is done using the expenditure incurred during a given financial period for delivery of the service. Total expenditure during given financial period is divided by total number of services delivered during that period. This is comparatively easier to do but it is difficult to arrive at the unit cost of a specific disease or procedure since the expenditure of a period covers many types of services and estimating what one of these services consumed may not be accurate.

Bottom-up Method

Bottom-up micro-costing is widely considered more appropriate as it considers, all relevant cost components utilized for patient groups or subgroups. This costing methodology has feasibility issues as it is very elaborate and time consuming, besides other challenges like non-availability of records in hospitals. In countries like India, researchers usually have to trade-off between accuracy and feasibility.

Mixed Method

Many a times, mix of top-down and bottom-up methodology is used to ascertain the unit cost of healthcare services. Top down approach is adopted for shared resources and those resources, which contribute a small proportion of overall unit cost (e.g., overheads); whereas, bottom-up approach is used for resources which are exclusive for a given service or contribute a large proportion of the overall cost (e.g., human resource).

Findings can be documented. It can include details about share of different resources in total cost, segregation according to type of facility, occupancy rates and location, etc. Details of methodology, perspectives used, assumptions and limitations of the costing exercise should also be incorporated in the report. Sensitivity analysis will add to quality of study by adjusting results to variation due to salaries across the states, rates of procurement of drugs, etc.

Concept of Discounting, Inflation and Reference Case

Discounting

Discounting is a process intended to adjust costs borne in future or past to today's equivalent costs or present value of resource. It also helps to adjust the value of costs and outcomes which occur in different time periods.

Cost analyses should account for the effect of the passage of time on the value of costs and outcomes. Costs and outcomes that occur in the future usually have less present value than costs and outcomes realized today. Discounting reflects the time preference for benefits earlier rather than later; it also reflects the opportunity costs of capital, i.e., whatever returns on investment that could have been gained if resources had been invested elsewhere. Thus, costs and outcomes should be *discounted* relative to their present value (e.g., at a rate of 3% or 5% per year).

Discounting allows comparisons involving costs and benefits that flow differently over time. DHR recommends discounting at the rate of 3%.

Inflation

Inflation is a quantitative measure of the rate at which the average price level of a basket of selected goods and services in an economy increases over some period of time. Cost analyses should also correct for the effects of inflation (which is different from the time preference accounted for by discounting), such as when cost or cost-effectiveness for one year is compared to another year. If original price of asset and year of purchase is available, adjustment for inflation can be done using GDP deflator or Consumer Price Index.

Reference Case

The reference case is a set of guidance for how economic evaluation should be conducted and will help in standardization of economic evaluations. The reference case for economic evaluation indicates that all available evidence relevant to the decision problem should be included.

Studies considered in the HTA process might present differences in terms of methodological approaches and reporting. This is unavoidable, as different methods will be more appropriate to specific research questions (and their corresponding field of enquiry), available data, resources and time. This is a big challenge for any country wanting to develop a workable HTA system.

Cost analysis and Interpretation

Enter data in Excel. Check the data for format (e.g., units) and completeness, remove irrelevant data. All recurrent and capital costs should be apportioned rationally across the services provided in given healthcare facility using time allocation studies (for salaries) or number of patients (e.g., for overheads). During analysis of capital assets, depreciate the cost and also annualize the same over period of its expected life. Adjust costs for inflation using GDP deflator or Consumer Price Index. If costs are being estimated from clinical trial data, modelling may be used to extrapolate costs beyond end-point of the trial. All assumptions, extrapolations and steps of analysis should be documented to improve transparency of analysis.

Sensitivity analysis will add to quality of study by adjusting results to variation due to salaries across the states, rates of procurement of drugs, etc. Any estimate of costs, outcomes, and other variables used in a cost analysis is subject to some uncertainty. Therefore, sensitivity analysis should be performed to determine if plausible variations in the estimates of certain variables thought to be subject to significant uncertainty affect the results of the cost analysis. A sensitivity analysis may reveal, for example, that including indirect costs, or assuming the use of generic as opposed to brand name drugs in a medical therapy, or using a plausible higher discount rate in an analysis changes the cost-effectiveness of one intervention compared to another.

Findings can be documented. It can include details about share of different resources in total cost, segregation according to type of facility, occupancy rates and location, etc. Details of methodology, perspectives used, assumptions and limitations of the costing exercise should also be incorporated in the report. Sensitivity analysis will add to quality of study by adjusting results to variation due to salaries across the states, rates of procurement of drugs, etc.

Steps for Costing Exercise

For the costing exercise to be streamlined and to address the needs of stakeholders, a clear work plan needs to be followed. Inadequately planned costing exercises can lead to repeated visits to healthcare facilities or collection of irrelevant data. Broadly, the step wise approach given below can be followed.

1. Outline aims and objectives of costing exercise and make a list of services/packages whose costing is planned,
2. Decide perspective. It is important to identify the perspective from which you are assessing the technology, the societal perspective or the health systems perspective.
3. Select costing methodology. Costing methodology (such as top-down/bottom-up/mixed methodology) should be selected based on priorities of all the stakeholders and resources available. Time horizon, approach for data collection (prospective/retrospective) and data period (year/month) should be well-defined.
4. Select sample. Identify sample for fetching costing data. For example, sample of service providers based on location (rural/urban), level of healthcare facility (primary/secondary/tertiary), occupancy rates and quality of service (NABH or other quality accreditation) and or patients characteristics (age, severity of disease), etc.
5. Prepare data collection tools. Enumerate all resources being used in costing exercise. Data on volume/number of resources needed for the costing should be identified and the unit cost of each resource used should be collected, so that total expenditure can be calculated.
6. Collect data. Data collection should be started from those resources, which make major proportion of total cost. Data can be collected from various cost centers by assessing health records (e.g., IPD records), accessing administrative databases (e. g., stock registers of equipment and furniture, bills paid during given financial year, etc.), patient interviews, staff interviews, etc. Any missing data can be substituted by consultation of expert panel (e.g., average life of equipment can be obtained from store in charge and OT technician, based on their experience). Estimation of infrastructure costs should be done by making some realistic assumptions or proxies as data pertaining to cost of construction or renovation is usually not available.
7. Analyze the data
8. Report finding in HTA outcome report.

KEY POINTS

- Healthcare costing distinguishes between the actual cost to providers and the price paid by users, stressing accurate cost measurement for effective health program evaluation.
- There are various costing approaches and perspectives for estimating healthcare costs and how different viewpoints affect economic evaluations in healthcare.
- There are various healthcare costs (like direct, indirect, capital) and different ways to calculate them, we need to decide based on their uses and challenges.
- A step-by-step guide for a thorough healthcare costing process, from planning and data collection to analysis and reporting.

BIBLIOGRAPHY

1. Department of Health Research. HTA Manual. [Internet]. Available from: https://htain.icmr.org.in/images/pdf/htain%20manual.pdf
2. Drummond MF, Sculpher MJ, Claxton K, Stoddart GL, Torrance GW. Methods for the economic evaluation of health care programmes. Oxford: Oxford University Press; 2015.
3. Sharma D. Reference case for undertaking economic evaluation for HTA in India. 2020. Unpublished.
4. Wilkinson T, et al. The International Decision Support Initiative Reference Case for Economic Evaluation: An Aid to Thought. Value in Health. 2016;19.
5. Wonderling D. Introduction to health economics. McGraw-Hill Education (UK); 2011.

CHAPTER 39

Micro and Macro Health Economics

Sarit Kumar Rout, Sudhir Prabhu H, Chandralekha Kona

"To understand the economy, you only need to understand how people make decisions: with emotions and irrationalities, not as the textbooks assume, with rational calculus."
—Richard Thaler

BACKGROUND

Resources are scarce and we have multiple objectives. The subject matter of economics deals with how to allocate scarce resources among multiple objectives in order to achieve maximum satisfaction, or welfare. This involves choice. Societies have to make choices about how to allocate scare resources for the production of health services, and how to distribute these services. These choices are the discipline of health economics

Definitions

- Microeconomics is simply the study of individual actions- for instance study of individual firm, prices, wage and revenue.
- Microeconomics is study of aggregate or the whole economy–national income, total employment aggregate supply and aggregate demand.

Differences (Table 1)

Table 1: Difference in characteristics of between microeconomics and macroeconomics.

Characteristics	Microeconomics	Macroeconomics
Area of interest	Demand for health/production of health/cost of health service delivery of an individual, household or a particular hospital	Aggregate demand, supply of health, improving health status of the population, investment in health, and its linkage with GDP, health to wealth and wealth to health
Scope	Demand for healthcare and what influences the demand for health, how health is produced by a hospital and what is cost of producing an unit of health services, what is the price of unit of healthcare service	Influences aggregate demand for healthcare, knowing about the people's demand, whether healthcare should be provided by market, regulations, whether to invest on child immunization or cancer care. Return on investment or how much to invest on health (proportion of GDP)

Data

The following are the sources for data

Primary Data
- Individual household survey
- Costing data from health facilities/other departments

Secondary Data
- Large sample surveys–NSSO, NFHS
- Data from IRDA
- Time series data on SRS and census
- Health budget and expenditure data
- GDP report, NHA report
- RBI and World bank reports

Research (Table 2)

Microeconomic Research
- Uses individual level data like socioeconomic indicators, healthcare demand and utilization, accessibility and availability of healthcare services to analyze the impact on individuals/households/communities, cost data.
- Cost of illness studies, CEA, equity analysis and wealth quantiles.

Macroeconomic Research
- Uses secondary data and run mathematical model and econometrics by using various techniques such as correlation, multiple regressions models, diseases models to get aggregate state/country level impact/results.
- E.g., infectious disease modelling—COVID-19 related prediction
- Budget impact analysis, public expenditure analysis
- Health economics map is depicted in **Fig. 1.**

Table 2: Difference between microeconomics and macroeconomics.

Microeconomic	*Macroeconomic*
• Mortality and morbidity	• Impact on productivity
• Direct medical costs (drugs, OPD visits, Hospitalization)	• GDP losses/gains
• Out of pocket payments	• Impact on human capital
• Travel costs and funeral costs	• Impact on total budget (budget impact)
• Presenteeism and absenteeism for firm and individual	• Capital formation
• Care–giving needs	

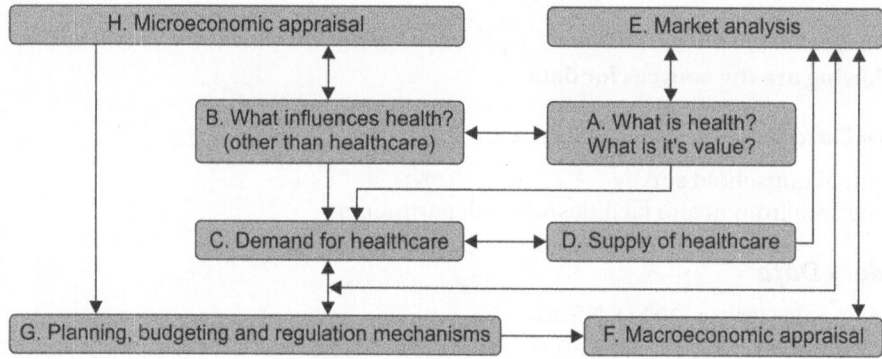

Fig. 1: Health economics map.

KEY POINTS

- Health economics explores how to best use limited resources for health services and the choices involved.
- It examines individual health needs and costs (microeconomics) and overall health investments and economy-wide impacts (macroeconomics).
- Research in this field uses surveys and national data to understand health costs and impacts at both personal and broader levels

BIBLIOGRAPHY

1. Harlin BO, Desselberger U. The financial burden of rotavirus disease in four countries of the European Union. Pediatr Infect Dis J. 2008;27:S20–7. Available from: www.webofscience.com/wos/woscc/fullrecord/WOS:000252144700004?SID=EUW1ED0F6Fv2TjyFYs6e2F9uNefa1
2. John RM. Price elasticity estimates for tobacco products in India. Health Policy Plan. 2008;23(3):200–9. doi: 10.1093/heapol/czn007
3. Kotsopoulos N, Connolly MP. Is the gap between micro- and macroeconomic assessments in health care well understood? The case of vaccination and potential remedies. J Market Access Health Policy. 2014;2(1). doi: 10.3402/jmahp.v2.23897

Introduction to HTA and Steps in HTA Protocol Development

Suthanthira Kannan, Komal Shah, Chandrlekha Kona

"Economics is a study of man in the ordinary business of life."
—*Alfred Marshall*

INTRODUCTION TO HTA

Health Technology Assessment (HTA) is a multidisciplinary process that summarizes information about the medical, social, economic, and ethical issues related to the use of a health technology in a systematic, transparent, unbiased, and robust manner. It aims to inform the formulation of safe, effective, health policies that are patient-focused and seek to achieve the best value. It involves a rigorous analysis of technical performance, clinical efficacy, safety, cost-effectiveness, organizational implications and societal aspects.

What is HTA?

HTA refers to the systematic evaluation of the properties and impacts of health technologies and interventions, including their direct and intended effects, as well as any indirect or unintended consequences, whether beneficial or harmful.

Importance of HTA

HTA plays a vital role in modern healthcare by assisting in decision-making processes related to technology adoption, reimbursement and research focus. It aids in:
- Evaluating the effectiveness and cost-effectiveness of technologies.
- Providing a basis for choices about which technologies to adopt.
- Ensuring that patient needs and preferences are considered.
- Guiding research and development in healthcare technologies.

Steps in HTA Protocol Development

HTA protocol development is a crucial part of the assessment process. It comprises several steps to ensure a thorough and unbiased assessment.

Step 1: Identifying the Research Question

The first step involves identifying and defining the research question that the HTA aims to answer. This includes understanding the technology, its intended use, the target population and the context in which it will be assessed.

Step 2: Conducting a Literature Review

A comprehensive literature review is conducted to gather existing evidence on the technology. This helps in understanding the current state of knowledge and identifying gaps that the HTA may fill.

Step 3: Assessment Methodology

The methodology for the HTA is then defined, including the selection of appropriate methods for assessing effectiveness, cost-effectiveness, and the social, ethical and legal aspects of the technology.

Step 4: Data Collection and Analysis

This step involves the collection and analysis of data related to the technology, including clinical trials, economic evaluations and patient surveys.

Step 5: Reporting and Dissemination

The final step involves summarizing the findings in a report and disseminating them to relevant stakeholders, including policymakers, healthcare providers, patients and the general public.

Checklist for All Factors to be Incorporated in the Health Technology Assessment Proposal

The health technology assessment (HTA) proposal must be meticulously crafted, considering various essential factors. The **objective** must clearly define the purpose of the HTA, such as contributing to evidence or informing adoption decisions. Identification of the principal audience, such as government, pharmaceutical companies, or patient groups, ensures that the assessment is tailored to the relevant stakeholders. The **perspective** should align with viewpoints like societal, healthcare system or insurer, while the targeted patient population must be specified by characteristics such as age, health status or gender. Relevant **comparators** and the embedding of technologies in clinical practice must be considered alongside a carefully planned timeline for completion, including data collection, analysis, and final report generation. The **time horizon** for the decision problem, relevant consequences, patient use, professional use and cycle length must be specified. Price level, resource use, equity considerations and social issues need to be carefully addressed. If a **budget impact analysis** is to be conducted, the level at which it will be undertaken should be specified. Provisions for additional analysis, ethical justification and proper acknowledgment of all reference materials must be included. Finally, any data collection tools being used, whether prevalidated or not, such as cost data collection tools or **Quality of Life questionnaires**, must be detailed in the annexures. This comprehensive approach ensures a robust and transparent HTA proposal that caters to the multifaceted nature of healthcare technology assessment.

Importance of HTA

HTA aims to provide evidence-based information to guide decisions and policy-making in healthcare. It supports the effective allocation of resources and ensures that technologies are assessed for their value, safety and suitability for specific healthcare settings.

> **KEY POINTS**
> - HTA is vital for healthcare decision-making to enhance healthcare quality and sustainability.
> - HTA is a systematic approach to assess health technologies, informing decisions on technology adoption, reimbursement, and research priorities, necessitating a well-planned and transparent protocol.
> - By linking research, policy, and practice, HTA ensures the delivery of safe, effective, and cost-efficient healthcare, aligning with patient needs and societal preferences.

BIBLIOGRAPHY

1. Indian Council of Medical Research. HTA Manual India. New Delhi: Indian Council of Medical Research; 2018.

Outcome Assessment in Economic Evaluation Studies

CHAPTER 41

Tanvi Kiran, Divya Sharma, Mohammad Waseem Faraz Ansari

> *"Good health is good economics; health is a precondition for economic prosperity."*
> —Margaret Chan

INTRODUCTION

Economic evaluation entails comparing the costs (inputs) and consequences (outcomes) associated with two or more alternative treatments or scenarios to determine the most efficient allocation of limited resources. To assess these interventions, the initial steps involve identifying, quantifying and assigning a value to their costs and outcomes.

The essential characteristics of an economic evaluation encompass the examination of both costs and outcomes, necessitating the comparison of at least two different strategies or interventions. Measuring costs in an economic evaluation is relatively straightforward, typically involving the measurement in a common currency. Costs and consequences in an economic evaluation depicted in **Fig. 1**.

However, a critical challenge in economic evaluation arises from selecting an appropriate outcome measure. Different interventions often yield outcomes that are expressed in diverse units of measurement. For instance, comparing the number of individuals screened for oral cancer in a screening program with the number of child deaths prevented through immunization involves units that are not directly comparable. Consequently, when the government faces a decision on where to allocate its resources between these programs, the task becomes complex due to the inherent disparity in outcome measures.

Outcome Assessment in Economic Evaluation

Outcome measures employed in economic assessments can typically be classified into one of the following categories **(Table 1)**.

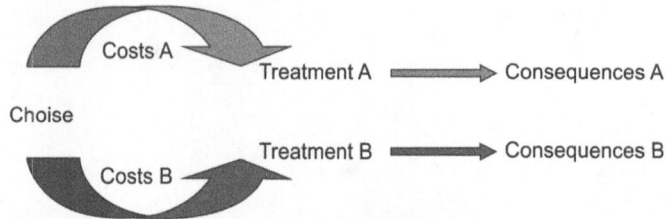

Fig. 1: Costs and consequences in an economic evaluation.

Source: Michael F. Drummond. Methods for the economic evaluation of health care programmes, 2nd edition, 1997

Chapter 41: Outcome Assessment in Economic Evaluation Studies

Table 1: Outcome measures in economic evaluation.

Health outcomes	Utility outcomes	Monetary outcomes
• Condition specific • Clinical endpoints • Survival • Mortality	• QALY • DALY	• Willingness to pay • Human capital approach

Health Outcomes

The following outcome measures are categorized under health outcomes:
- **Condition specific:** Specific outcomes related to a condition, such as smoking cessation rates or episode-free days for diseases like asthma or acid reflux.
- **Clinical endpoints:** Including measures like reduced cholesterol levels, the number of heart attacks or ulcers prevented, etc.
- **Survival:** To calculate the gained years of life. For example, life years they gained using antiretroviral therapy among HIV patients.
- **Mortality:** Number of deaths averted because of an intervention.

Health outcomes such as clinical endpoints are simple to assess but have drawbacks as they make comparisons between different healthcare treatments complex.

> We cannot make an informed decision based on these outcomes as they are not comparable.
> **Example:** It is not possible to directly compare reduced cholesterol levels with the number of heart attacks prevented because these two clinical endpoints are distinct from each other.

Survival, on the other hand, enables comparisons even between highly distinct therapies but is not without its challenges **(Fig. 2)**.

In order to facilitate comparisons among various healthcare regions, it is essential to establish a standardized measure. This measure should encompass both the effects of a treatment on a patient's life expectancy and its impact on their quality of life related to health. This quality of life is widely acknowledged as a critical indicator of treatment outcomes.

Hence, there is a growing trend in assessing outcomes across different diseases by incorporating quality measures that extend beyond clinical and mortality indicators.

Utility Outcomes

Now that we understand that summarizing health outcomes into a single effectiveness unit is challenging, it becomes evident that for the purpose of comparison, we need more standardized and one-dimensional outcome measures. These measures should also consider an individual's quality of life.

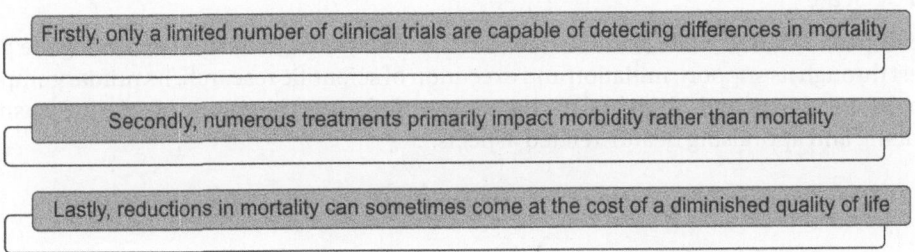

Fig. 2: Challenges associated with survival outcomes.

Two examples of such indicators, which combine morbidity and mortality into a single value, are:
1. Quality-Adjusted Life Years (QALYs)
2. Disability-Adjusted Life Years (DALYs)

Quality-Adjusted Life Years

QALYs represent the duration of life lived in a state of optimal health, encompassing both the quantity and quality of life. This means it considers not only how long an individual lives but also how well they live by factoring in both morbidity and mortality aspects of health. This is achieved by assigning a weight to each year based on the quality of life (utility) experienced during that year.

$$QALYs = Survival \times Utility\ Score$$

Utility score is measured between 0 and 1:
Where, 0 = Death and 1 = Perfect health

> **Exercise I: Calculation of QALYs**
> Calculate the QALYs for a person who is living for 75 years in perfect health.
> **Solution:** Life years lived = 75
> He has perfect health for 75 years (Utility Score = 1)
> $$QALYs\ Lived = 75 \times 1 = 75$$
> Calculate the QALYs for a person who is living for 70 years in perfect health. He has perfect health for 55 years and utility score of 0.6 for 15 years.
> **Solution:** If a person is living for 70 years
> Life years lived = 70
> QALYs lived = 55 × 1 + 0.6 × 15
>   = 55 + 9
>   **QALYs lived = 64**

In the exercise, we observed the utilization of utility scores in the computation of QALYs. These utility scores continually fluctuate as an individual's health state evolves over the course of their life. Now, let us delve deeper into the process of calculating these utility scores.

Scales to Measure Health States to Calculate Utility Score

Numerous organizations have designed a range of Quality of Life assessment scales, such as the World Health Organization Quality of Life Instrument (WHOQOL), the Global Quality of Life Scale, the Health-Related Quality of Life Scale (HRQOL) by the Center for Disease Control, and the EQ5D-5L scale. Among these, the most utilized scale is the EQ5D-5L, developed by the European Quality of Life (EuroQol) research foundation.

EQ5d-5L Scale

The European Quality of Life (EuroQol) research foundation is dedicated to serving the public interest through its support, initiation and execution of scientific research. Its primary emphasis lies in the creation of tools designed to characterize and assess health, particularly focusing on describing and appraising health-related aspects.

It introduced an instrument 5-level EQ-5D version- EQ-5D-5L (EuroQol- Five dimensions-Five levels) in 2009. The EQ-5D-5L essentially consists of the following:
- EQ Visual Analogue Scale (EQ VAS)
- EQ-5D descriptive system

EQ Visual Analogue Scale

The EQ VAS captures a patient's self-assessed health status using a vertical visual analog scale. This scale is marked with endpoints labeled as 'the best health you can imagine' and 'the worst health you can imagine.' The VAS serves as a quantitative means of measuring health outcomes that mirror the patient's personal evaluation.

EQ-5D Descriptive System

The descriptive system comprises five dimensions: mobility, self-care, usual activities, pain/discomfort, and anxiety/depression. Each dimension has five levels ranging from 1 to 5, where 1 is no problem and 5 is an extreme problem. A unique health state is defined by combining one level from each dimension. A value set is used to assign a numerical value to a particular health state.

Disability-Adjusted Life Years

DALYs quantify the combined impact of disease and injury by measuring the years of healthy life lost due to these conditions. Each DALY can be understood as a single year of healthy life lost. It comprises both Years of Life Lost and Years Lived with Disability. The disability score used in DALYs stands in contrast to that used in QALYs.

In this context, a disability weight of 0 represents perfect health, while a weight of 1 signifies death.

DALYs = Years of Life Lost (YLL) + Years Lived with Disability (YLD)

Monetary Outcomes

Monetary outcomes can provide a broader perspective on the economic impact of an intervention or policy. These allow for direct comparison of the costs and benefits of different interventions or programs. This comparability can be especially useful when evaluating interventions across various sectors or industries.

There are two main approaches used for valuation of outcomes in monetary terms:
1. **Willingness to pay approach:** It is alternatively known as Contingent Valuation. It entails determining the amounts that individuals express a willingness to pay in exchange for a reduced risk of alterations in the quality or duration of life (e.g., the willingness to pay for a percentage chance of experiencing a life free from cardiac symptoms or for improved air quality). Using this method, various effects, such as the disability days avoided or life-years gained, are translated into economic benefits.
2. **Human capital approach:** In this approach, each person is viewed as a source of production, and their worth is determined by their income. Sickness and mortality within the workforce represent a significant economic loss because they result in individuals losing their capacity to contribute time and productivity to work and other productive endeavors.

> **KEY POINTS**
> - This chapter has provided a comprehensive exploration of outcome assessment in economic evaluation studies.
> - Understanding the various outcomes and their valuation is a fundamental concept in the field of economic evaluations and it serves as the cornerstone for conducting different types of economic analyses.
> - To make meaningful comparisons, researchers need to use consistent outcome measures and valuations.
> - Understanding the outcomes and their valuation helps in making sense of the findings and communicating them to a broader audience.

BIBLIOGRAPHY

1. Basakha M, Soleimanvandiazar N, Tavangar F, Daneshi S. Economic value of life in iran: The human capital approach. Iran J Public Health. 2021;50(2):384–90.
2. EuroQol. EQ-5D-5L – EQ-5D [Internet]. [cited 2023 Oct 6]. Available from: https://euroqol.org/eq-5d-instruments/eq-5d-5l-about/
3. EuroQol. Valuation – EQ-5D [Internet]. [cited 2023 Oct 6]. Available from: https://euroqol.org/eq-5d-instruments/eq-5d-5l-about/valuation-standard-value-sets/
4. Johannesson M, Jönsson B, Karlsson G. Outcome measurement in economic evaluation. Health Econ. 1996;5(4):279–96.
5. Lorgelly PK, Lawson KD, Fenwick EAL, Briggs AH. Outcome measurement in economic evaluations of public health interventions: A role for the capability approach? Int J Environ Res Public Health. 2010;7(5):2274–89.
6. Saldivia S, Vicente B, Torres F. Measuring outcomes in economic evaluations. Rev Med Chil. 2010;138(Suppl. 2):79–82.
7. Salomon JA. Quality Adjusted Life Years [Internet]. 2nd edition. Vol. 5, International Encyclopedia of Public Health. Elsevier; 2016. 224–228 p. Available from: http://dx.doi.org/10.1016/B978-0-12-803678-5.00368-4
8. Stanford University. Health-Related Quality of Life Scale | SPARQtools [Internet]. [cited 2023 Oct 6]. Available from: https://sparqtools.org/mobility-measure/health-related-quality-of-life-scale/
9. Whitehead SJ, Ali S. Health outcomes in economic evaluation: The QALY and utilities. Br Med Bull. 2010;96(1):5–21.
10. World Health Organization (WHO). Disability-adjusted life years (DALYs) [Internet]. [cited 2023 Oct 6]. Available from: https://www.who.int/data/gho/indicator-metadata-registry/imr-details/158
11. World Health Organization (WHO). WHOQOL - Measuring Quality of Life| The World Health Organization [Internet]. [cited 2023 Oct 6]. Available from: https://www.who.int/tools/whoqol

CHAPTER 42

Sensitivity Analysis and Modeling

Komal Shah, A Akshay Subramanian, Sunhitha Velamala, Mohammad Waseem Faraz Ansari

"In the long term, the economy and the environment are the same thing. If it's unenvironmental it is uneconomical. That is the rule of nature."
—Mollie Beattie

INTRODUCTION

Sensitivity analysis is a financial model that determines how target variables are affected based on changes in other variables known as input variables. It is a way to predict the outcome of a decision given a certain range of variables. Sensitivity analysis is the study of how uncertainty in the output of a mathematical model or system can be divided and allocated to different sources of uncertainty in its inputs. It has evolved as an indispensable method for assessing the robustness and reliability of mathematical models used to understand the dynamics of diseases in populations. Early epidemiological models often simplified complex systems, assuming fixed values for various parameters. However, as the field advanced, researchers recognized the inherent uncertainties in these models, prompting the development of sensitivity analysis techniques.

Why is Sensitivity Analysis Required in Healthcare Sector?

- It helps to reduce the likelihood of undertaking bad projects while not failing to accept good projects.
- It discusses "how" and "how much" changes in the parameters of an optimization problem modify the optimal objective function value and the point where the optimum is attained.

Formula-Percentage Change In Output/Percentage Change of Input

For example, bookstore a sells all their books for the same price. By reviewing historical data, they know that if they increase the price of their book by 15%, that their sales fall by 30%.

Understanding Sensitivity Analysis

In this example, we will explore sensitivity analysis in the context of an infectious disease model.

Example scenario: Consider an epidemiologist developing a mathematical model to predict the spread of a novel infectious disease within a population. The model incorporates parameters such as the transmission rate, the incubation period, and the effectiveness of control measures.

Step 1: Identify Key Parameters

- **Transmission rate (β):** The rate at which the disease is transmitted from an infected person to a susceptible person.
- **Incubation period (α):** The time it takes for an infected individual to show symptoms.
- **Control measure effectiveness (γ):** The effectiveness of interventions, such as vaccination or social distancing, in reducing transmission.

Step 2: Define Plausible Ranges

For each parameter, define a plausible range based on existing literature, empirical data, or expert opinion.
- **Transmission rate (β):** Plausible range: 0.2–0.5 transmissions per person per day.
- **Incubation period (α):** Plausible range: 5–10 days.
- **Control measure effectiveness (γ):** Plausible range: 0.2–0.8 (where 1 indicates full effectiveness).

Step 3: Conduct Sensitivity Analysis

One-way Sensitivity Analysis

- Vary one parameter while keeping others constant.
- For instance, vary the transmission rate (β) and observe its impact on the total number of infected individuals.
- **Result:** The model is highly sensitive to changes in transmission rate, with higher rates leading to a substantial increase in the number of infections.

Multi-way Sensitivity Analysis

- Simultaneously vary transmission rate (β) and control measure effectiveness (γ) to examine their combined effects.
- **Result:** Identifying scenarios where the transmission rate has a more significant impact, even when control measures are partially effective.

Threshold Analysis

- Determine the minimum vaccination coverage (γ) required to achieve herd immunity and prevent sustained transmission.
- **Result:** Illustrate the critical threshold for vaccination coverage needed to control the outbreak.

Step 4: Interpret Results

- Understand which parameters have the most significant impact on model outcomes.
- Identify scenarios where the model predictions are most sensitive to parameter variations.
- Inform decision-makers about key factors influencing the spread of the disease and guide intervention strategies.

In this example, sensitivity analysis helped the epidemiologist understand the model's sensitivity to variations in transmission rate, incubation period, and control measure effectiveness. This information is crucial for refining the model, informing public health strategies, and communicating the uncertainties associated with predictions. Sensitivity analysis enhances the transparency and reliability of epidemiological models, making them valuable tools for evidence-based decision-making in the face of infectious disease outbreaks.

Methodologies in Sensitivity Analysis

Deterministic Sensitivity Analysis
- One way sensitivity analysis
- Multi way sensitivity analysis
- Threshold analysis

Probabilistic Sensitivity Analysis
- Monte Carlo simulation
- Latin hypercube sampling
- Bootstrapping

Global Sensitivity Analysis
- Variance based sensitivity analysis
- Morris method

Bayesian Sensitivity Analysis
- Bayesian model averaging
- Prior sensitivity analysis

Structural Sensitivity Analysis
Model structural uncertainty

Meta-Analysis and Systematic Reviews
Application of Sensitivity Analysis (advantages of sensitivity analysis)
- Model robustness assessment
- Identification of key parameters
- Resource allocation
- Uncertainty qualification
- Optimization of control measures
- Policy decision support
- Model validation
- Scenario planning

Disadvantages
- Complexity and interpretation
- Assumption dependency
- Data limitation
- Limited to modelled factor
- Quantification challenges

Modeling in Economic Evaluation

Utilizing Decision Trees for Economic Evaluations in Healthcare
- **Overview:** In the realm of health economics, decision trees are pivotal. They provide a structured approach to evaluating and comparing different healthcare strategies, considering both their financial and clinical outcomes.

- **Fundamentals:** At its core, a decision tree is a schematic that maps out various decision paths and their probable outcomes. Each decision leads to a series of potential events, represented by branches, culminating in different endpoints or outcomes. These outcomes are quantified in terms of both health consequences and economic costs.
- **Practical Illustration:** Imagine a scenario where a healthcare provider must decide whether to implement a new screening program for a chronic illness. The decision tree would display options like conducting or skipping the screening. Each choice leads to different pathways, including possible detection of the illness, subsequent treatments, and varied health outcomes, each with associated costs and probabilities.

Markov Models: A Dynamic Approach in Health Economic Analysis

- **Introduction:** Markov models are indispensable in health economics, particularly for analyzing diseases that progress over time. They offer a dynamic framework to study the long-term implications of medical interventions.
- **Essence:** A Markov model is composed of distinct health states and the likelihood of transitions between these states over specified time intervals. It accounts for the evolving nature of healthcare scenarios, attaching costs and health outcomes to each state.
- **Applied example:** Consider the management of a progressive disease like hypertension. The Markov model would include states such as 'Normal Blood Pressure', 'Elevated Blood Pressure', and 'Hypertensive Crisis'. The model would assess the transitions among these states over time, factoring in interventions like medication or lifestyle modifications and their impact on health outcomes and healthcare expenditures.

KEY POINTS

- Sensitivity analysis in epidemiology stands as a testament to the field's commitment to precision, transparency, and adaptability.
- It enables researchers to unravel the complexities of health-related phenomena and contribute to the improvement of public health on a global scale.
- Decision trees and Markov models are vital tools in health economics, used to evaluate the financial and clinical outcomes of healthcare strategies.
- While decision trees map out the consequences of immediate healthcare decisions, Markov models analyze long-term implications of diseases and treatments over time.

BIBLIOGRAPHY

1. Azreena E, Juni MH, Manaf R, Juni M, Muhamad H, Juni. Methodological approaches in health economic evaluation. Int J Public Health Clin Sci. 2017;4.
2. Caro JJ, Briggs AH. Sensitivity analysis and the expected value of perfect information. Med Decis Making. 1999;19(4):411-4. doi: 10.1177/0272989X9901900412.
3. Heesterbeek H, Anderson RM, Andreasen V, et al. Modeling infectious disease dynamics in the complex landscape of global health. Science. 2015;347(6227):aaa4339. doi: 10.1126/science.aaa4339.
4. Hutubessy R, Chisholm D, Edejer TT, WHO-CHOICE. Generalized cost-effectiveness analysis for national-level priority-setting in the health sector. Cost Eff Resour Alloc. 2003;1(1):8. doi: 10.1186/1478-7547-1-8.

CHAPTER 43

Budget Impact Analysis

Somen Saha, Kedar Mehta

> *"Economics is everywhere, and understanding economics can help you make better decisions and lead a happier life."*
> —Tyler Cowen

INTRODUCTION

Budget impact analysis (BIA) is a method for economic evaluation of healthcare technologies. It assesses the financial consequences of the introduction of a new healthcare technology in a specific setting in the short-to-medium term.

A cost-effectiveness analysis provides information on whether a health technology is value for money. A cost-effectiveness threshold is used to objectively inform whether a technology should be considered cost effective, by considering both affordability and societal preferences (willingness to pay). However, this is not telling us whether the use of such technology will be financially sustainable given current real budget of the healthcare system (at local, regional or national level) and/or patients. Such a question may be answered by undertaking a budget impact analysis, which estimates the financial consequences of increasing uptake of a health technology in a target disease population over the near future (3–5 years).

In addition to cost data, as for cost-effectiveness analysis, populating budget-impact models requires epidemiological inputs, to define the target patient population, provider choices which define the current distribution of treatment alternatives, and expected uptake of the health technology being assessed.

Recommendation for BIA by Department of Health Research

Perspective

A BIA from the budget holder's or payer's perspective should be done for two scenarios: current existing share of budget holder and out-of-pocket expenditure (OOPE) as well as a scenario where universal access to services would be guaranteed by the budget holder without any OOPE.

Time Horizon

The time frame chosen for the BIA should conform to the requirements and budgeting process of the budget holder as well as the time it takes for a new technology to reach its optimum or desired coverage. Present results for a minimum of 1 year to a maximum of 5 years.

Eligible Population

BIA population is defined as an open cohort; patients may enter and leave throughout the time horizon of the analysis.

The top-down approach is considered preferable and should be used. Top-down approach starts from the total population size and applies the epidemiological data and information on restrictions/eligibility to estimate the number of patients eligible for treatment at every year of the analysis. Since this approach breaks down the estimation of the target population in subsequent steps, it is very transparent and allows for inclusion of projections in demographic and epidemiology over time.

Scenarios to be Compared

Two scenarios should be compared: The current mix of interventions and future mix of interventions for the eligible population.

The current treatment mix should represent an accurate description of the current situation in terms of currently available healthcare technologies in real practice. It may include a number of different health-technologies, no intervention or alternative treatment strategies corresponding to the condition/disease of interest. The future mix of interventions should represent routine care for the target population following the introduction of the new intervention. It should therefore include the new intervention in addition to any of the current mix interventions which are predicted to remain alternative treatment options in the future.

Coverage mix and Uptake of the new Intervention

Assumptions of the coverage can be made based on: International data where the technology or a similar technology has already been introduced; and expert opinion.

Discounting and Inflation

Discounting is not recommended as BIA aims to present the actual financial implications required to deliver the new intervention over each year of the analysis. Thus, in BIA costs should be presented as real costs at each subsequent year of the analysis.

Current price should be used to present the prices of resource use at each year of the analysis. Inflation will apply only to updated costs/prices of resources used in the model at the current price level.

Approach to Budget Impact Modeling

Clinical data on the natural disease history, efficacy and safety of all health-technologies considered in the analysis should be used to develop a decision analytical modeling approach (e.g., decision-tree or Markov model).

Costing Approach

Financial or economic costing approach should be followed depending on the mechanism of service provisioning, whether supply or demand side provisioning.
- Budget impact analysis should consider resource use and costs directly associated with the condition for which the intervention is designed and other costs resulting from the intervention.
- Only costs from the selected perspective, which are incurred during the time horizon of the analysis should be included.

- Costs such as direct costs such as acquisition/administration costs for health intervention, adverse event-related costs, follow-up/monitoring cost for disease management and when relevant, subsequent treatments costs.
- The analysis should include only costs which is relevant for the budget holder based on perspective including the valuation of resources spent by the patients at the prices which the payer would pay.

Presentation of Results

- Results should be presented in total as well as year wise budget impact spread across the chosen time horizon.
- Results should be disaggregated by the type of budget holder, type of resource use (capital as well as recurrent). For example, infrastructure, equipment, health technology/drugs, human resources, consumables, any maintenance cost.
- It should represent both monetary as well as natural units for resource use should be given.

Uncertainty Analysis

Deterministic sensitivity analysis and scenario analysis should be carried out.

KEY POINTS

- Budget impact analysis evaluates the financial impact of new health technologies, guiding decisions on their adoption and funding.
- It compares current and future healthcare scenarios over 1–5 years, considering patient numbers and treatment options from both healthcare payer and patient perspectives.
- BIA uses models to predict costs and effects of treatments, focusing on direct healthcare costs and presenting them in current value terms.
- Results show total and yearly financial impacts, with analyses to account for possible variations and uncertainties.

BIBLIOGRAPHY

1. Bilinski A, Neumann P, Cohen J, Thorat T, McDaniel K, Salomon JA. When cost-effectiveness interventions are unaffordable: Integrating cost-effectiveness and budget impact in priority setting for global health programs. PLoS medicine. 2017;14(10).
2. Briggs A, Sculpher M, Claxton K. Decision Modelling for Health Economic Evaluation. Oxford: Oxford University Press; 2006.
3. Chugh Y, Francesco M D, Prinja S. Framework for budget impact analysis: Recommendations for India.

CHAPTER 44

Drawing up the Protocol for an Economic Evaluation Study

Farah Naaz Fathima, Chandralekha Kona

"Health is not just an expense, but an investment in a productive and prosperous future."
—*Unknown*

INTRODUCTION

Drawing up a protocol is the first step in conducting an economic evaluation. A well-written protocol provides a framework for conducting the study, addresses ethical considerations, contributes to the scientific rigor, and overall quality of the research, and supports the decision-making process. In the context of economic evaluations, a well-written protocol is indispensable for the credibility, transparency, and reproducibility.

This chapter explains the steps in writing up a protocol for an economic evaluation.

Title

To formulate a robust economic evaluation protocol, the first step involves the creation of a study title. During the title composition process, attention is required to two key considerations. Firstly, the study should be distinctly categorized as an economic evaluation by incorporating terms such as economic evaluation, cost-effectiveness analysis, or costing. This necessitates the explicit inclusion of phrases like cost utility analysis, cost-benefit analysis, cost of illness study, or cost description, analysis, aligned with the specific type of economic evaluation being conducted.

Secondly, a crucial aspect of the title involves the explicit specification of the interventions under scrutiny. The essence of economic evaluation lies in the comparison and contrast of two or more interventions, aiding in the determination of the most cost-effective course of action. As a result, the title should clearly explain what you are comparing and which interventions are being examined in the economic evaluation process.

Introduction

In the introduction section of the protocol, it is essential to delineate the context, articulate the research question, summarize existing knowledge on the topic, and identify gaps in the current evidence. In addition, the practical relevance for decision-making by either policy or practice should be clearly stated. The fundamental purpose of conducting an economic evaluation is to facilitate decision-making, aiding in the selection of multiple options. If the rationale behind the economic evaluation and its application to specific decision-makers or scenarios is not articulated, the introduction remains incomplete.

The objective of the economic evaluation should be clearly stated. Employing the PICO acronym, typically used for setting objectives in interventional studies, provides a suitable framework for outlining the methods in an economic evaluation study. In this framework, "P" refers to either patients or population intervention, and "I" and "C" indicate the elements under comparison. "O" represents the outcome, which varies depending on the type of economic analysis being conducted. The different types of outcomes in economic evaluation studies have been detailed in the preceding chapter.

Methods

Perspective

A unique aspect of economic evaluation studies is considering the "perspective" from which the analysis is conducted. This is a key detail to include in the protocol. Perspective, indicates whose viewpoint the study represents and can be explained using the concept of the four Ps. These include Patient, Provider, Payer and Population.

The first "P" stands for the patient's viewpoint, where costs and outcomes are looked at from the perspective of individuals dealing with health conditions. This involves considering out-of-pocket expenses and other indirect costs incurred by patients related to their health condition.

The second "P" refers to the provider, which could be a hospital or healthcare facility. When a patient is treated at a hospital, various costs come into play, such as salaries, equipment, infrastructure, and space expenses. If the study focuses on these costs, it adopts a provider perspective.

The third aspect involves the payer, typically represented by insurance companies. These entities extensively utilize economic evaluation data and employ various modeling techniques to determine the premiums that individuals need to pay. Insurance companies are particularly interested in understanding the costs incurred by hospitals or patients. Therefore, an economic evaluation can be conducted from the perspective of the payer.

The fourth element is the population, also known as the societal perspective. When adopting a societal perspective, the economic evaluation considers two or more viewpoints, which could be from the patient, provider, or payer perspective. If the study encompasses multiple perspectives, it is termed a population or societal perspective.

Time Horizon

In all economic evaluation studies, it is crucial to address the concept of a time horizon, which pertains to the duration over which outcomes and costs are calculated. The significance of the time horizon in economic evaluation lies in its impact on decisions made at a specific point in time, influencing net intervention effects and resource utilization well into the future. Therefore, in an economic evaluation, it is essential to specify the time horizon, whether it spans a few years, perhaps five or ten, or if the modeling extends over a lifetime.

The UK's National Institute for Health and Care Excellence (NICE) generally favors a lifetime horizon, but sensitivity analysis may involve testing intermediate time horizons of 5-10 years using more robust data. Employing a long-term time horizon often involves extrapolating cohort experiences into the future, assuming sustained intervention efficacy.

One of the unique aspects of economic evaluation studies is the ability to utilize modeling to predict future outcomes and costs. This predictive capability allows for decision-making based on assumptions about how events will unfold over time. From a modeling perspective, this entails projecting current health states and care costs, estimating transitions between health states, and associated outcomes and costs at various time points as specified by the time horizon of the study. Discounting future costs and health outcomes is also a common practice.

The choice of the time horizon in economic evaluations depends on factors such as the nature of the disease, the type of intervention, and the analysis's purpose. Chronic conditions requiring ongoing medical management may necessitate longer time horizons, while shorter ones may be suitable for acute conditions with less significant long-term consequences. It's crucial to maintain consistency in the time horizon for both costs and health outcomes.

Costing

The protocol for a costing study should prominently feature a crucial step: a comprehensive description of the costs involved. The four essential steps in costing necessitate careful consideration. Firstly, the costs must be identified. Following identification, the subsequent steps involve measuring the costs, assigning a value to them, and ultimately applying discounting. Each of these steps will be briefly explored.

Identification of Costs

The initial step involves the identification of costs in an economic evaluation. The costs incurred during the analysis can be categorized into direct, indirect, or intangible costs.

Direct costs are those incurred due to a direct association with disease conditions or treatments. Direct medical costs encompass expenses for medicines, investigations, hospital admissions, and any procedural costs incurred. Direct nonmedical costs include expenditures such as travel costs for each hospital visit or health checkup and cost incurred due to specific dietary requirements related to the disease.

The second category of costs is the indirect cost, which is incurred by both the patient and the caregiver and can be elucidated in terms of productivity losses. When a patient undergoes a health checkup or is admitted to a hospital, their ability to perform regular work is compromised, resulting in a loss of productivity. This encompasses both paid and unpaid work. Additionally, when a patient visits a hospital, there may be a caregiver accompanying them, incurring productivity losses. Quantifying and converting these losses into costs is imperative.

The third category consists of intangible costs, which encompass the cost of pain and the cost of suffering. Quantifying and measuring these costs is particularly challenging.

Measuring the Costs

After costs have been identified, the subsequent step involves measuring them. Various techniques can be employed for this purpose. One approach is the utilization of cost interviews, typically conducted through a questionnaire administered to either the patient or the healthcare provider. Questions may involve inquiries about travel expenses and medication costs, which can be cross-verified through prescriptions, bills, or accounts. Alternatively, examining hospital purchase department records and invoices provides additional insights. Another method is a cost diary, particularly useful for measuring indirect costs wherein patients are asked to maintain a record of different costs incurred. Time-motion studies can also be conducted to quantify costs, assigning a monetary value to them. Additionally, databases maintained by care providers, hospitals, insurance companies, or national databases offer valuable secondary data sources for measuring costs. The choice of measurement technique depends on the nature of the cost. A combination of the above methods may be employed when dealing with multiple costs. It's crucial to determine the most suitable approach for each cost type in the study. Sometimes, conducting a small survey may be necessary to identify costs specific to the study.

When crafting the protocol, it is crucial to ensure that the units in which costs are measured are explicitly stated. While comprehending costs in Indian rupees may be straightforward, if the intention is to publish the research in an international journal, conversion into US dollars may be necessary. Clearly specifying the chosen unit, whether it is Indian rupees or US dollars, is of paramount importance. Additionally, details on the conversion rate and the specific year for which the rate is applicable should be included in the protocol.

Valuing of Costs

Once costs have been identified and measured, the subsequent step involves valuing the costs. Valuing, in this context, entails estimating the worth of each resource, where value is synonymous with worth. All costs which cannot be measured directly need to be valued.

There are some points to consider while valuation of resources. The first is the decision to whether to assess the cost or consider the price. Another factor to be considered is shadow costing. Shadow costing involves assigning a cost to resources that may not have a market rate. For instance, determining the cost of the time a housewife spends caring for a child with AR requires a method of costing. A value can be assigned, even in such cases, through the utilization of shadow costing. Opportunity costs refer to the cost of the next best option that was not chosen.

Two other concepts to consider are incremental costs and marginal costs. Marginal cost is the cost of adding one additional unit of output. For instance, if you've trained ten health workers, the cost of training the 11th health worker would be considered the marginal cost—representing the cost of one additional unit of output. On the other hand, incremental cost is the cost associated with adding a new variety or expanding the product. For example, if your health worker is already skilled in the management of respiratory illnesses in children, and you decide to teach them a new skill like Kangaroo Mother Care, the cost of teaching this new skill would be an incremental cost. Incremental cost is incurred when adding a new variety or type of output. In summary, one additional unit of output is the marginal cost, while adding a new variety of outcome constitutes the incremental cost. Details of which estimation is planned for the study should be included in the protocol.

There are two commonly used approaches for valuation: the human capital approach and the frictional cost approach. In the human capital approach, the economic value to society is estimated by considering the market rate for a healthy individual of the same age and gender. This often involves calculating the salary or days of productivity lost multiplied by the average earnings per day.

On the other hand, the frictional cost approach suggests that when a disease or problem occurs, a system aims to restore it to its original productivity. The cost of productivity loss is calculated, again multiplied by the average value. To illustrate this, consider the example of valuing the time of a housewife caring for an elderly person or a child with a disability. Frictional cost could be determined by evaluating how much she would be paid for such activities if done for someone else, or alternatively, how much it would cost to hire someone for the same tasks. In an economic evaluation protocol, it is essential to specify the techniques used for valuing costs that cannot be directly measured, whether through the human capital or frictional cost method.

Discounting

Having identified, measured, and valued the costs, the subsequent step involves discounting. Discounting is necessary when dealing with chronic diseases such as diabetes and hypertension that span an extended period. When the time horizon of the study exceeds one year, discounting is incorporated into the analysis.

The rationale behind discounting lies in the recognition that costs may be incurred both presently and in the future. The value of, for example, 100 rupees today is considered more significant than the value of the same amount ten years later. Discounting involves adjusting all costs and effects to their current value, creating a level playing field for comparison. A mathematical formula is applied to calculate the discounted rate.

$$\text{Net present value} = \frac{\text{value in time}}{(1 + R)^t}$$

where
"R" represents the rate, usually ranging between three percent to five percent in most health economic evaluation studies, "t" is the number of years

While computer software can be utilized for this purpose, grasping the conceptual essence is crucial—the conversion of costs and effects occurring at different times into their present values.

Outcome Assessment

Depending on the type of economic evaluation being conducted, outcomes may either be measured or valued. In a cost-effectiveness analysis, outcomes are measured in natural units. On the other hand, in a cost-utility analysis or a cost-benefit analysis, outcomes need to be converted into utilities or monetary terms, a process referred to as valuation. Various techniques are available for valuation.

In a cost-utility analysis, outcomes require conversion into a "health utility." A utility is a value between zero and one assigned to an individual's health state. Health utility values range from 0.0 to 1.0, where 0.0 signifies death, 1.0 signifies perfect health, and negative values indicate health states worse than death. These values have clinical significance, providing a standardized metric for measuring outcomes. This allows for meaningful comparisons across different diseases and interventions. A higher utility value indicates a better quality of life.

For example, envision an individual on a typical day. If asked about their well-being, the health utility value might be seven or eight. However, if experiencing a severe migraine the utility value on that day could be two or three.

Various methods exist for measuring health utilities, including the use of specific instruments tailored for conditions like diabetes and asthma, as well as population-based instruments designed for specific age groups such as adolescence. Additionally, health utilities can be measured based on the condition or problem under consideration. Specific instruments and generic instruments, both direct and indirect, are available.

Direct methods include the use of specific preference-based measures like the Visual Analog Scale, Standard Gamble, and Time Trade-off. These measures are employed to calculate health utilities, which, when converted, contribute to the outcome in utility analysis. Indirect methods involve the use of multi-attribute health status classification questionnaires such as the Health Utility Index, EuroQol (EQ-5D-5L).

Upon obtaining a utility value, the next step is to convert it into a Quality Adjusted Life Years (QALY). One QALY, represents one year spent in perfect health. By multiplying the number of years by the utility value, you can obtain the qualities at different points in time. Subsequently, the qualities for different interventions can be calculated, facilitating a comparison to determine which intervention yielded more qualities.

Modeling

A model is essentially a simplified representation of reality, serving to depict complex scenarios which may unfold over several years with various potential outcomes. There are two main types of modeling techniques: decision tree model and Markov state transition model.

In a decision tree model, the focus is typically on acute outcomes, while a Markov's model delves into chronic outcomes. In your protocol, you must provide a description of the specific type of model being employed.

Once the model has been described, it is imperative to outline the analytics and assumptions. Projected outcomes over specific timeframes, such as 5–10 years, are inherently based on assumptions. Data for feeding into the model is obtained through a literature review, and the outcomes are contingent on these assumptions. Variations in the measure of a variable may arise from different literature sources or databases. Conducting a sensitivity analysis becomes essential in such scenarios to assess the outcomes corresponding to different levels found in literature. This involves examining the effects of varied inputs into the model. Uncertainty, once again, serves to elucidate the potential impact on the model should the situation undergo changes. In the protocol, a detailed description of the assumptions, heterogeneity and distribution effects used is essential. Furthermore, the analytics employed, such as log transformation or statistical techniques for data, should be clearly delineated. Furthermore modeling is a fascinating process conducted using computer programs. Understanding the fundamental concepts enables one to input the necessary variables into the system, utilizing the chosen software for modelling. Emphasizing the importance of accurately feeding the right input variables, which must be detailed in the protocol, is crucial.

Audience

The primary purpose of conducting an economic evaluation is decision-making. Therefore, it is imperative to specify in the protocol the individual or entity responsible for making decisions, the initiator of the study, and the intended audience. The protocol should also elucidate how engagement with the audience, ultimately making the decisions, will be facilitated.

Ensuring Quality in Research Studies

Equator Network, focuses on enhancing the quality and transparency in health research, provides valuable checklists for researchers when drafting protocols or for reviewers assessing the quality of a manuscript. Checklist for explanation and elaboration of evaluation studies (CHEERS) guidelines are specific for economic evaluations and comprises 28 items.

In conclusion, a meticulously crafted protocol ensures clarity, transparency, and quality in economic evaluations, facilitating meaningful decision-making

---

KEY POINTS

- Protocols in economic evaluations provide a structured framework ensuring ethical rigor, credibility, and transparency, which are vital for study reproducibility and integrity.
- A clear title categorizes the study type and compares interventions, while the introduction sets the research context, articulates the question, and highlights its relevance to policy and practice.
- Methods should detail the analytical perspective, time horizon, costing approach, and outcome assessment, using appropriate units, discount rates, and health utility values.
- Describe the chosen model and its inputs and assumptions, and identify the decision-makers and audience to ensure the study's findings are relevant and actionable.
- Employ quality checklists like CHEERS guidelines to uphold high standards in the economic evaluation process.

BIBLIOGRAPHY

1. Gheorghe A, Kyte D, Calvert M. The need for increased harmonisation of clinical trials and economic evaluations. Expert Rev Pharmacoecon Outcomes Res. 2014;14(2):171-3.
2. Haas M, Hall J. The Economic Evaluation of Health Care. Health Inf Manag J. 1998;28:169-72.
3. Hoomans T, Severens J. Economic evaluation of implementation strategies in health care. Implement Sci. 2014;9.
4. Lessard C. Complexity and reflexivity: Two important issues for economic evaluation in health care. Soc Sci Med. 2007;64(8):1754-65.
5. Shemilt I, Mugford M, Drummond M, Eisenstein E, Mallender J, McDaid D, Vale L, et al. Economics methods in Cochrane systematic reviews of health promotion and public health related interventions. BMC Med Res Methodol. 2006;6(55).
6. Walker S, Griffin S, Asaria M, Tsuchiya A, Sculpher M. Striving for a Societal Perspective: A Framework for Economic Evaluations When Costs and Effects Fall on Multiple Sectors and Decision Makers. Appl Health Econ Health Policy. 2019;17:577-90.

SECTION 6

Systematic Review and Meta-analysis

SECTION OUTLINE

- **Chapter 45:** Systematic Review and Meta-analysis: Rationale
- **Chapter 46:** Writing a Good SRMA Research Question
- **Chapter 47:** Protocol Writing in Systematic Review and Meta-analysis
- **Chapter 48:** Search Strategy in Systematic Review and Meta-analysis
- **Chapter 49:** PRISMA Flowchart
- **Chapter 50:** Data Extraction
- **Chapter 51:** Introduction to RevMan in Systematic Review and Meta-analysis
- **Chapter 52:** Choosing the Measures of Effect in Systematic Review and Meta-analysis
- **Chapter 53:** Principles of Meta-analysis in Systematic Review and Meta-analysis
- **Chapter 54:** Risk of Bias Assessment for Systematic Reviews
- **Chapter 55:** The GRADE Tool for Rating Certainty in Evidence and Recommendations

CHAPTER 45

Systematic Review and Meta-analysis: Rationale

Pankaj Bharadwaj, Sourav Basu, Ashwini Lonimath

"Half of what you'll learn in medical school will be shown to be either dead wrong or out of date within five years of your graduation; the trouble is that nobody can tell you which half – so the most important thing to learn is how to learn on your own." —David Sackett

INTRODUCTION

With the volume of research literature growing at an ever-increasing rate, it is impossible for individual decision makers to assess this vast quantity of primary research to enable them to make the most appropriate healthcare decisions that do rather than do any harm. Studies are of varying quality and their findings are often conflicting. Some studies have been too small and their results too imprecise to be useful in real life.

The current era of medicine is called as "evidence based medicine (EBM)." Goal of EBM is to solidify scientific foundations and to reduce medical uncertainties in clinical decision making. It seeks to discover best course of care for the patient and integrates clinical experience and patient values with the best available research information. It is a movement which aims to increase the use of high-quality clinical research in clinical decision making. It "converts the abstract exercise of reading and appraising the literature into the pragmatic process of using the literature to benefit individual patients while simultaneously expanding the clinician's knowledge base."

One of the greatest achievements of evidence-based medicine has been the development of systematic reviews and meta-analyses, methods by which researchers identify multiple studies on a topic, separate the best ones and then critically analyze them to come up with a summary of the best available evidence.

Systematic reviews address a need for health decision makers like clinicians, researchers and public health professionals to be able to access high quality, relevant, accessible, and up-to-date information to take informed decisions. They aim to minimize bias using prespecified research questions and methods that are documented in protocols and by basing their findings on reliable research.

These are to be conducted by a team that includes domain expertise and methodological expertise, who are free of potential conflicts of interest. People who might make—or be affected by—decisions around the use of interventions should be involved in important decisions about the review. Good data management, project management and quality assurance mechanisms are essential for the completion of a successful systematic review.

However, SRMA comes with certain challenges and weaknesses. Reviews are of different types, like literature/narrative/critical review. These are based on prior beliefs, often not replicable or updated which might lead to missing small but important findings. When different reviewers reach different conclusions times the heterogeneity is not addressed.

Systematic Review

It is a review that is conducted according in clearly stated, scientific research methods, and is designed to minimize biases and errors inherent to traditional, narrative reviews.

It collates all empirical evidence that fits prespecified eligibility criteria to answer a specific research question. It clearly states objectives with predefined eligibility criteria for studies and has explicit, reproducible methodology. It is a systematic search that attempts to identify all studies and assessment of the validity of the findings of the included studies (e.g., risk of bias). It involves systematic presentation, and synthesis, of the characteristics and findings of the included studies and minimizes bias.

A systematic review is a more scientific method of summarizing literature because specific protocols are used to determine which studies will be included in the review.

Traits of a good Systematic Review (Fig. 1)

* It starts with a specific question.
* Includes thorough literature search.
* Refining the search by applying predetermined inclusion and exclusion criteria.
* Extracts the appropriate data.
* Assesses their quality and validity.
* Synthesizes, interprets, and reports data.

Significance of Systematic Reviews

Systematic reviews should be undertaken by a team. Working as a team not only spreads the effort but ensures that tasks such as the selection of studies for eligibility, data extraction and rating the certainty of the evidence will be performed by at least two people independently, minimizing the likelihood of errors. Review teams must include expertise in the topic area under review.

It can be original Research, a part of Post Graduate Thesis, future research agenda for securing funding. It will establish clinical, or cost effectiveness & provides best evidence to clinical intervention and policy decision.

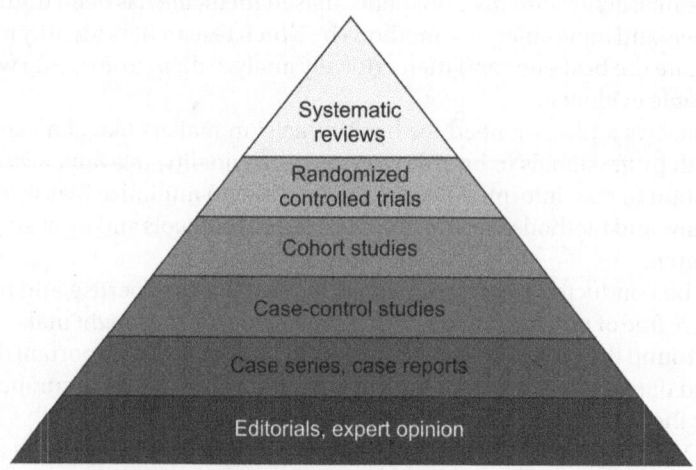

Fig. 1: Hierarchy of evidence.

Benefits of Systematic Review

Save Readers Time

They are an efficient way of bringing together a whole body of research to answer a specific question. This saves readers time and expertise required to locate and appraise research, as well as interpret results.

Provide Reliable Evidence

They present a more reliable picture of the available evidence than any single study, which may or may not have found similar results to other studies on the same question. They aim to present an unbiased, comprehensive picture of all the available evidence, which can then be used to support decisions in healthcare.

Resolve Inconsistencies

They can resolve inconsistencies in practice caused when single studies produce conflicting results.

Identify Gaps

They highlight areas where there is not enough evidence and can identify gaps in knowledge which can be used to guide future research efforts.

Meta-analysis

Meta-analysis is the use of statistical methods to summarize the results of independent studies. It is a statistical technique for combining the results of independent, but similar, e.g., studies to obtain an overall estimate of treatment effect **(Figs. 2 and 3)**. While all meta-analyses are based on systematic review of literature, not all systematic reviews necessarily include meta-analysis. For performing a meta-analysis, a statistician or an epidemiologist should be part of team during all phases of the study.

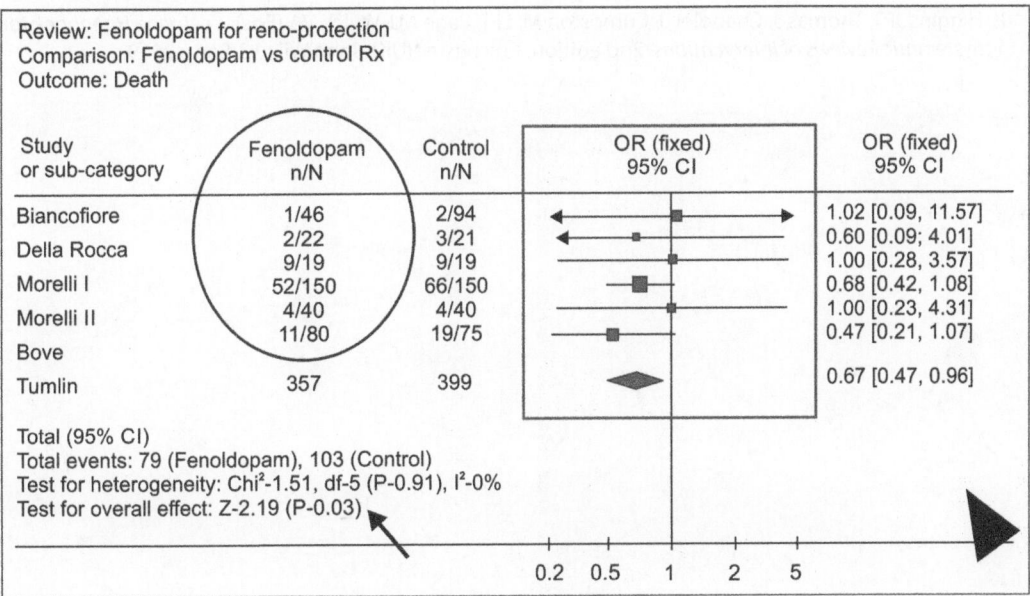

Fig. 2: Forrest plot.

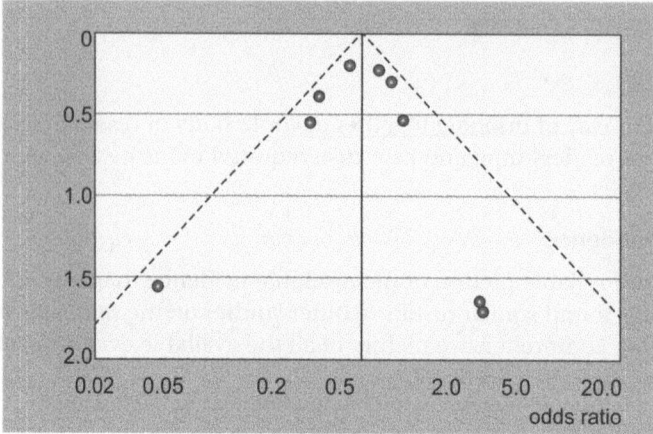

Fig. 3: Funnel plot.

KEY POINTS

- Evidence-based medicine combines the best research with clinical expertise and patient values to make healthcare decisions.
- Systematic reviews are detailed studies that gather and analyze all relevant research to provide clear, unbiased health information.
- Effective reviews are well-planned, thoroughly researched, and carefully analyze data to ensure accurate health advice.
- Meta-analysis are techniques which pools data from several studies to give a more precise understanding of treatment effects.

BIBLIOGRAPHY

1. Higgins JPT, Thomas J, Chandler J, Cumpston M, Li T, Page MJ, Welch VA (Eds). *Cochrane Handbook for Systematic Reviews of Interventions*. 2nd edition. Chichester (UK): John Wiley & Sons; 2019.

Writing a Good SRMA Research Question

Sourav Basu, Ashwini Lonimath, Pankaj Bharadwaj

> *"A well-posed question is the half of knowledge."* —Charles P. Kettering

INTRODUCTION

In systematic reviews and meta-analyses, formulating a clear, focused, and relevant research question is a foundational step that guides the entire review process. The question directs the identification, selection, and synthesis of evidence to answer a specific research inquiry. A well-articulated research question is crucial as it sets the scope and objectives of the review, facilitating a structured and systematic approach to gathering and analyzing data.

Step: Choosing a Research Question?

"A well-developed and answerable question is the foundation for any systematic review". The most useful reviews are those, that change clinical practice (or confirm value of current practice), those that provide evidence on interventions to improve public health.

Formulating the Question

There are Four basic components that must be incorporated in the research question (PICO).
1. P - Specification of type of person (patients with a specific disease condition, high-risk population such as pregnant women or the elderly).
2. I - Types of exposure (risk factor, prognostic factor, intervention, diagnostic test).
3. C - Definition of control groups.
4. O - Specifications of outcomes

An example of a poorly formulated question:
Are anticoagulant agents (type of exposure) useful in patients who have had a stroke (type of person)?

An example of a well-formulated question:
- Do anticoagulant agents (type of exposure) Improve outcomes (outcomes) in patients with acute ischemic stroke (type of person) compared with no treatment (type of control)?
- **Type of exposure**—(anticoagulant agents) unfractionated heparin, low molecular weight heparin, heparinoids, oral anticoagulants.
- **Outcomes**—Death, disability, major hemorrhage, recurrent stroke, DVT.
- **Type of person**—(acute ischemic stroke) clinical diagnosis +/- CT, age, sex, severity, outpatient/inpatient, those within 48 hours of stroke onset.
- **Type of control**—No anticoagulation
- **Type of study**—RCT, other designs.

Some More Examples

1. What is the prevalence of metabolic syndrome among the adult population in India?
2. Are children with Type 1 diabetes who have insulin injections at decreased risk for diabetic ketoacidosis compared with those who use an insulin pump?
3. What is the effect of flax seed oil consumption on blood pressure among patients with metabolic syndrome and related disorders?
4. Can menstrual cup be a better alternative in menstrual hygiene management compared to existing methods amongst adolescent girls in rural India?

Other Question Frameworks

The PEO question Framework

It is useful for qualitative research topics. PEO questions identify three concepts: population, exposure, and outcome **(Table 1)**.

Research Question: *What challenges with breastfeeding are experienced by mothers with postnatal depression?*

Table 1: PEO framework.

Element	Definition	Example
Population	Who is my question focused on?	Mothers
Exposure	What is the issue I am interested in?	Postnatal depression
Outcome	What, in relation to the issue, do I want to examine?	Challenges with breastfeeding

The SPIDER Question Framework

It is useful for qualitative or mixed methods research topics focused on "samples" rather than populations. SPIDER questions identify five concepts: sample, phenomenon of interest, design, evaluation, and research type **(Table 2)**.

Research question: *What are the experiences of recently diagnosed patients with diabetes mellitus in attendance of diabetes related health education classes?*

The ECLIPSE Framework

It is useful for qualitative research topics investigating the outcomes of a policy or service. ECLIPSE questions identify six concepts: expectation, client group, location, impact, professionals, and service **(Table 3)**.

Table 2: SPIDER framework.

Element	Definition	Example
Sample	Who is the group of people being studied?	Recently diagnosed patients with Diabetes Mellitus
Phenomenon on interest	What are the reasons for behavior and decisions?	Attendance at Diabetes health education classes
Design	How has the research been collected (e.g., interview and survey)?	Interviews
Evaluation	What is the outcome being impacted?	Experiences
Research type	What type of research (qualitative or mixed methods)?	Qualitative studies

Table 3: ECLIPSE framework.

Element	Definition	Example
Expectation	What are you looking to improve or change? What is the information going to be used for?	To increase access to peer education programs
Client group	Who is the service or policy aimed at?	Patients with hypertension
Location	Where is the service or policy located?	Primary healthcare settings
Impact	What is the change in service or policy that the researcher is investigating?	Clients have access to a peer education program
Professionals	Who is involved in providing or improving the service or policy?	Nursing and medical professionals
Service	What kind of service or policy is this?	Provision of a peer education program

Research Question: *How can I increase access to peer education programs for patients with hypertension in primary healthcare settings?*

KEY POINTS

- A good research question is crucial in studies because it defines the study's focus and how to collect and analyze data. It should be clear and direct to make a significant impact.
- A research question should include four key parts: the population studied, the intervention or factor being examined, the comparison group, and the outcomes expected. This makes the question precise and useful.
- Different types of research need different question structures. PICO is for quantitative studies, PEO for qualitative research, SPIDER for detailed sample studies, and ECLIPSE for evaluating policies or services. Each structure helps make the research question clear and relevant.

BIBLIOGRAPHY

1. Brannon PM, Taylor CL, Coates PM. Use and applications of systematic reviews in public health nutrition. Annu Rev Nutr. 2014;34:401-19. doi: 10.1146/annurev-nutr-080508-141240.
2. Chung KC, Burns PB, Kim HM. Clinical Perspective: A Practical Guide to Meta-Analysis. J Hand Surg [Am]. 2006;31A(10):1671.
3. Creating PRISMA Compliant Flow Diagrams. YouTube [Internet]. 2021 Aug 16; [cited 2023 Dec 25]. Available from: https://www.youtube.com/watch?v=IySomccfnFE.
4. Duke University Medical Center Library. Asking the Clinical Question: A Key Step in Evidence-Based Practice [Internet]. Durham (NC): Duke University Medical Center; [cited 2023 Dec 25]. Available from: https://guides.mclibrary.duke.edu/sysreview/question and https://libguides.uky.edu/ld.php?content_id=48868183.
5. Higgins JPT, Thomas J, Chandler J, Cumpston M, Li T, Page MJ, Welch VA (Eds). Cochrane Handbook for Systematic Reviews of Interventions version 6.4 (updated August 2023). Cochrane; 2023. Available from: www.training.cochrane.org/handbook.
6. Margaliot Z, Chung KC. Systematic Reviews: A Primer for Plastic Surgery Research. PRS J. 2007;120(7):1840.
7. Page MJ, Moher D, Bossuyt PM, Boutron I, Hoffmann TC, Mulrow CD, McKenzie JE. PRISMA 2020 explanation and elaboration: updated guidance and exemplars for reporting systematic reviews. BMJ. 2021;372.
8. PRISMA 2020: updated guidelines for reporting systematic reviews and meta-analyses. YouTube [cited 2023 Dec 25]. Available from: https://www.youtube.com/watch?v=Y-fu00PSm9o.
9. PRISMA Statement. PRISMA 2020 expanded checklist [Internet]. [cited 2023 Dec 25]. Available from: http://www.prisma-statement.org/documents/PRISMA_2020_expanded_checklist.pdf.
10. PRISMA Statement. PRISMA Flow Diagram [Internet]. [cited 2023 Dec 25]. Available from: http://www.prisma-statement.org/PRISMAStatement/FlowDiagram?AspxAutoDetectCookieSupport=1.

CHAPTER 47

Protocol Writing in Systematic Review and Meta-analysis

Manoj Kumar Gupta, Dewesh Kumar, Suthanthira Kannan

> *"Protocol writing in systematic reviews and meta-analyses is akin to laying the blueprint for a house. It necessitates meticulous planning and foresight, ensuring that every analysis conducted is objective, transparent, and replicable, thereby paving the way for robust conclusions and impactful insights."*

BACKGROUND

The task of conducting a systematic review and meta-analysis involves a complex and rigorous process to compile and analyze data from multiple studies to arrive at a consolidated scientific understanding. Before embarking on this journey, it is essential to create a detailed protocol that serves as a roadmap for the review. This protocol establishes a pre-defined plan for the systematic review, reducing bias and enhancing the reliability and validity of the findings. In health research, the importance of such protocol writing cannot be overstated, given the necessity for accuracy and precision in data interpretation that can potentially affect clinical decisions and public health policies.

The elements of a systematic review protocol should be clearly defined in line with the preferred reporting items for systematic reviews and meta-analyses protocol (PRISMA-P) guidelines. A well-written protocol should include an introduction, objectives, eligibility criteria, information sources, search strategy, study selection, data extraction, quality assessment, data synthesis, and a plan for assessing the risk of bias.

Introduction

This section should provide the background of the study, outlining the context and significance of the research topic. The research question should be specific, relevant, and framed according to the population, intervention, comparison, outcome, and study (PICOS) design. For instance, a protocol for a systematic review on diabetes management might explore: *"What is the effectiveness of lifestyle interventions compared to medication in managing type 2 diabetes in adults?"*

Objectives

This section should clearly state the purpose of the review. For instance, the objective could be *"to assess the effectiveness of lifestyle interventions compared to medication in managing type 2 diabetes in adults."*

Eligibility Criteria

This section outlines the inclusion and exclusion criteria for studies to be considered in the review. These could include aspects like study design, participants' characteristics, type of intervention, outcome measures and language of publication.

Information Sources and Search Strategy

Here, the databases and other sources to be searched should be identified, such as PubMed, Cochrane Library, Web of Science, etc. The search strategy should include the keywords and Medical Subject Headings (MeSH) terms to be used. For our diabetes example, MeSH terms might include "Diabetes Mellitus, Type 2", "Life Style", "Drug Therapy", etc.

Study Selection

This section outlines the process for selecting studies from the search results. Typically, this includes initial screening of titles and abstracts, followed by full-text reviews. Any disagreements would be resolved by consensus or by a third reviewer.

Data Extraction

Here, the process for extracting necessary data from the selected studies is defined. Data items could include study characteristics, participant details, intervention and comparator details, and outcome measures.

Quality Assessment

The quality of the studies to be included in the review will be assessed using appropriate tools like the Cochrane Risk of Bias tool for randomized trials or the Newcastle-Ottawa Scale for observational studies.

Data Synthesis

This section explains the process for synthesizing the data extracted from studies. For a meta-analysis, this would involve statistical methods for pooling results from different studies. Heterogeneity will also need to be assessed using I^2 statistics.

Risk of Bias Assessment

Lastly, the protocol should also outline how the risk of bias in the included studies will be assessed. Tools like the Cochrane Risk of Bias Tool or the Risk of Bias in Non-randomized Studies - of Interventions (ROBINS-I) can be used.

The development and registration of the systematic review protocol is a crucial first step to ensure transparency and rigor in health research. This step-wise, methodical approach allows for the objective evaluation of evidence, making it a powerful tool in the evidence-based medicine toolkit.

Here are a few examples to illustrate how risk of bias assessment is performed in actual systematic reviews and meta-analyses.

Example 1: Assessment in a Drug Efficacy Study

A systematic review investigating the efficacy of a particular drug might utilize the Cochrane Risk of Bias tool to assess the included randomized controlled trials (RCTs). The assessment might reveal that some studies didn't adequately blind participants, thereby introducing a risk of performance bias.

Example 2: Assessment in a Dietary Intervention Study
A meta-analysis exploring the effects of a dietary intervention on cardiovascular outcomes could employ the ROBINS-I tool to assess nonrandomized studies. The assessment might find a high risk of bias due to confounding, as some studies did not adequately control for other dietary factors that could influence cardiovascular health.

Example 3: Assessment in a Surgical Intervention Study
A systematic review examining the outcomes of a surgical intervention may use the Newcastle-Ottawa Scale to assess the risk of bias in cohort studies. The assessment might show a low risk of bias in the selection and comparability of cohorts, but a high risk of bias in the assessment of outcomes due to lack of blinding.

Example 4: Assessment in a Psychological Therapy Study
A meta-analysis studying the impact of psychological therapies on depression might use the GRADE approach to assess the overall quality of evidence. The assessment might reveal inconsistency across studies due to varying levels of treatment fidelity and adherence.

KEY POINTS

- Creating a detailed plan before starting a systematic review or meta-analysis is essential for a reliable and unbiased study, especially in health research.
- A good plan follows a set structure, like PRISMA-P guidelines, outlining everything from the research question to how data will be analyzed, ensuring a thorough and systematic review.
- Evaluating the risk of bias in studies is crucial to ensure the review's findings are trustworthy and based on high-quality data.

BIBLIOGRAPHY

1. Higgins JP, Thompson SG, Deeks JJ, Altman DG. Measuring inconsistency in meta-analyses. BMJ. 2003;327(7414):557-60. doi: 10.1136/bmj.327.7414.557.
2. Higgins JPT, Green S (Eds). Cochrane Handbook for Systematic Reviews of Interventions Version 5.1.0 [updated March 2011]. The Cochrane Collaboration, 2011. Available from www.handbook.cochrane.org.
3. Liberati A, Altman DG, Tetzlaff J, et al. The PRISMA statement for reporting systematic reviews and meta-analyses of studies that evaluate health care interventions: Explanation and elaboration. J Clin Epidemiol. 2009;62(10):e1-e34. doi:10.1016/j.jclinepi.2009.06.006
4. Moher D, Shamseer L, Clarke M, et al. Preferred reporting items for systematic review and meta-analysis protocols (PRISMA-P) 2015 statement. Systematic Reviews. 2015;4(1):1. doi:10.1186/2046-4053-4-1
5. O'Connor D, Green S, Higgins JP. Defining the review question and developing criteria for including studies. Cochrane Handbook for Systematic Reviews of Interventions. 2008;5(1):81-94.
6. Sterne JA, Hernán MA, Reeves BC, et al. ROBINS-I: A tool for assessing risk of bias in non-randomised studies of interventions. BMJ. 2016;355:i4919. doi:10.1136/bmj.i4919
7. Wells GA, Shea B, O'Connell D, et al. The Newcastle-Ottawa Scale (NOS) for assessing the quality of nonrandomised studies in meta-analyses. Ottawa Hospital Research Institute. http://www.ohri.ca/programs/clinical_epidemiology/oxford.asp

CHAPTER 48

Search Strategy in Systematic Review and Meta-analysis

Akhil Dhanesh Goel, Medha Mathur, Suthanthira Kannan

> *"We can't find any answers without first living the questions."*   Rainer Maria Rilke

INTRODUCTION

A systematic review and meta-analysis involve a meticulous approach to identifying, selecting and critically appraising relevant research while collecting and analyzing data from the studies included in the review. The search strategy is pivotal to this process, ensuring that all relevant studies are captured, thus enabling a comprehensive synthesis of evidence.

Meaning of Search Strategy

The search strategy within the context of systematic reviews and meta-analyses refers to the systematic method of locating pertinent studies from databases and other resources to be included in the review.

The Significance of Search Strategy

The importance of an accurate search strategy cannot be understated. It helps ensure the inclusion of all relevant studies, thereby minimizing bias and provides a complete and robust examination of the available evidence.

Developing a Search Strategy

Key Concept Identification

The initial phase involves forming the research question using the Population, Intervention, Comparison, Outcome (PICO) structure.

Using the research question, "How effective is cognitive behavioral therapy (CBT) for depression treatment?" as an example, the PICO could be:
- **Population:** Patients diagnosed with depression.
- **Intervention:** Cognitive behavioral therapy.
- **Comparison:** Conventional treatment or absence of treatment.
- **Outcome:** Reduction in symptoms of depression.

Identifying Keywords and Search Terms

Following this, the identification of relevant keywords and search terms linked to the key concepts is necessary. For the example given, potential keywords might include 'depression', 'cognitive behavioral therapy', 'treatment', 'effectiveness', among others.

Selecting Databases and Other Sources

The appropriate databases and resources for searching need to be chosen. The choice could range from PubMed, Cochrane Library, PsycINFO, to Embase. Manual searching in specific journals and scrutinizing reference lists from identified studies may also be required.

Conducting the Search

The identified keywords and search terms are then used in executing the search. Boolean operators like AND, OR, NOT are often utilized to enhance the search process. For example, the search string could be constructed as: (Depression AND "cognitive behavioral therapy" AND treatment AND effectiveness).

Recording the Search

This phase involves the documentation of the used databases, search terms, the number of located records, and reasons for excluding certain studies.

Selection of Studies and Data Collection

Once the relevant studies have been identified, they need to be screened for relevance, and pertinent data are collected for the review. This selection process usually involves an initial scan of the titles and abstracts, followed by an in-depth review of the full texts. The collected data often encompass study characteristics, population data, interventions, outcomes, and results.

Evaluating Study Quality

The quality of the included studies is then evaluated using specific tools, such as the Cochrane Risk of Bias tool for randomized controlled trial or the Newcastle-Ottawa Scale for observational studies.

Data Synthesis and Analysis

The final step encompasses the synthesis of the collected data and the execution of the meta-analysis if it is applicable. The synthesis of data could involve a narrative synthesis or a quantitative synthesis (meta-analysis) if the studies are sufficiently homogeneous.

Example 1: Investigating the efficacy of a drug treatment for diabetes
- **Keywords and phrases:** Initial keyword and phrase identification might include "Diabetes Mellitus," "Drug Treatment," "Metformin," "Glycemic Control," etc.
- **Database selection:** Utilize databases like PubMed, Scopus, and Web of Science for a broad coverage of medical literature.
- **Boolean operators:** Employ Boolean operators to refine the search, e.g., ("Diabetes Mellitus" AND "Drug Treatment" AND "Metformin").
- **Filters and limits:** Apply filters such as publication date (e.g., published in the last 10 years), language (e.g., English), and study type (e.g., randomized controlled trials).
- **Manual searching:** Manually search the reference lists of identified articles for additional relevant studies.

Example 2: Examining the impact of physical activity on cardiovascular health
- **Keywords and phrases:** Initial keywords and phrases might include "Physical Activity," "Exercise," "Cardiovascular Diseases," "Heart Health," etc.
- **Database selection:** Utilize databases like PubMed, Cochrane Library, and CINAHL to access a broad spectrum of health-related literature.
- **Boolean operators:** Use Boolean operators to combine terms, e.g., ("Physical Activity" OR "Exercise") AND ("Cardiovascular Diseases" OR "Heart Health").
- **Filters and limits:** Apply filters such as age group (e.g., adults), publication type (e.g., peer-reviewed articles), and publication date (e.g., published in the last 5 years).
- **Snowball searching:** Check the cited references in the included studies to identify other potentially relevant studies.

KEY POINTS
- The process of systematic review and meta-analysis is cyclical, with each step in continuum with the next.
- It necessitates careful planning and execution to guarantee the accuracy of the review's findings.

BIBLIOGRAPHY
1. Higgins JPT, Thomas J. "Co-ordinating editor's perspective on PICO". Cochrane Database Syst Rev. 2020.
2. Page MJ, McKenzie JE, Bossuyt PM, Boutron I, Hoffmann TC, Mulrow CD, et al. "The PRISMA 2020 statement: An updated guideline for reporting systematic reviews." BMJ. 2021.
3. Moher D, Liberati A, Tetzlaff J, Altman DG. "Preferred reporting items for systematic reviews and meta-analyses: The PRISMA Statement." PLoS Med. 2009.

CHAPTER 49

PRISMA Flowchart

Padmavathi S, Suthanthira Kannan, Akhil Dhanesh Goel, Sourav Basu

"Searching for answers is not merely about finding them but about learning and growing along the way. It's in the pursuit that wisdom lies, not just the conclusions."

INTRODUCTION

A transparent, complete, and accurate account of why the systematic review (SR) was done, what the authors did (such as how studies were identified and selected) and what they found (such as characteristics of contributing studies and results of meta-analyses) is necessary. It ensures a SR is valuable to users such as patients, healthcare providers, researchers, and policy makers. Transparent reporting enables others to replicate the methods used in the review, which can facilitate attempts to verify or reproduce the results. Efforts to standardize and improve the reporting of systematic reviews resulted in the publication of the PRISMA statement (2009) with its accompanying explanation and elaboration document.

SRMA Reporting: Transparent?

Page and colleagues evaluated epidemiological and reporting characteristics of a random sample of 300 systematic reviews of biomedical research indexed in MEDLINE in February 2014. They found that in at least a third of the reviews there was no information on eligible publication types, the years of coverage of the search, the methods used to collect data and appraise studies or the funding source of the review. Out of 300, 87 (29%) SRs reported using a reporting guideline (e.g., PRISMA, MOOSE). The purpose of these guidelines was frequently misinterpreted; in 45/87(52%) of these SRs, it was stated that the reporting guideline were used to guide the conduct and not the reporting of the SR.

PRISMA

Preferred reporting items for systematic reviews and meta-analyses (PRISMA) is a protocol for conducting and reporting systematic reviews and meta-analyses. It is a valuable tool to ensure transparency, completeness, and clarity in systematic reviews and meta-analyses. The PRISMA 2020 update is a considerably expanded version of the original (2009); it includes standards and examples for the 27 original and 13 additional reporting items that capture methodological advances and may enhance the replicability of reviews. This article will discuss the significance of the PRISMA, its components, and how to construct and use one for systematic reviews and meta-analyses.

Systematic Reviews and the role of PRISMA

PRISMA, since its inception in 2009, was designed to help authors to prepare coherent transparent accounts of their SRs and its recommendations, organize and standardize the reporting of the SRs.

The latest PRISMA 2020 was designed especially for SRs of studies evaluating Health Interventions. However, the checklist items are equally applicable to social or educational interventions as well.

PRISMA: A Brief Summary

The Preferred Reporting Items for Systematic Reviews and Meta-Analyses (PRISMA) was published in 2009. It is an evidence-based, minimum set of items, for reporting in systematic reviews (SR) and meta-analyses (MA) and aims to "facilitate transparent and complete reporting of SRs". The latest update is the PRISMA 2020. It has 7 sections, and 27 items, as distributed in the adjacent **Table1**. Some items have sub-items **(Fig. 1)**.

Table 1: PRISMA checklist components.

Section	No. items
Title	1
Abstract	1
Introduction	2
Methods	11
Results	7
Discussion	1
Other information	4

Learning About Prisma

Guidance material is available in the form of open-access articles, video tutorials, guidance manuals, tools for assessing SRs and exploring the PRISMA checklist and the expanded PRISMA checklist. Resources for deconstructing your SR, item by item, from the PRISMA checklist and reading statement papers about each aspect of your SR. Using

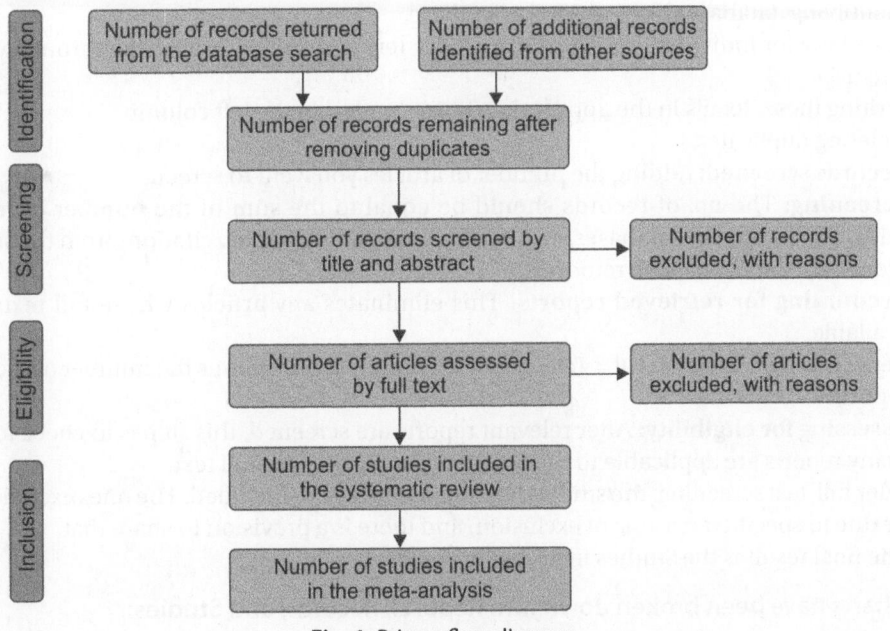

Fig. 1: Prisma flow diagram.

relevant PRISMA extensions, which facilitate reporting of different aspects of SRs, such as: individual patient data, scoping reviews, PRISMA flowchart templates or creating your own flowchart.

PRISMA Flowcharts

The PRISMA flowcharts **(Flowchart 1)** are simple 'box and arrow' based flowcharts that visualize the checklist into a clean and rapidly digestible format.

There are inputs, outputs, and edges or arrows indicating the flow of information. Boxes or 'nodes' contain brief summaries of the numbers of records included, excluded at each stage.

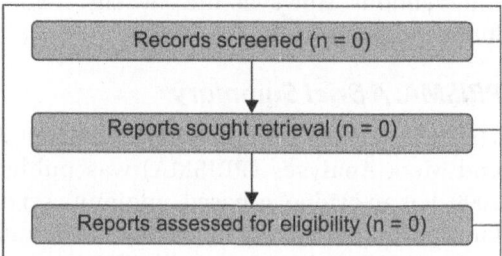

Flowchart 1: PRISMA flow charts.

The flowchart is divided into three stages:
1. **Identification:** To identify which records have been included in the database, accounting for any duplicates, sources of the records, if available
2. **Screening:** The records incorporated into the database are then screened for eligibility, and whether their reports have been retrieved or not.
3. **Result (included):** The final stage is filtering the reports which have been included as studies for the SR after their identification and screening.

*n indicates the number of records/reports/studies, depending upon the SR and the respective stage of the chart.

Understanding the Steps to Create a PRISMA Flowchart (Fig. 1)

1. Choosing the template or format of the flowchart maker.
2. Identifying databases like PubMed or embase.
3. Searching for individual records through key terms, abstract, or filtering through year or language.
4. Writing these details in the appropriate boxes 'nodes' in the left column
5. Deleting duplicates.
6. **Records screened:** Adding the number of articles you want to screen.
7. **Screening:** The no. of records should be equal to the sum of the number of records initially identified in databases, and if there are any overlapping citations from the sources identified, they should be removed.
8. **Accounting for retrieved reports:** This eliminates any articles whose full text is not available.
9. Reports sought for retrieval = Total no. of Screened records minus the number of excluded reports.
10. **Assessing for eligibility:** After relevant reports are screened, this step is to check for how many reports are applicable to the SR after screening of the full text.
11. After full-text screening, the studies become eligible to be included. The ones excluded can be due to specified reasons of exclusion, and there is a provision to share that.
12. The final result is the Studies included in the SR.

Flowcharts have been broken down into Reports, Records, and Studies:

❖ **Report:** A document (paper or electronic) supplying information about a particular study. It could be a journal article, preprint, conference abstract, study register entry, clinical study

report, dissertation, unpublished manuscript, government report or any other document providing relevant information.
- **Record:** The title or abstract (or both) of a report indexed in a database or website (such as a title or abstract for an article indexed in Medline). Records that refer to the same report (such as the same journal article) are "duplicates"; however, records that refer to reports that are merely similar (such as a similar abstract submitted to two different conferences) should be considered unique.
- **Study:** An investigation such as a clinical trial, that includes a defined group of participants and one or more interventions and outcomes. A "study" might have multiple reports. For example, reports could include the protocol, statistical analysis plan, baseline characteristics, results for the primary outcome, results for harms, results for secondary outcome, and results for additional mediator and moderator analyses.

Using the Flowchart

Two user-friendly ways of creating comprehensive and aesthetically organized flowcharts are:
1. Using one of the 4 existing templates available on the PRISMA website, as per the type of searches and sources used
2. Using the evidence synthesis hackathon (ESH) online PRISMA flowchart creator tool, found on the link: https://www.eshackathon.org/software/PRISMA2020.html
   - Working on the R Package on GitHub to edit and code the flowchart
   - Downloading the CSV file which contains the Microsoft Excel template
   - Working directly on the ESH website, in the tab of "Create Flow Diagram"

The PRISMA Flowchart Templates (Fig. 2)

PRISMA offers easy-to-use, user-friendly templates, accessed in .Word files.
- Clicking on the blue hyperlinks in the image at http://prisma-statement.org/PRISMAStatement/Flow Diagram downloads the templates.
- The PRISMA website has 4 available templates, depending upon the type of review and the sources:

Using Templates (Fig. 3)

The four templates provided by PRISMA can be downloaded as word attachments from the PRISMA website. These are ready to use flowcharts that can be filled with the relevant details of the three stages and based on whether the studies have been sourced from databases and registers or from other sources. The Word Template cannot 'AutoSum' or indicate any discrepancies in the numbers. Thus the author is recommended to manually double-check all information.

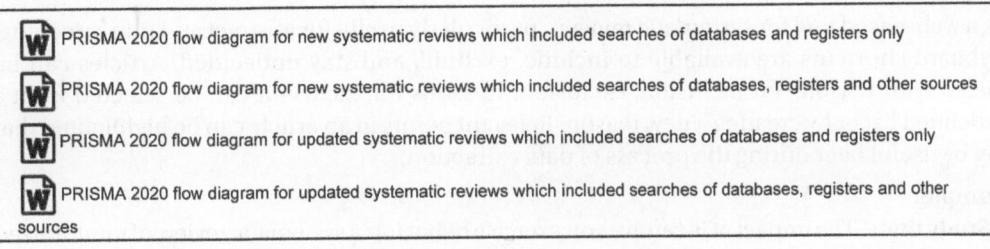

Fig. 2: PRISMA flow charts templates.

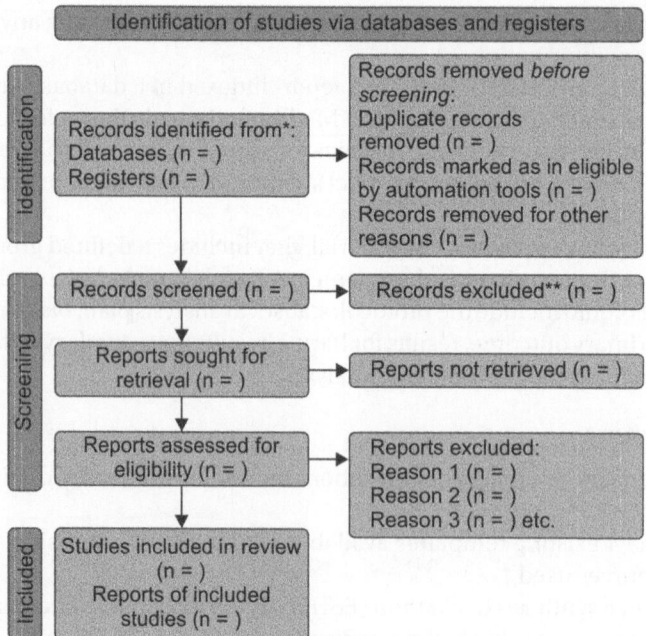

Fig. 3: Use of prisma template.

Using the GitHub R Package

The GitHub file can be accessed on: https://github.com/nealhaddaway/PRISMA2020. This method allows for greater control over the customization and aesthetics of the flowchart. It requires a proficiency in the use of the software R.

Using the .csv Template

The Excel file in a .csv extension can be downloaded from: https://estech.shinyapps.io/prisma_flowdiagram/_w_2d8fbf24/PRISMA.csv

This method also provides a template, however, building it in Microsoft Excel allows for more customization and tabulation, such as Autosum; compared to the Word templates Proficiency in the use of Excel is required.

Using the Website Tool

Probably one of the most user-friendly and simple tools to create the flowchart is the ESH. Simply click on the "Create Flow Diagram" tab and fill in the details in the left column. It also allows for downloading of the flowchart in multiple formats, like interactive HTML,. PNG,. PDF, etc.

Using Rayyan

It is a web-based tool for systematic reviews, particularly useful for abstract and title screening. Keyboard shortcuts are available to include, exclude, and stay undecided. Articles can be labeled with reasons for inclusion, exclusion. Reasons for exclusion can be selected from a predefined list or by creating a new reason. Relevant points in an article can be highlighted that may be useful later during the process of data extraction.

Example:
- **Study title:** "The impact of incentives on exercise behavior: a systematic review of randomized control trials."

- ❖ **DOI link:** https://doi.org/10.1007/s12160-013-9577-4
- ❖ **Background:** The effectiveness of reinforcing exercise behavior with material incentives is unclear.
- ❖ **Purpose:** To conduct a SR of existing research on material incentives for exercise, organized by incentive strategy.
- ❖ **Methods:** 10 studies conducted between Jan 1965 and June 2013 assessed the impact of incentivizing exercise compared to nonincentivized control.
- ❖ **Results:** There was significant heterogeneity between studies regarding reinforcement procedures and outcomes. Incentives tended to improve behavior during the intervention, whilst findings were mixed regarding sustained behavior after incentives were removed.

Example: Flowchart (Fig. 4)

- ❖ The total records identified here are: 1,873
- ❖ Additional Records: 8
- ❖ Total records after Duplicates removal: 1,492
- ❖ Records screened: 1,492
- ❖ Records excluded: 1,467
- ❖ Full-text accessed for eligibility: 27
- ❖ Full-texts excluded with reasons: 18
- ❖ Studies included in qualitative synthesis: 10
- ❖ Studies included in quantitative synthesis (meta-analysis): N.A.

Scope of the PRISMA

The PRISMA 2020 statement provides updated reporting guidance for systematic reviews that reflects advances in methods to identify, select, appraise, and synthesize studies. The PRISMA 2020 statement has been designed primarily for systematic reviews of studies that evaluate the effects of health interventions, irrespective of the design of the included studies. However, the

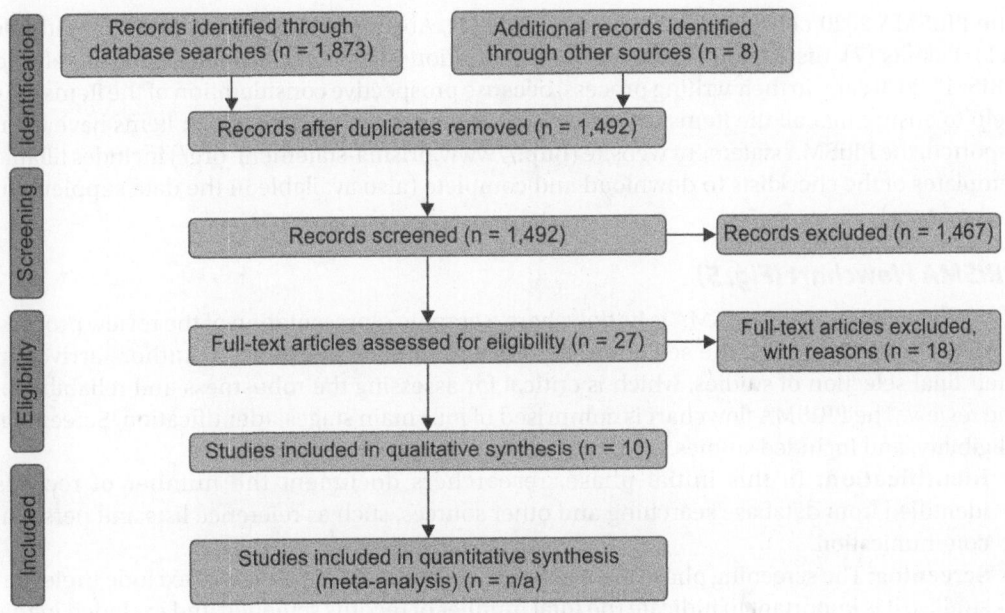

Fig. 4: Example flowchart.

Table 2: PRISMA extensions.

Acronym	PRISMA extension	Year
PRISMA-E	PRISMA for systematic reviews with a focus on health equity	2012
PRISMA for Abstracts	Reporting systematic reviews in journal and conference abstracts	2015; 2020a
PRISMA-P	PRISMA for systematic review protocols	2015
PRISMA-NMA	PRISMA for network meta-analyses	2015
PRISMA-IPD	PRISMA for individual participant data	2015
PRISMA-Harms	PRISMA for reviews including harms outcomes	2016
PRISMA-DTA	PRISMA for diagnostic test accuracy	2018
PRISMA-ScR	PRISMA for scoping reviews	2018
PRISMA-A	PRISMA for acupuncture	2019
PRISMA-S	PRISMA for reporting literature searches	2021

PRISMA 2020 checklist items are applicable to reports of systematic reviews evaluating other interventions (such as social or educational interventions), and many items are applicable to systematic reviews with objectives other than evaluating interventions (such as evaluating etiology, prevalence or prognosis). PRISMA 2020 can be used for original systematic reviews, updated systematic reviews, or continually updated ("living") systematic reviews.

PRISMA Extensions (Table 2)

Extensions to the PRISMA 2009 statement have been developed to guide reporting of network meta-analyses, meta-analyses of individual participant data, systematic reviews of harms, diagnostic test accuracy studies, and scoping reviews and protocol.

PRISMA 2020 Checklist

The PRISMA 2020 checklist has 27 items – Title (1), Abstract (1), Introduction (2), Methods (11), Results (7), discussion (1) and other information (4). We recommend authors refer to PRISMA 2020 early in their writing process, because prospective consideration of the items may help to ensure that all the items are addressed. To help keep track of which items have been reported, the PRISMA statement website (http://www.prisma-statement.org/) includes fillable templates of the checklists to download and complete (also available in the data supplement on bmj.com).

PRISMA Flowchart (Fig. 5)

A crucial component of PRISMA is its flowchart, a graphic representation of the review process. It allows readers to track the selection process and understand how the authors arrived at their final selection of studies, which is critical for assessing the robustness and reliability of the review. The PRISMA flowchart is comprised of four main stages: Identification, Screening, Eligibility, and Included studies.

- **Identification:** In this initial phase, researchers document the number of records identified from database searching and other sources, such as reference lists and personal communication.
- **Screening:** The screening phase involves reviewing titles and abstracts to exclude irrelevant studies. It is important to indicate the total number of records screened and excluded in this phase.

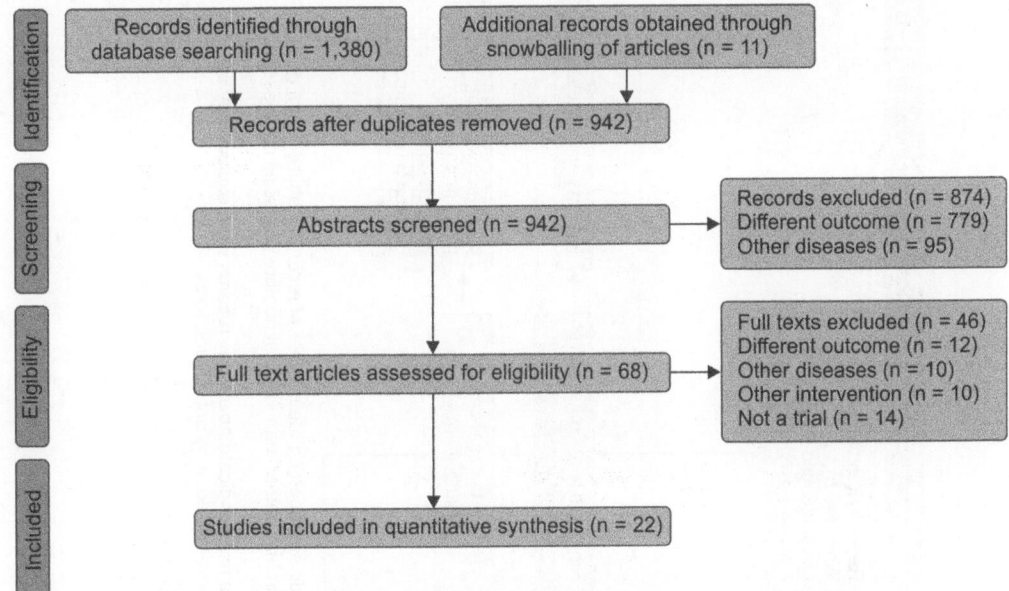

Fig. 5: Example for PRISMA flowchart.

- ❖ **Eligibility:** This step includes a thorough assessment of the full-text articles for their suitability for inclusion. Here, researchers should report the number of full-text articles assessed for eligibility and reasons for exclusions.
- ❖ **Included studies:** The final section provides the number of studies included in the qualitative synthesis (systematic review) and/or quantitative synthesis (meta-analysis).

We will provide an example of how the PRISMA flowchart might be used. Krishnamoorthy Y, et al. conducted a systematic search to find studies that compared the effectiveness of financial incentives with usual or standard care for improving any part of the HIV care continuum from the dates of database inception until July 2019. They identified a total of 1,380 citations and after removal of duplicates from multiple databases, 942 records were screened for title, abstract and keywords. They retrieved 68 relevant studies and full-text of these articles were assessed for eligibility criteria. Finally, they analyzed data from 22 studies with 38,119 participants satisfying the inclusion criteria **(Fig. 5)**.

Figure 6 depicts the new design of the PRISMA 2020 Flowchart template.

Constructing the PRISMA Flowchart

When constructing a PRISMA flowchart, researchers should accurately report the numbers associated with each phase of the study selection process. Consistency and clarity are vital in representing the process faithfully. Any exclusions must be justified and reasons for exclusion at the eligibility stage should be detailed.

Using the PRISMA Flowchart

In utilizing the PRISMA flowchart, researchers are encouraged to adhere strictly to the guidelines and report the details at each stage of the review process. It is also important to use the PRISMA flowchart in conjunction with the PRISMA checklist, which provides a detailed guide on other aspects of conducting and reporting a systematic review and meta-analysis.

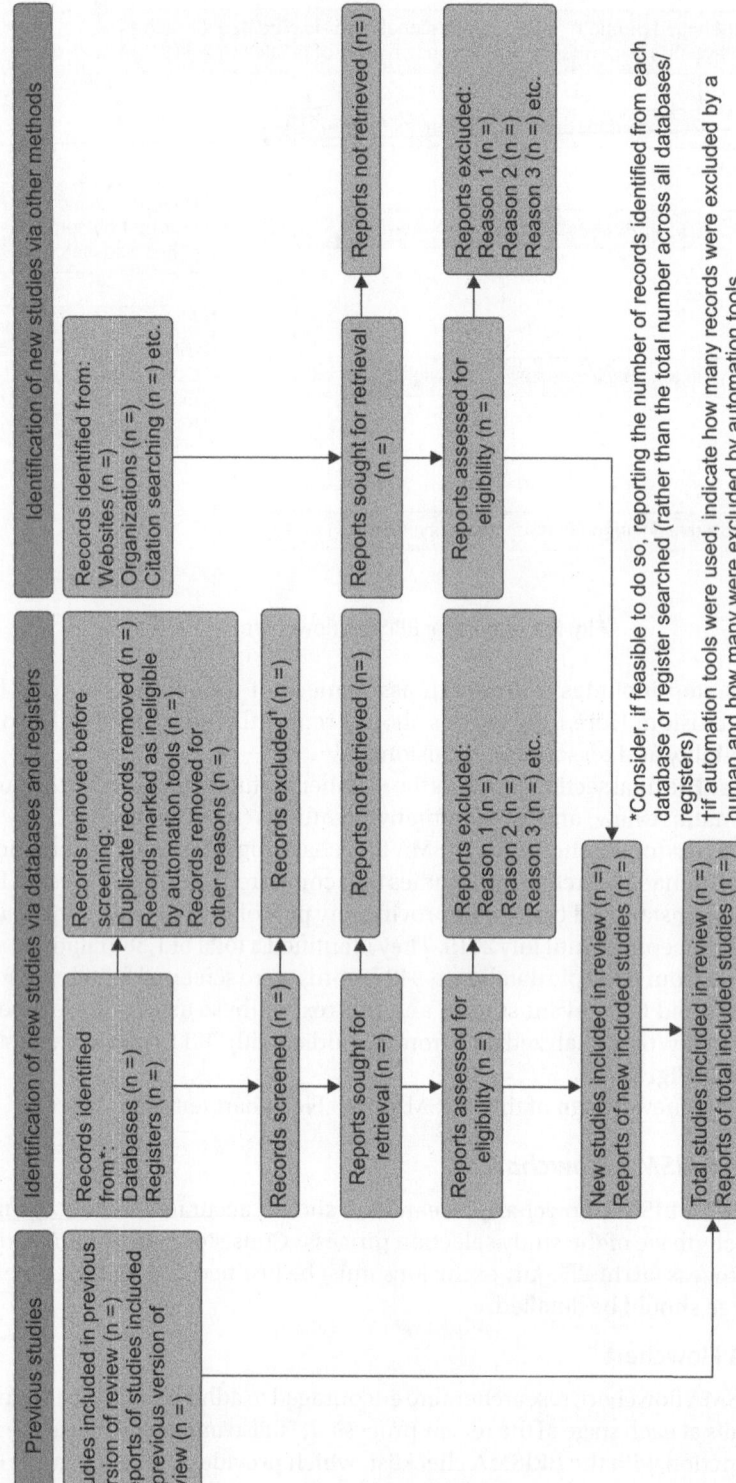

Fig. 6: PRISMA 2020 flowchart template new design.

Limitations

Reporting of many SRs remains poor despite the availability of the PRISMA statement since 2009.
- Some authors may still be unaware of PRISMA or assume that they already know how to report a SR completely.
- The extent to which journals endorse PRISMA is highly variable, with some explicitly requiring authors to submit a completed checklist at the time of manuscript submission, others only recommending its use in the instructions to authors and many not referring to it at all.
- Also, some PRISMA items include multiple elements (e.g., item 7 asks authors to describe the databases searched, whether authors were contacted to identify additional trials, the years of coverage of the databases searched, and the date of the last search). Some authors may assume that they have adequately addressed an item if they report at least one element.

PRISMA checklists evaluate how completely an element of review conduct was reported, but do not evaluate the caliber of conduct or performance of a review. Thus, review authors and readers should not think that a rigorous systematic review can be produced by simply following the PRISMA 2020 guidelines.

KEY POINTS

- By providing a clear, step-by-step pathway, PRISMA enhances transparency and facilitates a comprehensive understanding of the methodology.
- As such, it should be seen as a fundamental tool in the conduct and reporting of systematic reviews and meta-analyses.

BIBLIOGRAPHY

1. Higgins JPT, Thomas J, Chandler J, Cumpston M, Li T, Page MJ, Welch VA (editors). Cochrane Handbook for Systematic Reviews of Interventions version 6.3 (updated February 2022). Cochrane, 2022. Available from www.training.cochrane.org/handbook.
2. Kolaski K, Logan LR, Ioannidis JPA. Guidance to best tools and practices for systematic reviews. Syst Rev. 2023;12:96. https://doi.org/10.1186/s13643-023-02255-9
3. Krishnamoorthy Y, Rehman T, Sakthivel M. Effectiveness of Financial Incentives in Achieving UNAID Fast-Track 90-90-90 and 95-95-95 Target of HIV Care Continuum: A Systematic Review and Meta-Analysis of Randomized Controlled Trials. AIDS Behav. 2021;25:814-25. https://doi.org/10.1007/s10461-020-03038-2
4. Moher D, Liberati A, Tetzlaff J, Altman DG, The PRISMA Group. Preferred Reporting Items for Systematic Reviews and Meta-Analyses: The PRISMA Statement. PLoS Med. 2009;6(7):e1000097. https://doi.org/10.1371/journal.pmed.1000097
5. Page MJ, Altman DG, Shamseer L, McKenzie JE, Ahmadzai N, Wolfe D, et al. Reproducible research practices are underused in systematic reviews of biomedical interventions. J Clin Epidemiol. 2018;94:8–18.
6. Page MJ, McKenzie JE, Bossuyt PM, Boutron I, Hoffmann TC, Mulrow CD, et al. The PRISMA 2020 statement: an updated guideline for reporting systematic reviews. BMJ. 2021;372:n71. doi:10.1136/bmj.n71
7. Page MJ, Shamseer L, Altman DG, Tetzlaff J, Sampson M, Tricco AC, et al. Epidemiology and Reporting Characteristics of Systematic Reviews of Biomedical Research: A Cross-Sectional Study. PLoS Med. 2016;13(5):e1002028. doi:10.1371/journal.pmed.1002028
8. PRISMA Flow Diagram. PRISMA. Available from: http://www.prisma-statement.org/PRISMAStatement/FlowDiagram.

Data Extraction

Suthanthira Kannan, Rashmi Kundapur

> *"The important thing is not to stop questioning. Curiosity has its own reason for existing."*
> —Albert Einstein

INTRODUCTION

Data extraction is the process of identifying and collecting relevant information from each study included in a systematic review and meta-analysis. This information is used to provide a detailed summary of the characteristics of each study and to calculate the effect sizes for the meta-analysis.

The process of data extraction is critical to the validity and reliability of a systematic review and meta-analysis. If the data is extracted incorrectly or incompletely, the results of the meta-analysis may be biased or inaccurate. Therefore, it is essential to follow a standardized approach to data extraction that ensures the accuracy and completeness of the data.

We will provide a detailed overview of the process of data extraction in systematic reviews and meta-analyses. We will discuss the steps involved in data extraction, the tools and resources that can be used to facilitate the process, and the challenges and limitations of data extraction.

Steps in Data Extraction

Data extraction involves a series of steps that are designed to ensure the completeness and accuracy of the data. The steps involved in data extraction are as follows:

Step 1: Develop a Data Extraction Form

The first step in data extraction is to develop a data extraction form. This form is a template that is used to collect relevant information from each included study. The data extraction form typically includes the following sections:

- **Study characteristics:** This section includes information about the study design, sample size, study population, and setting.
- **Intervention characteristics:** This section includes information about the intervention(s) being studied, including the type of intervention, the duration of the intervention and the frequency of the intervention.
- **Outcome measures:** This section includes information about the outcome measures used in the study, including the primary and secondary outcomes, the time points at which outcomes were assessed and the statistical information about the outcomes (e.g., mean, standard deviations, effect sizes).

- **Risk of bias assessment:** This section includes an assessment of the risk of bias in each study, using a standardized tool such as the Cochrane Risk of Bias tool.

Step 2: Conduct the Data Extraction

Once the data extraction form has been developed, the next step is to extract the data from each included study. This process involves a detailed review of the full-text articles and the collection of relevant information.

Data extraction should be conducted independently by two reviewers to minimize the risk of errors and bias. Discrepancies in the extracted data should be resolved through discussion and consensus.

Step 3: Verify the Data Extraction

After the data has been extracted from each included study, it is important to verify the accuracy and completeness of the data. This involves checking that all the relevant information has been included in the data extraction form and that there are no errors or inconsistencies in the data.

Step 4: Enter the Data Into a Database

The final step in data extraction is to enter the extracted data into a database. The database is used to facilitate the analysis of the data and to generate summary statistics and effect sizes for the meta-analysis.

Several tools and resources are available to facilitate the data extraction process, including:

- **Covidence:** Covidence is an online platform that simplifies the screening, data extraction, and synthesis of studies for systematic reviews. It is a user-friendly tool that enables reviewers to manage the systematic review process in one place, facilitating collaboration among team members. Covidence also provides features such as duplicate screening, customizable forms, and real-time tracking of progress.
- **Rayyan:** Rayyan is another online tool that simplifies the screening process for systematic reviews. It enables reviewers to upload articles and manage the screening process in a collaborative environment. Rayyan has a range of features, including AI-assisted screening, full-text review, and real-time tracking of progress.
- **JBI SUMARI:** JBI System for the Unified Management, Assessment, and Review of Information (SUMARI) is a comprehensive systematic review software that facilitates the review process from protocol development to publication. It includes features such as data extraction, meta-analysis and risk of bias assessment, making it a one-stop solution for systematic review management.
- **Excel:** Excel is a widely used data extraction tool, particularly for small-scale reviews. It allows reviewers to create customized data extraction forms and store data in a spreadsheet format. While it may require more manual effort than other tools, Excel is widely accessible and allows reviewers to customize the data extraction process to their needs.
- **DistillerSR:** DistillerSR is a web-based platform that facilitates the entire systematic review process, including screening, data extraction, and synthesis. It includes advanced features such as machine learning, full-text screening, and real-time collaboration, making it a powerful tool for large-scale reviews.
- **Cochrane data extraction forms:** Cochrane collaboration provides a range of data extraction forms for different types of studies, including randomized controlled trials, observational studies and diagnostic test accuracy studies. These forms are available online

and are designed to be comprehensive and user-friendly, enabling reviewers to extract data efficiently and accurately.
- **PRISMA checklist:** The Preferred Reporting Items for Systematic Reviews and Meta-Analyses (PRISMA) checklist is a widely used tool for reporting systematic reviews and meta-analyses. It includes a checklist of 27 items that reviewers should report in their review, including the data extraction process. The PRISMA checklist serves as a useful guide for reviewers to ensure that they have reported their review comprehensively and transparently.

In conclusion, the data extraction process is crucial for systematic reviews and meta-analyses, and several tools and resources are available to facilitate this process. Choosing the right tool depends on the scale of the review, the level of customization required and the reviewer's preferences. It is essential to choose a tool that simplifies the data extraction process while ensuring accuracy and transparency.

Common Issues in Systematic Reviews and Meta-analysis

There are a number of common issues that can arise in data extraction for systematic reviews and meta-analyses. These include:
- **Incomplete or missing data:** Studies may not report all of the data that is needed for a systematic review or meta-analysis. This can make it difficult to draw accurate conclusions about the evidence.
- **Inconsistency in data reporting:** Studies may report data in different ways, making it difficult to compare results. This can be a particular problem when studies are from different countries or cultures.
- **Bias in data extraction:** The person extracting the data may introduce bias into the study if they are not careful. This can be avoided by using a standardized data extraction form and by having two people extract the data independently.

There are a number of things that can be done to overcome these issues. These include:
- **Developing a clear and comprehensive data extraction form:** The data extraction form should be developed in consultation with experts in the field and should be piloted on a small number of studies before it is used for the main study.
- **Using standardized data extraction procedures:** The data extraction procedures should be standardized as much as possible to reduce the risk of bias. This includes using a consistent approach to coding data and to resolving any discrepancies.
- **Having two people extract the data independently:** This can help to identify any errors or inconsistencies in the data extraction.
- **Using statistical methods to deal with missing data:** There are a number of statistical methods that can be used to deal with missing data. These methods should be chosen carefully to ensure that they do not introduce bias into the study.

By following these steps, it is possible to reduce the risk of errors and bias in data extraction for systematic reviews and meta-analyses

Here are some additional tips for overcoming common issues in data extraction:
- *Be clear about the purpose of the systematic review or meta-analysis:* This will help you to identify the key pieces of information that you need to extract from the studies.
- *Use a standardized data extraction form:* This will help to ensure that you extract the same information from each study.
- *Be careful not to introduce bias into the data extraction process:* This can be done by using a systematic approach and by being transparent about your methods.
- *Check the data for accuracy:* This can be done by using a second person to extract the data independently or by using statistical methods to identify errors.

Advantages of Data Extraction

- **Standardization of information**: Data extraction allows for the standardization of information collected from different studies, making it easier to compare and analyze data across a wide range of research.
- **Enhanced accuracy**: By following a structured data extraction process, researchers can minimize errors, ensuring the accuracy and reliability of the data collected.
- **Reproducibility**: Data extraction facilitates the reproducibility of the review, as it allows other researchers to follow the same procedure and compare their results.
- **Efficient synthesis**: It enables efficient synthesis of data from multiple studies, which is essential for drawing more reliable conclusions, especially in meta-analyses where quantitative synthesis is performed.
- **In-depth analysis**: Data extraction allows for an in-depth analysis by ensuring that all relevant data, including subgroup data and covariates, are meticulously collected.
- **Quality assessment**: It allows for quality assessment of the included studies, which is essential for evaluating the strength of the evidence.
- **Transparent reporting**: Data extraction promotes transparent reporting by providing a clear record of the data collected, including where it was obtained from and how it was analyzed.
- **Time-efficiency**: Although labor-intensive, a well-structured data extraction process can streamline the review process and save time in the long-term by reducing the likelihood of errors that need to be corrected later on.
- **Facilitates meta-analyses**: In meta-analyses, data extraction is crucial for obtaining the necessary statistical information needed to perform pooled analyses across studies.
- **Evidence summarization**: It enables summarization of evidence in a systematic and organized manner, which is crucial for informing policy, practice and further research.

KEY POINTS

- Data extraction in systematic reviews and meta-analyses is crucial for accuracy and reliability, involving steps from developing a form to entering data into a database.
- Tools like covidence and Excel aid this process.
- Common issues include incomplete data and bias, which can be mitigated through standardized forms and independent extraction.
- The process enhances accuracy, allows quality assessment, and facilitates efficient data synthesis for evidence-based conclusions.

BIBLIOGRAPHY

1. Cochrane Community. Cochrane data extraction templates [Internet]. [cited Year Month Day]. Available from: https://community.cochrane.org/review-production/cochrane-data-extraction-templates
2. Covidence. About Covidence [Internet]. [cited Year Month Day]. Available from: https://www.covidence.org/about
3. DistillerSR. About DistillerSR [Internet]. [cited Year Month Day]. Available from: https://www.evidencepartners.com/products/distillersr-systematic-review-software/about/
4. Moher D, Liberati A, Tetzlaff J, Altman DG, PRISMA Group. Preferred reporting items for systematic reviews and meta-analyses: The PRISMA statement. PLoS Med. 2009;6(7):e1000097. Available from: https://doi.org/10.1371/journal.pmed.1000097
5. Ouzzani M, Hammady H, Fedorowicz Z, Elmagarmid A. Rayyan: A web and mobile app for systematic reviews. Syst Rev. 2016;5(1):210. Available from: https://doi.org/10.1186/s13643-016-0384-4

Introduction to RevMan in Systematic Review and Meta-analysis

CHAPTER 51

Mahalaqua Nazli Khatib, Dhanajayan, Rashmi Kundapur

"We are drowning in information but starved for knowledge."   —John Naisbitt

INTRODUCTIN OF REVMAN

The Review Manager (RevMan) software is a widely used tool developed by the Cochrane Collaboration for conducting systematic reviews and meta-analyses. Designed to facilitate rigorous and comprehensive evaluations of healthcare interventions, the software is particularly lauded for its user-friendly interface and specialized functions tailored for both narrative and statistical synthesis of research data.

RevMan enables researchers to organize their data systematically, providing various options for data input, analytical methods and output formats. One of its key features is its ability to perform complex statistical analyzes, such as meta-analyses, without requiring the user to have an extensive background in statistics. This makes it an invaluable asset for clinicians, researchers and policy-makers looking to make evidence-based decisions.

Importance of RevMan

RevMan is user-friendly software that simplifies the process of creating and maintaining systematic reviews. It supports data entry, the management of included and excluded studies, synthesis of the evidence (including meta-analysis), and the presentation of results.

Key Features of RevMan

Data Entry and Management

RevMan allows authors to enter and manage the studies and data used in their review. This includes key characteristics of studies, risk of bias assessments and numerical data for meta-analysis.

Statistical Analysis

RevMan is equipped with statistical tools that facilitate the execution of meta-analysis. It calculates standard metrics such as risk ratios for dichotomous data and mean differences for continuous data, along with their 95% confidence intervals. Furthermore, it can generate forest plots to visualize the results of the meta-analysis (Borenstein et al., 2011).

Presentation of Results

RevMan assists in organizing and presenting results of the review in a clear and standardized format, which promotes understanding and reproducibility.

Getting Started with RevMan

Using RevMan requires some understanding of systematic reviews and meta-analysis methodology. The software can be freely downloaded from the Cochrane website and extensive user guides are available to assist new users. It is important to note that while RevMan is a powerful tool, it's just one component of a systematic review and meta-analysis, and its use should be coupled with rigorous methodological practices.

Limitations of RevMan

While RevMan is a valuable tool for systematic review authors, it has some limitations. It does not directly support network meta-analyses or certain complex statistical analyses. Moreover, it does not conduct literature searches or screening, and these tasks need to be performed using other resources and tools.

Example 1: Analyzing Treatment Effects Across Multiple Studies

A researcher wants to compare the efficacy of Drug A versus Drug B in treating hypertension. They collect data from 10 randomized controlled trials and input these into RevMan. The software helps them perform a meta-analysis, using fixed or random-effects models, to determine which drug is more effective based on pooled data.

Example 2: Subgroup Analysis

A team is investigating the effectiveness of a specific diet plan on weight loss. They have data separated by age groups and gender. Using RevMan, they can perform subgroup analyses to determine if the diet plan is more effective in certain demographics.

Example 3: Sensitivity Analysis

Researchers are unsure about the quality of some studies included in their systematic review of smoking cessation interventions. RevMan allows them to conduct sensitivity analyses, wherein they can exclude these lower-quality studies and examine how this impacts the overall results.

Example 4: Forest Plots

A meta-analysis is conducted to assess the efficacy of different types of surgical interventions for knee pain. The researchers use RevMan to generate forest plots, which visually display the effectiveness of each type of surgery, alongside the associated confidence intervals and degree of heterogeneity.

Example 5: Integration with GRADE

After performing a meta-analysis on the effectiveness of vaccinations in preventing a certain disease, the team uses the integrated GRADEpro tool within RevMan to assess the quality of evidence. This helps in providing a more comprehensive and transparent review.

Example 6: Narrative Synthesis

In some instances, the studies being reviewed are too heterogeneous for statistical synthesis. In such cases, RevMan also offers features that aid in narrative synthesis, where findings from different studies can be qualitatively compared and contrasted.

Example 7: Reporting and Publication

Once the analysis is complete, researchers can use RevMan's various reporting options to generate tables, summaries, and charts that are publication-ready and meet the guidelines set by Cochrane and other bodies for systematic reviews.

> **KEY POINTS**
> - RevMan is a critical tool in the execution of systematic reviews and meta-analyses.
> - By facilitating data entry, management, statistical analysis and presentation of results, it makes the process more efficient and accessible.

BIBLIOGRAPHY

1. Borenstein M, Hedges LV, Higgins JPT, Rothstein HR. "Introduction to Meta-Analysis." John Wiley & Sons, 2011.
2. Cochrane. "Review Manager (RevMan)." [Online] Available at: https://training.cochrane.org/online-learning/core-software-cochrane-reviews/revman, 2020.
3. Page MJ, McKenzie JE, Bossuyt PM, Boutron I, Hoffmann TC, Mulrow CD, et al. "The PRISMA 2020 statement: An updated guideline for reporting systematic reviews." BMJ. 2021.

Choosing the Measures of Effect in Systematic Review and Meta-analysis

Jaykaran Charan, Deepthi R, Suthanthira Kannan

"Choosing the right measures of effect in systematic reviews and meta-analyses is not just a statistical endeavor; it is the cornerstone of translating data into actionable healthcare insights."

INTRODUCTION

Systematic reviews and meta-analyses are widely recognized as the highest level of evidence in scientific research. These powerful tools provide comprehensive and reliable summaries of existing evidence on a specific topic. One of the most crucial aspects of conducting a systematic review or meta-analysis involves selecting an appropriate measure of effect.

Understanding Measures of Effect

A measure of effect is a statistical value that provides an estimate of the magnitude of a relationship between an intervention or exposure and an outcome. Various measures of effect exists, including risk ratios, odds ratios, hazard ratios, mean differences, standardized mean differences and correlation coefficients. Each has different implications and is appropriate for different types of data and research questions.

Choosing the Right Measure of Effect

The choice of effect measure largely depends on the nature of the data being analyzed, the research questions being addressed, and the type of outcome.

Binary Outcomes

For binary outcomes (events that either occur or not), the risk ratio, odds ratio and risk difference are typically used. The risk ratio (or relative risk) is the ratio of the probability of the event occurring in the exposed group to the probability in the control group. The odds ratio compare the odds of an event occurring in the treated group to the odds in the control group. Risk difference is the absolute difference in risk between the experimental and control groups.

Continuous Outcomes

When outcomes are continuous (e.g., blood pressure, weight), the mean difference or standardized mean difference is usually used. The mean difference is simply the difference in means between two groups. When different studies use different scales, the standardized mean difference, also known as Cohen's d, is used.

Time-to-Event Outcomes

For outcomes that involve time to an event (like survival analysis), hazard ratios are typically used.

The Implication of the Measure of Effect on Interpretation

Different measures of effect not only affect the analysis but also the interpretation and communication of results. Relative measures (like risk ratios and odds ratios) usually overstate the effect compared to absolute measures (like risk difference). The choice between presenting absolute or relative effect measures depends on the context and the intended audience of the research.

Combining Different Measures of Effect in Meta-analysis

In some cases, studies included in a meta-analysis may use different measures of effect. Researchers may need to convert these measures to a common metric using statistical transformations. However, it is important to remember that conversion methods have limitations and may introduce some degree of bias.

KEY POINTS

- Choosing the appropriate measure of effect is a vital step in the systematic review and meta-analysis process.
- The choice should be guided by the type of data, the nature of the outcome, and the research question.
- It should also consider the implications for the interpretation and communication of the research findings.

BIBLIOGRAPHY

1. Borenstein M, Hedges LV, Higgins JP, Rothstein HR. Introduction to meta-analysis. Wiley; 2011.
2. Deeks JJ, Higgins JP, Altman DG. Analysing data and undertaking meta-analyses. In: Cochrane Handbook for Systematic Reviews of Interventions. 2019;241-84.
3. Higgins JPT, Thomas J, Chandler J, Cumpston M, Li T, Page MJ, Welch VA (Eds). Cochrane Handbook for Systematic Reviews of Interventions. 2nd edition. Chichester (UK): John Wiley & Sons; 2019.

Principles of Meta-analysis in Systematic Review and Meta-analysis

Vikas Yadav, Pentapati Siva Santosh Kumar, Suthanthira Kannan

> *"In the realm of systematic reviews, meta-analysis serves as the mathematical lens through which the complexity of multiple studies can be synthesized into a coherent understanding, guiding evidence-based practice and policy."*

INTRODUCTION

Meta-analysis is a statistical methodology that combines results from multiple studies to generate a single estimate of the major effect, providing a comprehensive and quantitative overview of the available evidence.

The Rationale of Meta-analysis

The motivation for performing a meta-analysis stems from the recognition that individual studies may not offer sufficient statistical power to detect effects or may report conflicting results. By synthesizing data across studies, meta-analysis increases statistical power and provides a more precise estimate of the effect size.

Key Principles of Meta-analysis

Comprehensive Literature Search and Selection

A thorough search strategy is crucial to identify all potential studies, thus reducing the risk of selection bias. An inclusive and robust selection process ensures that the meta-analysis includes all relevant studies on the topic.

Standardization and Data Extraction

Data extracted from each study must be standardized to allow comparison and aggregation. The effect size, variance and standard error are commonly used metrics.

Statistical Combination of Results

This is the core of a meta-analysis. Using statistical methods, results from individual studies are combined to calculate an overall effect size. Both fixed-effects and random-effects models can be used, depending on the assumption about the underlying true effect sizes.

Heterogeneity Assessment

Heterogeneity refers to the variability in study outcomes beyond what would be expected due to sampling error alone. The presence of significant heterogeneity may suggest that the effect size varies across studies. Tools such as the I^2 statistic and Cochran's Q can assess heterogeneity.

Interpretation and Presentation of Results

Results from a meta-analysis should be interpreted cautiously, considering potential sources of bias and heterogeneity. Typically, results are presented as forest plots, which provide a visual representation of the estimated effect size and its confidence interval for each study and the combined effect size.

Criticisms and Limitations of Meta-analysis

While meta-analysis is a powerful tool, it is subject to several limitations. These include publication bias, where studies with negative findings are less likely to be published and the "apples and oranges" criticism, where studies that are too dissimilar are combined. These and other limitations should be considered when interpreting results.

KEY POINTS

- Meta-analysis is a key component of systematic reviews that offers the ability to synthesize evidence quantitatively.
- It requires careful planning, rigorous execution, and cautious interpretation.

BIBLIOGRAPHY

1. Borenstein M, Hedges LV, Higgins JP, Rothstein HR. "Introduction to Meta-Analysis". Chichester, UK: Wiley; 2009.
2. Higgins JP, Thomas J, Chandler J, Cumpston M, Li T, Page MJ, Welch VA (Eds). "Cochrane Handbook for Systematic Reviews of Interventions". Cochrane; 2020.
3. Higgins JP, Thompson SG. "Quantifying heterogeneity in a meta-analysis". Stat Med. 2002;21(11):1539-58.
4. Sutton AJ, Duval SJ, Tweedie RL, Abrams KR, Jones DR. "Empirical assessment of effect of publication bias on meta-analyses". BMJ. 2000;320(7249):1574-7.

CHAPTER 54

Risk of Bias Assessment for Systematic Reviews

Manya Prasad, Rivu Basu

"Risk of bias assessment isn't merely a procedural step in systematic reviews; it's the bedrock on which the integrity of conclusions rests, ensuring that evidence guides practice, not bias."

INTRODUCTION

Systematic reviews represent the best quality evidence for answering clinical questions, attempting to synthesize the complete body of evidence on a given clinical question. However, the validity of the results of a systematic review and meta-analysis depends on the validity of the included studies. Indeed, if the included studies employ methods that introduce bias, then what the systematic review and meta-analysis will synthesize is also an invalid pooled estimate.

The pertinent question to ask here is: did the included studies take adequate measures in their methodology to reduce bias? An apt acronym to describe the issue is 'GIGO', i.e., Garbage in = Garbage Out **(Fig. 1)**. Indeed, if the primary studies in the systematic review are rife with bias, what the meta-analysis will churn out will also be a biased estimated.

From a practical standpoint, risk of bias assessment involves the critical appraisal of methodology of included studies, done with the help of various tools specific to study design.

Risk of bias can arise from various sources, including selection bias, performance bias, detection bias, attrition bias, reporting bias, and other biases related to the study design or

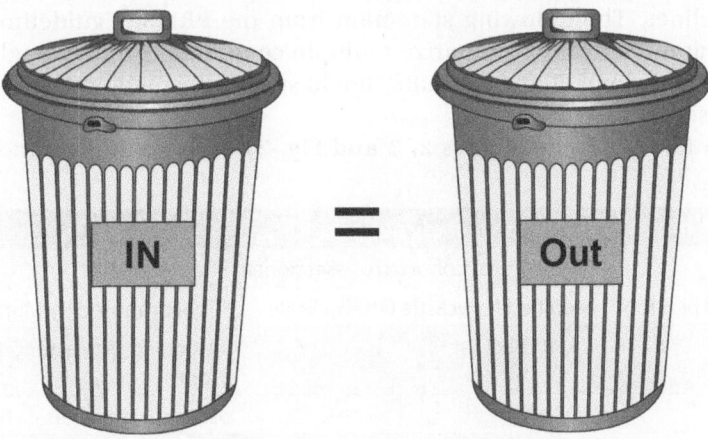

Fig. 1: 'GIGO'- Garbage in = Garbage Out.

execution. Assessing the risk of bias will enable reviewers to draw accurate conclusions from the synthesized evidence.

Risk of Bias Assessment Tools

Several tools and frameworks are available to assess the risk of bias in individual studies included in systematic reviews. Commonly used tools include the Cochrane Risk of Bias Tool, the Newcastle-Ottawa Scale, the ROBINS-I tool for nonrandomized studies, and the QUADAS-2 tool for diagnostic accuracy studies. These tools provide a structured approach for reviewers to evaluate different aspects of study quality and potential bias across domains such as selection, performance, attrition, detection, and reporting bias. The most widely used tool for clinical trials is the Cochrane Collaboration's Risk of Bias tool, which provides a standardized approach to evaluate seven specific domains of bias: random sequence generation, allocation concealment, blinding of participants and personnel, blinding of outcome assessment, incomplete outcome data, selective outcome reporting and other sources of bias.

The tool to be used for risk of bias assessment on primary studies depends on the study design being assessed. **Table 1** below mentions a few risk of bias tools for various study designs.

Calibration Exercise

A calibration exercise may be carried out before the actual risk of bias assessments are made for the systematic review. This will help to minimize discrepancy in interpretation and reporting of the standardized tools. As a calibration exercise, reviewers may assess risk of bias for one or two papers in duplicate, and a third reviewer may discuss the conflicts with both reviewers.

Reporting Risk of Bias Assessment

Transparent reporting of risk of bias assessments is essential for readers to understand the limitations and potential biases in the synthesized evidence. Systematic reviews should clearly present the results of risk of bias assessments, including tables or graphs summarizing the ratings for each included study. Additionally, reviewers should discuss the implications of the risk of bias assessments in the interpretation of the review findings, emphasizing the potential impact on the overall conclusions.

Tools that summarize the assessments as an overall score are discouraged as per the PRISMA guidelines. The following statement from the PRISMA guidelines pertains to this: 'scales that numerically summarize multiple components into a single number are misleading and unhelpful. Rather, authors should specify the methodological components that they assessed.'

Below are a few examples **(Tables 2, 3 and Fig. 2)** of the presentation of risk of bias assessments.

Table 1: Few risk of bias tools for various study designs.		
RCT	Case control/cohort/cross-sectional	Case series
Cochrane risk of bias tool	Modified Newcastle Ottawa Scale	Tool proposed by Murad et al
RoB 2	CASP checklist	Modified McMaster Critical Review form
Jadad scale	ROBINS-I	JBI critical appraisal checklist
		NIH quality scale for case series

Table 2: Adjusted for invasive mechanical ventilation; use of methylprednisolone and APACHE II score at baseline; height adjusted for other co-interventions such as TCZ, antivirals, anticoagulation, HCQ, vasopressor use; dialysis requirement, etc.

Study	Adequate sequence generation	Allocation concealment	Blinding	Incomplete data addressed	Free of selective reporting	Free of other bias	% of yes answers
Lekovic et al. 2000	Yes	Unclear	Yes	Unclear	Unclear	Yes	50%
Velasquez-Plata et al. 2002	Yes	NA	Yes	Unclear	No	Yes	50%
Zucchelli et al. 2003	Yes	Yes	Yes	Unclear	Yes	Yes	83.3%
Gurinsky et al. 2004	Yes	Unclear	Yes	Yes	Unclear	Yes	66.6%
Sculean et al. 2005	Yes	Unclear	Unclear	Yes	Yes	Yes	66.6%
Bokan et al. 2006	Yes	Yes	Yes	Unclear	Unclear	Unclear	50%
Kuru et al. 2006	Yes	Unclear	Yes	Yes	Yes	Yes	83.3%
Guida et al. 2007	Yes	NA	No	Yes	No	Yes	50%
Yilmaz et al. 2010	No	No	Yes	Yes	Yes	Yes	66.6%
Meyle et al. 2011	Yes	Yes	Yes	Yes	Yes	Yes	100%
Cortellini and Tonetti 2011	Yes	Yes	Unclear	Yes	Yes	Yes	83.3%
De Leonardis and Paolantonio 2013	Yes	Yes	Yes	Yes	Yes	Yes	100%

N/A—not available

Reporting Risk of Bias Assessment for Various Outcomes

The risk of bias assessments must be provided for each outcome. This is because risk of bias differs depending on the outcome. For instance, blinded outcome assessment may not have much of an effect on an outcome such as mortality. Mortality is a 'hard' outcome and is not vulnerable to misclassification by outcome assessors. On the other hand, if it is a subjective outcome, such imaging by ultrasound or quality of life scale, risk of bias is more relevant in unblinded assessments. Thus, reviewers must make it clear which outcome the risk of bias assessment is presented for and possibly report separate assessments for each outcome.

Table 3: Propensity matched controls high risk for O2 requirement; low risk for survival.

Study (reference)	From the same population	Assessment of exposure	Outcome present at start	Adjustment	Assessment of prognostic factors	Assessment of outcome	Adequate followup	Co-interventions similar
Rasheed 2020	Definitely low	Definitely low	Definitely low	Definitely high	Probably high	Probably high	Probably low	Probably high
Abolghasemi 2020	Definitely low	Definitely low	Definitely low	Definitely high	Definitely high	Definitely high	Probably low	Probably high
Omrani 2020	Definitely low	Definitely low	Definitely low	Definitely low	Definitely low	Probably high	Probably low	Probably high
Rogers 2020	Definitely low	Definitely low	Definitely low	Definitely low	Definitely low	Definitely low	Probably low	Definitely high
Salazar E 2020	Definitely low	Definitely low	Definitely low	Definitely low	Definitely low	Probably high	Probably low	Definitely high
Xia 2020	Definitely low	Definitely low	Definitely low	Definitely high	Definitely high	Probably high	Probably low	Definitely high
Liu 2020	Definitely low	Definitely low	Definitely low	Definitely low[3]	Definitely low	Definitely low	Probably low	Definitely high

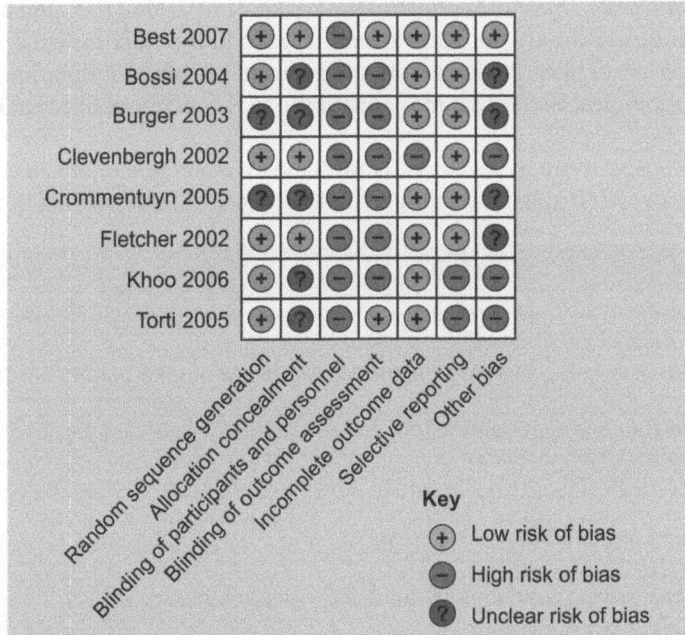

Fig. 2: High risk of bias for respiratory support and viral clearance; low risk for survival.

Reliability of Risk of Bias Assessment

Assessing risk of bias in included studies is often subjective. Despite using standardized tools and criteria, individual reviewers may interpret and apply the guidelines differently. For this reason, the risk of bias assessment is typically performed in duplicate by two independent reviewers. The reviewers assign a judgment of low, high, or unclear risk of bias for each domain based on predefined criteria based on the tool being used. Discrepancies between reviewers are resolved through discussion or by involving a third reviewer.

High level of agreement between the two reviewers will provide reassurance that the risk of bias assessment is reliable. There are various ways of measuring agreement between the reviewers. Reviewers may report percent agreement, or alternatively, the kappa statistic. The kappa statistic would provide a measure of agreement between two reviewers over and above that which is present by chance.

Other Sources of Bias in Systematic Reviews

The overall risk of bias in the systematic review depends on a number of other factors, apart from risk of bias. Included amongst these are heterogeneity, indirectness, publication bias and imprecision. These concepts are discussed briefly in the chapter on the GRADE tool.

Challenges in Risk of Bias Assessment

Assessing the risk of bias is a complex task that can be influenced by several challenges. One challenge is the availability and accessibility of information. Some studies may not provide sufficient details on their methods and procedures, making it difficult to assess the risk of bias accurately. In such cases, reviewers may need to contact study authors for additional information or make conservative judgments based on the available data.

Furthermore, the risk of bias tools often do not cover all areas that threaten internal validity. For example, change in primary outcome is not included in the Cochrane risk of bias tool and may be reported as 'other bias'. Reviewers should be aware of these limitations and consider all additional methodological issues that may contribute to risk of bias while reading the primary study.

Furthermore, sensitivity analyses can be conducted to assess the impact of studies with high risk of bias on the overall results, providing a more nuanced understanding of the evidence.

> **KEY POINTS**
>
> - **Critical evaluation:** Assessing the risk of bias in systematic reviews is crucial for evaluating the quality and reliability of the included studies.
> - **Accuracy:** It aids in ensuring that the synthesized evidence accurately mirrors the true effects of the subject matter.
> - **Reduction of erroneous conclusions:** This assessment helps in reducing the likelihood of drawing incorrect conclusions from the data.
> - **Systematic approach:** Employing a systematic and transparent approach to risk of bias assessment is essential.
> - **Enhanced credibility:** Through meticulous risk of bias assessment, reviewers can enhance the credibility of the systematic reviews.
> - **Valid results:** This process contributes to the validity of the systematic reviews.
> - **Evidence-based decision-making:** Ultimately, rigorous risk of bias assessment aids in evidence-based decision-making within healthcare.

BIBLIOGRAPHY

1. Guyatt GH, Oxman AD, Vist GE, Kunz R, Falck-Ytter Y, Alonso-Coello P, Schünemann HJ; GRADE Working Group. GRADE: An emerging consensus on rating quality of evidence and strength of recommendations. BMJ. 2008;336(7650):924-6.
2. Higgins JPT, Green S (editors). Cochrane Handbook for Systematic Reviews of Interventions Version 5.1.0 [updated March 2011]. The Cochrane Collaboration, 2011. Available from www.handbook.cochrane.org.
3. Moher D, Shamseer L, Clarke M, Ghersi D, Liberati A, Petticrew M, et al. Preferred reporting items for systematic review and metaanalysis protocols (PRISMA-P) 2015 statement. Syst Rev. 2015;4:1.
4. The Evidence-Based Medicine Working Group; edited by Gordon Guyatt, Drummond Rennie. Users' Guides to the Medical Literature: A Manual for Evidence-Based Clinical Practice. Chicago, IL: AMA Press, 2002.

The GRADE Tool for Rating Certainty in Evidence and Recommendations

CHAPTER 55

Manya Prasad, Rivu Basu

> "The GRADE tool doesn't just rate the quality of evidence and strength of recommendations; it serves as a compass in the complex landscape of healthcare decision-making, pointing the way toward evidence-based, patient-centered solutions."

INTRODUCTION

Grading of recommendations assessment, development, and evaluation (GRADE) tool, a systematic approach used to assess the certainty of evidence and strength of recommendations in healthcare guidelines. The GRADE methodology aims to enhance transparency, consistency and rigor in evaluating evidence and informing clinical decision-making. This chapter describes the key components of the GRADE tool, including the factors considered in assessing evidence quality, the process for rating certainty, and the implications for developing recommendations.

In the field of healthcare, making informed decisions that are evidence-based is crucial for providing optimal patient care. Medical research produces a vast amount of evidence, ranging from observational studies to randomized controlled trials (RCTs). However, not all evidence is of the same quality and recommendations based on weak or uncertain evidence can lead to suboptimal outcomes. Therefore, there is a need for a systematic and transparent approach to assess the certainty of evidence and develop reliable recommendations. The GRADE provides a transparent approach to rating the strength of evidence and certainty in recommendations for any given clinical question.

With respect to systematic reviews and meta-analyses, GRADE rates the complete body of evidence on a given clinical question. Typically, this body of evidence is present in the form of a systematic review and meta-analysis, which in turn informs the guideline development. Quite often, in the absence of a recent and updated systematic review on a clinical question, agencies such as the World Health Organization (WHO), commission a systematic review by a group of methodologists.

It was in the year 2000 that the GRADE working group began to meet. This group was comprised of experts in the field of clinical epidemiology, methodologists and guideline developers. The first paper that described the approach appeared in the British Medical Journal in 2004.

Since its inception, the GRADE system has since gained widespread recognition and adoption, with over 110 organizations worldwide adopting it. Included amongst these are the WHO, CDC, NHS, cochrane collaboration, and many leading medical associations and societies. Electronic textbooks such as UpToDate and Dynamed have tens of thousands of graded recommendations using this approach.

Limitations of Traditional Approaches to Evidence Grading

Traditionally, guideline development has often lacked a systematic and transparent approach to rating the strength of evidence that informs the guidelines. The following are key to ensuring that the guidelines development process is trustworthy:
❖ Appropriate panel
❖ Conflict of interest exclusion or management
❖ Systematic review of best evidence
❖ Rating of quality of evidence
❖ Transparent presentation of review results
❖ Explicit values and preferences
❖ Rating strength of recommendations
❖ Optimal presentation

The traditional approaches have often lacked these key properties, thus raising uncertainty about the guideline development process. The GRADE approach attempts to meet the requirement for all of these key issues.

Importance of Assessing Certainty in Evidence for Informed Decision-Making

The cartoon (**Fig. 1**) depicts the importance of rating the strength of recommendations. The statement spoken by the weatherman depicts that one can state the likelihood of rain, but it is possible that there may be no confidence in that likelihood assessment. Similarly, one may estimate the likelihood of an outcome occurring with regard to any clinical question; however, one can either be very confident in the measure of that likelihood or not confident at all.

This encapsulates the difference between assessing the likelihood of something happening, and the confidence in that assessment. The GRADE approach addresses this concept and takes into consideration a number of factors in rating the certainty in outcomes and strength of recommendations. GRADE recognizes that high-quality evidence does not necessarily translate to strong recommendations and vice versa.

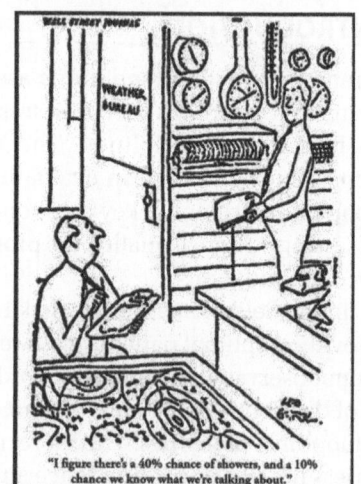

Fig. 1: Cartoon, depicts the importance of rating strength of recommendations.

Framework for Rating Strength (Certainty/Confidence) of Evidence

It provides a structured framework for evaluating and grading the quality of evidence, considering factors such as study design, risk of bias, inconsistency, indirectness, imprecision, and publication bias. This systematic approach ensures a comprehensive evaluation of the evidence base.

One can think about the certainty or confidence in the evidence as being on a continuum, ranging from very confident to not confident at all.

Within this continuum, the GRADE system has four categories, which are arbitrary but have the advantage of simplicity. The four categories are high, moderate, low and very low.

High Certainty

High certainty indicates that the available evidence provides a high level of confidence in the estimate of the effect. High-certainty evidence comes from well-conducted studies with consistent results and minimal risk of bias, and it is unlikely that further research will significantly change the confidence in the estimate.

Moderate Certainty

Moderate certainty suggests that the available evidence is sufficient to support a conclusion, but further research may still impact the confidence in the estimate. Moderate-certainty evidence may arise from studies with limitations, inconsistencies, possibility of bias, lack of high-quality evidence, etc.

Low Certainty

Low certainty implies that the available evidence is limited and the true effect may be substantially different from the estimate. This may be due to serious methodological flaws, inconsistency in results, indirectness of evidence, imprecision, or a high risk of bias. Additional research is likely to have an important impact on the confidence in the estimate.

Very Low Certainty

Very low certainty indicates that the available evidence is insufficient to support any firm conclusions. Very low-certainty evidence arises from studies with major methodological limitations, inconsistent or contradictory results, sparse evidence or a high risk of bias. The true effect is often unknown and future research is expected to have a significant impact on the confidence in the estimate. For this category, values and preferences of patients are a major consideration.

Upgrading or Downgrading Certainty (Table 1)

Study Design

The study design is an important factor in assessing evidence quality. Randomized controlled trials are generally considered higher quality compared to observational studies due to their rigorous methodology, random allocation and control of confounding factors. However, not all RCTs are of equal quality and well-conducted observational studies can also provide valuable evidence.

Downgrading Evidence

By default, bodies of evidence that arises from RCTs start out as high certainty and observational studies start out as low certainty. However, a number of factors may result in rating up or rating down of certainty in evidence. A detailed discussion of all these factors are beyond the scope of this chapter and only a brief description is mentioned below. These factors that can rate down certainty in evidence are:

Risk of Bias

The risk of bias refers to the potential for systematic errors in the design or conduct of a study that can lead to biased results. Assessing the risk of bias involves evaluating key aspects such

Table 1: Grade's approach to rating quality of evidence.

1. Establish initial level of confidence		2. Consider lowering or raising level of confidence		3. Final level of confidence rating
Study design	Initial confidence in an estimate of effect	Reasons for considering lowering or raising confidence		Confidence in an estimate of effect across those considerations
		Lower if	Higher if*	
Randomized trials	High confidence	Risk of Bias Inconsistency	Large effect Dose response	High ⊕⊕⊕⊕
		Indirectness Imprecision Publication bias	All plausible confounding and bias would reduce a demonstrated effect or ∀ would suggest a spurious effect if no effect was observed	Moderate ⊕⊕⊕
Observational studies	Low confidence			Low ⊕⊕
				Very low ⊕

*Upgrading criteria are usually applicable to observational studies only

as random sequence generation, allocation concealment, blinding, completeness of outcome data, selective reporting and other sources of bias. Studies with a low risk of bias are considered to have higher internal validity and thus higher evidence quality.

Inconsistency

Inconsistency refers to the degree of variation in the results across different studies. If multiple studies on the same research question produce consistent findings, it increases confidence in the evidence. Inconsistency can arise due to differences in study populations, interventions, comparators, outcomes measured or the study design. The issue of inconsistency has been addressed in previous chapters in the context of heterogeneity. The assessment is made by visual inspection of forest plots (to check overlap of confidence intervals and closeness of point estimates) or using statistical methods (I-squared statistic).

Indirectness

Indirectness refers to the extent to which the available evidence directly addresses the research question of interest. This can occur when the study population, intervention, comparison or outcomes differ from those of interest. Indirect evidence may still be informative, but it decreases the certainty of the findings. GRADE evaluates the relevance and applicability of the evidence to the target population or intervention.

Imprecision

Imprecision refers to the degree of uncertainty around the effect estimates. Wide confidence intervals or small sample sizes may indicate imprecision, limiting the certainty of the evidence. GRADE considers the precision of the effect estimates, the statistical significance and the clinical importance of the findings.

Publication Bias

Publication bias occurs when studies with positive or statistically significant results are more likely to be published than studies with negative or nonsignificant results. This can introduce bias in the available evidence base, as it may not represent the full range of study findings. GRADE recommends assessing and addressing publication bias to minimize its impact on evidence certainty.

GRADE uses a structured approach to evaluate these factors and assign a rating of high, moderate, low, or very low certainty to the evidence. Each of these factors—study design, risk of bias, inconsistency, indirectness, imprecision, and publication bias—leads to downgrading of evidence.

Upgrading Evidence

Factors that may lead to upgrading of evidence from observational studies include:

Large Magnitude of Effect

A large magnitude of effect observed in the available evidence may lead to upgrading the certainty of evidence, indicating greater confidence in the estimate. When a very large effect is observed in a very short span of time, high quality evidence may be obtained even from observational studies. For example, Epinephrine for anaphylactic shock, Frusemide for pulmonary oedema, total hip replacement, etc.

Dose-response Gradient

The presence of a dose-response relationship, where increasing exposure or intervention leads to a proportional increase or decrease in the effect, may result in upgrading the certainty of evidence.

Linking Evidence Certainty to Recommendation Strength

GRADE recognizes that the certainty of evidence should be directly linked to the strength of recommendations. Recommendations should be based on the best available evidence and reflect the level of confidence in the evidence. Higher certainty evidence warrants stronger recommendations, while lower certainty evidence may result in weaker or conditional recommendations.

Considerations in Determining Recommendation Direction and Strength

Several key considerations inform the determination of recommendation direction (favorable or unfavorable) and strength (strong or weak):

Balance of Benefits and Harms

The balance between the anticipated benefits and potential harms of an intervention or action is a crucial consideration. If the benefits substantially outweigh the harms, a favorable recommendation may be warranted. Conversely, if the harms outweigh the benefits, an unfavorable recommendation may be appropriate.

Values and Preferences

Values and preferences of individuals or populations affected by the recommendation play a significant role. Recommendations should be aligned with the values, priorities, and expectations of the target population. GRADE encourages explicit consideration of values and preferences in the formulation of recommendations.

Resource Implications

Resource implications refer to the costs, availability and feasibility of implementing the recommended intervention. The economic impact and resource allocation considerations should be taken into account, especially when resources are limited. Recommendations should consider the cost-effectiveness and sustainability of interventions.

Feasibility

The feasibility of implementing the recommended intervention in real-world settings is an important consideration. Practical aspects such as logistical challenges, healthcare infrastructure and human resources should be assessed. Recommendations should be feasible and practical for implementation.

Rating Recommendations as Strong or Weak

GRADE utilizes a system for rating recommendations as strong or weak:

Strong Recommendations

Strong recommendations are issued when the desirable effects of an intervention clearly outweigh the undesirable effects or when the undesirable effects clearly outweigh the desirable effects. Strong recommendations are applicable to most individuals or populations and should be followed as a standard of care.

Weak Recommendations

Weak recommendations are made when the desirable and undesirable effects are closely balanced, or the available evidence is of low certainty. Weak recommendations recognize that different options may be appropriate for different individuals or situations. Shared decision-making, considering individual values and preferences, is essential for weak recommendations.

Example 1: Smoking cessation programs
- **Evidence**: Multiple high-quality RCTs show that a specific smoking cessation program significantly increases the quit rates among smokers.
- **GRADE rating**: Strong recommendation, as the evidence quality is high and the benefit clearly outweighs the risk.

Example 2: Use of antibiotics for viral infections
- **Evidence**: Numerous studies indicate that antibiotics are ineffective against viral infections and can contribute to antibiotic resistance.
- **GRADE rating**: Strong recommendation against the use of antibiotics for treating viral infections.

Example 3: Surgical intervention for lower back pain
- **Evidence**: Mixed results from various studies, some showing moderate benefits but others showing little to no improvement, coupled with potential surgical risks.
- **GRADE rating**: Weak recommendation, given the uncertainty in benefit and potential for harm.

Example 4: Vitamin D supplements for general population
- **Evidence**: Some observational studies suggest a benefit in taking Vitamin D supplements, but RCTs provide inconsistent results.
- **GRADE rating**: Weak recommendation, as the quality of evidence is low and the net benefit is uncertain.

Example 5: Screening for prostate cancer
- **Evidence**: While screening can detect prostate cancer early, it also leads to overdiagnosis and overtreatment, subjecting patients to potential harm.
- **GRADE rating**: Weak recommendation, given the trade-offs between early detection and the risks associated with unnecessary treatments.

Example 6: Exercise for mental health
- **Evidence**: Multiple high-quality studies show consistent, significant improvements in mental health with regular exercise.
- **GRADE rating**: Strong recommendation for the incorporation of exercise in mental health treatment plans.

KEY POINTS

- The GRADE tool offers a systematic and transparent framework for assessing evidence quality and strength of healthcare recommendations, ensuring consistent and trustworthy evaluations.
- GRADE significantly influences healthcare guideline development and implementation, fostering consistency in evidence communication and integration across various healthcare settings.
- Continuously adapting to meet the evolving needs of evidence grading, GRADE undergoes ongoing developments to stay relevant and effective in the face of complex healthcare challenges.
- By providing a structured approach to evidence grading, GRADE shapes the field, ensuring healthcare decisions are based on the best available evidence, thereby improving healthcare outcomes.
- GRADE's ultimate aim is to enhance patient care by informing healthcare policies and practices with high-quality evidence, leading to better-informed decisions and improved patient outcomes.

BIBLIOGRAPHY

1. Alonso-Coello P, Schünemann HJ, Moberg J, et al. GRADE Evidence to Decision (EtD) frameworks: a systematic and transparent approach to making well informed healthcare choices. 2: Clinical practice guidelines. BMJ. 2016;353:i2089.
2. Alonso-Coello P, Schünemann HJ, Moberg J, et al. GRADE Evidence to Decision (EtD) frameworks for adoption, adaptation, and de novo development of trustworthy recommendations: GRADE-ADOLOPMENT. J Clin Epidemiol. 2017;81:101-110.
3. Atkins D, Eccles M, Flottorp S, et al. Systems for grading the quality of evidence and the strength of recommendations I: Critical appraisal of existing approaches The GRADE Working Group. BMC Health Serv Res. 2004;4(1):38.
4. Balshem H, Helfand M, Schünemann HJ, et al. GRADE guidelines: 3. Rating the quality of evidence. J Clin Epidemiol. 2011;64(4):401-6.
5. GRADE Working Group. GRADE Handbook. Updated October 2013. Available from: https://gdt.gradepro.org/app/handbook/handbook.html
6. Guyatt GH, Oxman AD, Kunz R, et al. GRADE guidelines: 7. Rating the quality of evidence—inconsistency. J Clin Epidemiol. 2011;64(12):1294-1302.
7. Guyatt GH, Oxman AD, Vist GE, et al. GRADE: An emerging consensus on rating quality of evidence and strength of recommendations. BMJ. 2008;336(7650):924-6.
8. Schünemann HJ, Cuello C, Akl EA, et al. GRADE guidelines: 18. How ROBINS-I and other tools to assess risk of bias in nonrandomized studies should be used to rate the certainty of a body of evidence. J Clin Epidemiol. 2019;111:105-14.
9. Schünemann HJ, Oxman AD, Brozek J, et al. Grading quality of evidence and strength of recommendations for diagnostic tests and strategies. BMJ. 2008;336(7653):1106-10.

Index

Page numbers followed by *f* refer to figure, *fc* refer to flowchart, and *t* refer to table.

A

Abstract 3, 6, 42, 215
    types of 6
    unstructured 7
Academic value, scholarly sources of 22
Accuracy 362
Acknowledgments 43, 52
Acronym 342
Action research 171, 175, 217
Adequate sequence generation 359
Adoption 255
Advanced statistics 136
Age distribution, stem and leaf plot for 116*f*
Agency's mission 277
Allocation concealment 359
Alternative healthcare actions, systematic comparison of 283
Analysis
    deductive 203
    stages of 207
    type of 285
    unit of 173
Analytical study
    classification of 59
    designs 59
Analyze public perception 206
Anaphylactic shock 367
Anemia, degrees of 147
Annualization 292
ANOVA
    assumptions for 137
    factorial 138
    limitations of 146
    one-way 137
    test
        broad classification of 137*fc*
        classification of 137
    two-way 138, 139
Anticoagulation 327, 359*t*
Antiretroviral treatment 238
    rural model of 241
Antivirals 359*t*
Appendices 51
Application, request for 277
Applied research 217
Appropriate study 30
Articles, number of 24
Attitudes 182
Autonomy, respect for 209
Auto-plagiarism 152
Average costs 291
Average earnings per day 317

B

Balanced counseling approach 258
Bar diagram 112
    component 113*f*
Basic research 217
Basic statistics 107
Bayesian sensitivity analysis 309
Behaviors 182
Benefits and harms, balance of 367
Berkson's bias 65
Bias 58
    address problems of 33
    assessment, reporting risk of 358
    at enrolment, avoid selection 74
    free of 359
    high risk of 361*f*
    in systematic reviews, sources of 361
    information 63
    observer's 33
    publication 367
    recall 29, 67
    researcher 178, 205
    response 33
    seasonal 106
    selection 33, 63
    survivorship 67
    tarmac 106
    tool, cochrane collaboration's risk of 358
    unclear risk of 361
Binary outcomes 353
Biomedical research, conduct of 249
Biostatistics 107
Blinding 86, 359
Block randomization 84*f*
Blood
    group, distribution of 113*f*
    pressure readings 119
    sugar
        estimates 121*t*
        values, distribution of 121*t*

Index

Boolean operators 23, 24, 335
Bottom-up method 292
Box and whisker plot 115, 115*f*
Broadcast media, writing for 274
Budget
    details 38
    impact analysis 300, 311
    impact modeling, approach to 312
Build research capacity 245

C

Calculate utility score 304
Calculate variance, steps to 120
Calibration exercise 358
Capital cost 291
Cardiovascular health 335
Care, standard of 368
Case
    control study 59
    histories observation 173
    series 56
Case study 55, 171, 175, 270
    and narratives 206
    collective 175
    instrumental 175
    intrinsic 175
Case-cohort study 72
    design 68, 68*f*
Case-control study 65
    advantages of 67
    design 65, 68
    limitations of 67
    measure in 66
Causality
    bias, reverse 63
    lack of 58
Central limit theorem 122
Centre for disease control 304
    and prevention 275
Cessation experiment trials 78
Chaos narrative 174
Chikungunya 147, 148
Child deaths, number of 302
Chi-square
    goodness 147
    points 148
Chi-square test 146, 147
    data requirement for 146
    logic of 146
    steps of 147
    types of 147
Civil registration system 235
Civil society and tuberculosis care 230
Clinical and health policy 11
Clinical endpoints 303
Clinical insights 57
Clinical trials, bias and confounding in 86

Closed cohort 71
Cluster randomized trials 84, 265
    problems with 266
Cluster sampling 102
Cochrane data extraction forms 347
Coding 185
    axial 204
    open 204
    selective 204
Cognitive scales 140
Cohort study 59, 71, 73
    analysis of 73
    design 70, 70*fc*
    results from 74
    retrospective 71
    steps of 71
    types of 71, 72
Co-interventions similar 360
Colaizzi model 207
Communicate findings 127
Communications 41
    short 41
Community
    engagement, principles of 249
    intervention trials 78
    level 243
Comparative research questions 12
Comparing two proportions 92
Comprehensive data extraction form 348
Comprehensive literature search and selection 355
Compute test statistic 141
Computer assisted
    software 203
    techniques 207
Conceptual context 177
Concurrently analyzed 173
Conduct data extraction 347
Confidence rating, final level of 366
Constant comparative method 206, 206*fc*
Constructing reality 171
Constructivism 171
Contamination 266
Content
    analysis 206
    need of 211, 216
Control measure effectiveness 308
Convenience sampling 103, 197
Cooperative agreements 278
Correlational studies 56
Cost
    and cost analysis, concept of 289
    benefit analysis 287
    identification of 316
    items 261
    minimization study 286
    outcome study 286
    types of 290

utility study 287
valuing of 317
Cost analysis 293
  studies 286
Cost-effectiveness analysis 287, 311
Costing 316
  approach 312
  approaches for 289
  exercise, steps for 294
  methodologies 292
Counseling skills, level of 259*f*
Covariance, analysis of 136
COVID-19
  outbreak 275
  surge 20
Creating opportunities 247
Credibility 178
Criterion sampling 196
Critical case sampling 196
Critical challenge 302
Critical evaluation 362
Critiques 179
Cross-sectional study 30, 59, 61
  descriptive 56
  design 61
  types of 62
Cultural domains 191

D

Daily health advice 275
Data 297
  analysis 28, 32, 62, 174, 185, 214, 218, 334
  availability 231
  cleaning 32
  collect and analyze 127
  discrete 111, 116
  dispersion of 119
  enter 347
  entry and management 350
  for accuracy 348
  graphical representation of 112
  grouping 204
  immersion in 204
  interpret 32, 185, 218
  management, good 323
  methods of presentation of 111*t*
  organization of 203
  primary 297
  quality 231
  reporting, inconsistency in 348
  secondary 297
  source of 241
  synthesis 331, 334
  transcribing 203
  triangulation 223
  type of 109*f*, 134
Data coding 204
  types of 204

Data collection 62, 213, 218
  and analysis 300
  and measurements 31
  assure confidentiality of 189
  context of 169
  method 172, 177
  and tools 37
Data extraction 331, 346, 355
  advantages of 349
  bias in 348
  form 346
  process 348
Data saturation 206
  collected until 173
Database selection 335
Deaths, number of 303
Decision theory 254, 269
Decision trees, utilizing 309
Declaration of Helsinki 209
Delphi technique 191
Dengue 147, 148
Descriptive statistics 107, 109, 110
Descriptive studies 55
  advantages of 58
  disadvantages of 58
  reporting guidelines for 57
  types of 55, 55*fc*
  uses of 57
Design 5
Deviation
  absolute 120
  from mean 120
  minus signs of 120
Dialysis requirement 359*t*
Dietary intervention study 332
Direct cost 290
Direct health care costs 290
Direct nonhealth care costs 290
Direct program relevance 245
Disability-adjusted life years 304, 305
Discussion
  checklist for 150
  components of 150, 150*f*
  effective 150
Disease 73
  etiology, studies of 29
Disney theme parks 238
DistillerSR 347
Document analysis 253
Dose-response gradient 367
Downgrading evidence 365
Dynamic programming 268, 269

E

Eclipse framework 328, 329*t*
Ecological studies 56

Economic
 analysis 261t
 conditions 48
Economic evaluation 281, 283, 284, 302
 approaches to 284
 basic framework of 284f
 complete 286
 costs and consequences in 302f
 modeling in 309
 studies
  assessment in 302
  protocol for 314
  types of 283, 285, 285t, 286f
Educational research 216, 218
 levels of 217
 reflects, history of 216
Effectively writing, steps of 50
Efficacy and effectiveness, comparison of 84f
Efficient synthesis 349
Electronic health records, adoption of 290
Element 328, 329
Eligibility
 assessing for 338
 criteria 331
Emphasizing participant perspective 189
Endline 259
Endpoint 5
Enhanced credibility 362
Epinephrine 367
Epistemological stance 169
Equator network website 150
Equivalence trial 29
Erroneous conclusions, reduction of 362
Error 91, 91f, 128
 types of 128t
Essential medicines, access to 236
Ethical concerns prevent random assignment 257
Ethical considerations 28, 32
Ethical principles 209
Ethical research, codes in 208
Ethics and consent 62
Ethnography 171, 173, 208
Evaluation studies guidelines, elaboration of 319
Evidence 368
 provide reliable 325
 summarization 349
 upgrading 367
Evidence-based
 decision-making 362
 medicine 35, 323
Excel 347
Experimental studies, types of 77
Exploratory nature 58
Exposure, assessment of 360
Extreme case sampling 196

F

Feasible 11
Federal agencies 278
Field intervention studies 229
Field trials 77
Financial donors 250
Financing 236
Fixed cost 291
Flowchart 339, 341f
Focus group discussion 182, 187, 187t
 conducting 183
 need for 182
Focus groups, number of 183
Forest plot 117, 117f, 325f, 351
Formative tools 168
Formulas presented 89
Formulate null 126
Formulating question 327
Foundation directory 278
Framing SMART objectives 17
Framingham cohort study 75
Free list 191
 technique 192
 uses of 192
Frequency
 distribution table 111, 111t
 polygon 114f
Frusemide 367
Full sentence titles 4
Fundamental research 217
Funding agencies 277, 278
Funding opportunities, online database of 278
Funnel plot 116, 326f

G

Game theory 254, 269
Gantt chart 39f, 251
Gaussian distribution 121
Geometric mean 118
Giorgi model 207
GitHub R package 340
Good research question, characteristics of 10
Good systematic review, traits of 324
Good title, components of 4
Good writing, tips for 25
Government agencies 278
Grounded theory 171, 172
 purpose of 173
Groups compared, number of 134

H

Hazard ratios 353
Health
 and care excellence 315

and hygiene practices, promotion of 275
care providers 259t
information systems 235
operational research 253
policies
   change in 36
   research to 46
programs 238
status, improving 233
wide range of 186
workforce 235
Health economic
   analysis 310
   map 298f
   perspectives in 289
Health system 233
   covering 233
   evaluation trials 78
   perspective 290
Health technology assessment 46, 47f, 281, 299, 300
   applications of 47, 48f
   proposal 300
      development 299
Healthcare
   decision-making processes 284
   economic evaluation in 283, 309
   ever-evolving landscape of 283
   interventions 284
   programs, economic evaluation of 283
   system
      complexity of 231
      modeling 271t
      simulation 271t
Hemoglobinometer, automated 20
Hermeneutic phenomenology 172
Heterogeneity
   assessment 356
   refers 356
Histogram 113
   depicting frequency 114f
Historical controls, before and after trial using 78
Historical research 176
Homogenous sampling 195
Homoskedasticity 137
Hospital
   admission rate bias 65
   purchase department records 316
Host community 249
Human capital approach 305
Human immunodeficiency virus treatment 241
Hypertension 317
   prevalence of 20
   status of 112
Hypothesis 127, 133, 134, 140, 177
   alternative 14, 91, 125, 126
   building 136
   complex 14

concept of 13
formulation of 218
generating 57
in research 13
simple 14
test, two-tailed 130f
testing 90, 125

I

Identify etiologic agents, trials to 78
Ill-health, financial consequences of 233
Incomplete data 348
   addressed 359
Inconsistency 366
In-depth
   analysis 175, 349
   interview 187, 187t
   understanding 58
In-depth interview guide
   components of 188
   preparing 188
Indirect cost 291
Inductive analysis 203
Inferential statistics 107, 109
Information 33
   dissemination 229
   power model 201f
   sources 152, 169
      and search strategy 331
   standardization of 349
   theory 268
Informed consent 250
Informed decision-making 364
Institutional Ethics Committee 251
Institutional regulations 152
Integer programming 269
Interim analysis 85
International Civil Society 250
International Federal Funding Agencies 278
Interpretivism 171
Interrogative title 4
Interval scale 110
Intervention amounted, total cost of 261
Interventional studies 28
Intervention-interacting domains, implementation of 245
Interview
   after 190
   arrangement for 189
   before 187
   duration of 189
   during 189
Interviewer, key skills of 189
Intracluster correlation 266f
Invasive mechanical ventilation, adjusted for 359t
Investigator triangulation 223
I-squared statistic 366

IUD
  insertion rate 260f, 261f
  knowledge, level of 259f
  services, change in quality of 260f

J

Journal 44

K

K way table 112t
Kangaroo mother care 317
Kappa statistic 361
Keywords 42
Knowledge
  lack of 242
  level of 259
Kolmogorov-Smirnov tests 132
Kruskal-Wallis test 132

L

Language and concepts forming theory 171
Leading questions 190
Learning about prisma 337
Life scale, global quality of 304
Line diagram 115, 115f
Linear programming 268
Literature review 22, 212
  matrix template 25t
Low calorie 140, 141
Low carbohydrate 140, 141
Low fat 140, 141
Lower back pain 368

M

Macro health economics 296
Macroeconomic 296t, 297t
  research 297
Malaria 147, 148
Male sterilizations per month, number of 265f
Mann-Whitney U test 132
Manuscript
  accepting and rejecting 43
  writing 41
Markov models 310
Markov process 268, 269
Marks obtained 119
Masking 86
Mass media campaign-condom use 263f, 264f
Matching controls 29
Maximum variation sampling 195
Mean deviation 119, 120
Means squares 142
Measure health states 304
Measuring costs 316
Media communication 273, 275
  writing for 273

Media writing 273
Medical arena, advancement in 221
Medical subject headings 8
Mendeley referencing software 153
Mental health, exercise for 369
Mesh data base 24
MeSH term 24
Meta-analysis 309, 325, 330, 348, 353-355
  criticisms of 356
  facilitates 349
  key principles of 355
  limitations of 356
  measures of effect in 354
  principles of 355
  protocol 330
  rationale of 355
  stems 355
Methodological triangulation 223
Methodological umbrella concerned 182
Methodology
  essentials steps of 27
  soundness of 249
Methylprednisolone, use of 359t
Micro health economics 296
Microeconomic 297t
  research 297
Missing data 348
Mixed method 28, 168, 223, 292
Mixed purposeful sampling 196
Mixed sampling
  designs 100
  methods 104
Modeling 271, 318
Monetary budgets 284
Monitoring health system's performance 233
Mortality 303, 305
Mosaic plagiarism 152
Multiphase sampling 105f
Multiple bar diagram 113f
Multiple effects, examination of 74
Multiple valid realities exist 171
Multistage purposeful random sampling 197
Multistage sampling 104f, 140

N

Narrative research 171, 174
Narrative synthesis 352
National Institutes of Health 278
National Policies 236
National stakeholders 250
National TB Programme 241
Natural experiments 78
Naturalism 171
Nested case-control study 69f, 72
  design 68
Network scheduling 268
New healthcare technology 311

Nominal group technique 191
Nonequivalent control group 262
Non-equivalent groups 256
Nongovernmental organizations, role of 246
Nonhypertensive 112
Noninferiority trial 29
Nonlinear programming 268, 269
Nonmaleficence 209, 250
Nonparametric test 132, 134
Nonprobability sampling 102
    designs 100
Nonrandom sampling 195
Nonrandomized concurrent trial 78
Nonstandard abbreviations 8
Normal distribution 121
    curve 122*f*
        characteristics of 121
        illustrating rejection 129*f*
Normative costing 289
Null hypothesis 14, 91, 125-127, 136, 147, 148
    testing, nonrejection regions for 129*f*
Nurenberg code 208

O

Observational studies 253
Odds ratios 353
One-tailed hypothesis test 130*f*
One-way analysis
    of covariance 139
    of variance 136
Open cohort 71
Operational research 28, 225, 227, 229, 238, 239, 249, 277
    application of 230
    enabling factors for 245
    ethical considerations in 250
    focuses 228
    funding opportunities in 277
    in health 253, 254
    qualitative analysis in 268
    scope of 242
    study 240*t*, 249*f*
        designs of 229
        categories of 229
Opportunistic sampling 196
Opportunity cost 291
Original objective 18
Out-of-pocket expenditure 311
Overhead costs 291

P

P value 143, 145
Pain relief, time to 145
Panic disorder 140
Paradigm shift 245
Parametric tests 134
Paraphrasing plagiarism 151
Partial economic evaluation 285
Participant selection 213
Participant's responses, documentation of 190
Participatory action research 176
Patient care, change in 36
PEO framework 328*t*
Percentage aware 259
Personal characteristics 213
Person-centeredness 235
Pertinent material 12
Phenomenology 171, 172, 206
Physical activity, impact of 335
Pictogram 114
    depicting frequency 114*f*
Pie diagram 112, 113*f*
Pilot study 33
Plagiarism 25, 151, 152
    amount of 152
    complete 151
    consequences of 152
    depends, consequences of 152
    direct 151
    in research, types of 151
    type of 152
Policy
    implications 51
    making 47
    options, critique of 51
    relevance 240
Policy brief
    effective 49
    executive summary 50
    objectives of 49
    template 50
    title 50
Policy-making
    factors affecting 48
    factors influencing 48*f*
Political activities 48
Polygon 114
Popular health issues 206
Population 4, 98, 333
    and sample 108*f*
    attributable risk 73
    mean, estimation of 92
    vs. sample 108*f*
Post-test design 257, 257*f*
Potential studies 355
Power of test 92
Practical illustration 310
Practical standpoint 357
Practice interview 188
Pragmatic costing 289
Precision analysis 90
Pre-conceived sampling frame 173
Preliminary research 11
Pre-post-test design 257*f*
Press release, writing for 274

Prevalence study 28, 61
Preventive trials 77
PRISMA 336, 337
    2020 checklist 342
    checklist components 337*t*
    extension 342, 342*t*
    flow diagram 337*f*
    scope of 341
    template, use of 340*f*
PRISMA flowchart 336, 338, 338*fc*, 342, 343, 343*f*
    templates 339
    constructing 343
        templates 339*f*
Probability sampling 100
Probe questions, use of 190
Productivity loss 292
Prospective cohort studies 71
    disadvantages of 74
Prospective evaluation, tool for 271
Prostate cancer, screening for 369
Protocol
    section of 314
    writing 35, 330
Pseudo-cohort study 64
Psoriasis and depression, cohort study of 75
Psychological therapy study 332
Public health
    improvement in 36
    messages 275
    perspective 290
    surveillance 57
Public opinion 48
PubMed
    creating search strategy in 24*t*
    search 24
Pulmonary oedema 367
P-value test 91

Q

Qualitative data 111
    management 207
    tabular representation of 112
Qualitative data analysis 203
    approaches in 203
    methods in 205
    models of 207
    stages in 203
Qualitative designs, need for 168
Qualitative enquiry, purpose of sampling in 194
Qualitative health 254
Qualitative methods 167, 168, 221, 221*t*
    assumptions underlying 169
    integration of 254
Qualitative modeling 271
Qualitative research 167, 169-171, 179, 221, 223, 253, 254
    components of 176

differs 170*t*
explores complex phenomena 211
future of 254
implementation of 254
in health care
    role of 167
    types of 171
in operational research 253
    role of 253
methodology 165
methods 221
    strengths of 222
practical applications of 221
report 211
    writing in 211
sampling in 194
techniques, common 253
types of 182
Qualitative studies 28
    analysis in 203
    ethical considerations in 208
    ethics in 203
Qualitative variables 109
    types of 110
Quality assessment 331, 349
Quality issues 243
Quality of life
    questionnaires 300
    scale, health-related 304
Quality patient care scale 18
Quality-adjusted life years 304
Quantitative approach 170*t*
Quantitative data 111, 133
    tabular representation of 110
Quantitative methods 168, 221, 221*t*
    integration of 254
Quantitative research 170, 223
    methodology 53
Quantitative study designs 27
Quantitative variable 110
    types of 110
Quasi-experiment 257, 257*t*
Quasi-experimental design 78
Quasi-experimental studies 256
    characteristics of 256
    role of 257
    types of 257
Quest narrative 174
Question
    closed-ended 188
    type of 30
Queuing theory 269
Quota sampling 103, 197

R

Random number table 83*t*, 101*f*
Random purposive sampling 197

Randomized controlled study 30
Randomized controlled trial 77, 79, 363
    crossover design of 82*fc*
    design 80*fc*
    factorial design of 83*fc*
    interpretation of 85
    two arm parallel group 82*fc*
Rapport building 189
Rating scales 32
Rating strength, framework for 364
Rayyan 340, 347
Real life examples 19, 86, 95, 185, 205, 219
Real-world
    applicability 58
    context 257
Record 339
    screened 338
Recording accurate outcomes 10
Recording search 334
Recurrent cost 291
Reference 43
    and experimental populations, selection of 81, 81*f*
    case 293
    list, elements in 153
    management software 153
Referencing and discussion 149
Referencing style 153
Registered patients only, sampling of 106
Relationship research questions 12
Report 338
Reporting
    and communication 62
    and dissemination 300
    and publication 352
    qualitative research, requirements of 211
    sample size calculations 93
Representative sample 99*f*
Representing information 149
Reproducibility 32, 349
Research 27, 297
    assistant 203
    conduct of 251
    design 27
    documents, familiar with 187
    domain 238, 239*f*
    failure and progress 13
    findings, transferability of 214
    implementation 238
    in education 216
    limitations of 214
    literature growing, volume of 323
    objective 14
    paper 3, 6
    problem 27, 31, 218
    protocol, components of 35, 36*t*
    purpose and focus 169
    regularly evaluate success of 246

    relationship 177
Research hypothesis 14
    importance of 13
    types of 14
Research methodology 125
    basics of 1
Research methods 221
    classified 218
Research question 10, 14, 176, 177, 242, 327-329
    address 177, 258
    and hypothesis, formulation of 10
    descriptive 12
    evaluate soundness of your 12
    examples, good and bad 12
    formulation 79
    identify 126
    strong 11, 11*t*
    types of 12, 30*t*
Research studies 16
    dissemination of findings of 251
    ensuring quality in 319
Resolve inconsistencies 325
Respiratory insufficiency 242
Respiratory support 361*f*
Restitution narrative 174
Retrospective cohort studies, disadvantages of 74
Review papers 41
Reviewing memos 185
Reviews and meta-analyses 336
RevMan 350
    limitations of 351
Risk factors trials 78
Risk of bias 361, 362, 365
    assessment 331, 347, 357, 361
    tools 358, 359
    tools 358*t*
Robust economic evaluation protocol 314
Rural health training center 29

S

Sample
    proportion 133
    selection 59
    unit 99
Sample size 25, 31, 37, 89, 199, 212
    calculation 89, 94*t*
        approaches to 90
        software for 94
    estimation 89, 91
Sampling
    advantages of 99
    basic concepts in 98
    basis of 99
    biases in 105
    decisions 177
    frame 99

Index

methods 100, 183, 194
   and errors 98
principles of 99
procedures, classification of 100*fc*
process of 194
purposive 103
techniques 31
SAT scores, standard normal distribution of 123*f*
Scientific contribution 36
Scientific discoveries 48
Scientific knowledge 11
Scientific research, anatomy of 149*f*
Screening tool, lack of 242
Search inputs 24
Search strategy 333
   developing 333
   meaning of 333
   significance of 333
Selecting databases 334
Selective reporting, free of 359
Sensitivity analysis 307, 309, 310, 351
   and modeling 307
   conduct 308
   deterministic 309
   methodologies in 309
   multi-way 308
   one-way 308
   probabilistic 309
   structural 309
   techniques, development of 307
   understanding 307
Sequencing theory 268
Service delivery 234
Shapiro-Wilk test 132
Short duration, missing cases of 106
Sickness 305
Similar words and relationship, clustering of 205
Simple bar diagram, elements of 112*f*
Simple random sampling 100
Simulation 269, 271
Smoking cessation programs 368
Snapshot study 28, 61
Snowball
   sampling 104, 196
   searching 335
Social and psychological structures 173
Social media, writing for 275
Social science research 58
Social seclusion 275
Social theory 221
Societal perspective 290
Socioeconomic status 111
Sociogram 184, 185*f*
Specific diet plan 351
SPIDER framework 328*t*
SPIDER question framework 328
Square deviation 120

Stakeholders 249
   and ethical concerns, role of 249
   knowledge regarding 249
Standard deviation 119
Standard error 123, 133
Standard normal
   curve 124*f*
   distribution 122
Standardized data extraction
   form 348
   procedures 348
Static-group comparison design 262, 262*f*
Statistical analysis 109, 350
Statistical averages and variation, measures of 117
Statistical errors, problem of 107
Statistical methodology 355
Statistical methods 348
Statistical significance, tests of 132
Statistical test 126
Statistics 107
   methods 108
Stem and leaf plot 115
Step wedge designs, rationale for 266*f*
Stock and flow notation 270*f*
Strategy selection 229
Stratified purposeful sampling 196
Stratified random sampling 102
Stressful life events 31
Study
   and data collection, selection of 334
   characteristics 346
   population in analytical studies, selection of 62*f*
   protocol, preparation of 80
   quality, evaluating 334
   selection 331
   subjects 30
   timeframe of 11
   type of 240, 327
Study design 25, 28, 37, 258, 365, 366
   choice of 30*t*
   classification of 28*fc*
   experimental 77
   in epidemiology, classification of 28
   specific to 94
   to adopt 30
   types of 29, 30*f*, 77, 94
Subgroup analysis 351
Subject matter, complexity of 218
Sudden infant death syndrome 147
Support programs 290
Surgical intervention study 332
Survival outcomes, challenges with 303*f*
Systematic approach 362
Systematic meta-analysis 321, 323
Systematic random sampling 101
Systematic review 309, 321, 323, 324, 330, 336, 348, 353, 355

and meta-analysis 333
benefits of 325
significance of 324
Systematic technique 191

T

Tabulated value 136
Tailed test 129
Technological changes 48
Templates 339
Temporal sequence, clarity of 73
Test
    hypothesis 125
    statistic 133, 134
    type of 134
Text smart 208
Thematic analysis 205, 205*fc*
Themes, levels of 204
Theoretical framework 176, 177
Theory 205, 254
    based sampling 196
    triangulation 223
Therapeutic agents, administration of 35
Therapeutic intervention 79
Threshold analysis 308
Time series
    analysis 256
    data 264
    design 263, 263*f*
Time-bound parts 17
Time-to-event outcomes 354
Title 5, 42, 314
    and abstract during publications, relevance of 8
    and abstract, need of 3
    compound 4
    contents of 5
    declarative 3
    neutral 3
    nominal 4
    suitable 6
    types of 3
    writing 5
Top-down method 292
Total hip replacement 367
Transmission rate 308
Transparency, lack of 179
Transparent reporting 349

Triangulation 223
    purpose of 224
    types of 223
True experiment 257*t*
t-tests 134
Two-tailed test 130
Typical case sampling 196

U

United Nations Children's Fund 278
United Nations Development Programme 278
United Nations Population Fund 278
Urban health training center 29
Utility outcomes 303

V

Valid results 362
Validity 32, 177
    lack of 58
Value theory 268
van Kaam model 207
Variable 107, 109
    cost 291
    types of 109*f*
Variation
    coefficient of 119
    source of 142, 143, 145
Verbatim 151
Verify data extraction 347
Very low certainty 365
Viral clearance 361*f*
Viral infections, antibiotics for 368
Visual analogue scale 305
Vitamin D supplements 368
Voice and body language, neutral tone of 189

W

Weakness 192, 193
Website tool 340
Wilcoxon signed-rank test 132
World Health Organization 278, 304
Writing research protocol, benefits of 35

Z

Z-tests 133